Perspectives on Complementary and Alternative Medicine

This book forms part of the core text for the Open University course K221 Perspectives on Complementary and Alternative Medicine and is related to other materials available to students, including two more texts also published by Routledge, Taylor & Francis:

- *Complementary and Alternative Medicine: Structures and Safeguards* (Book 2)
- *Perspectives on Complementary and Alternative Medicine* (Course Reader).

If you are interested in studying this course, or related courses, please write to the Information Officer, School of Health and Social Welfare, The Open University, Walton Hall, Milton Keynes MK7 6AA, UK.

Details are also given on the web page at www.open.ac.uk

Perspectives on Complementary and Alternative Medicine

Edited by Tom Heller, Geraldine Lee-Treweek, Jeanne Katz, Julie Stone and Sue Spurr (The Open University)

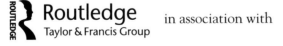 in association with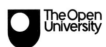

This book forms part of an Open University course K221 Perspectives on Complementary and Alternative Medicine. Details of this and other Open University courses can be obtained from the Course Information and Advice Centre, PO Box 724, The Open University, Milton Keynes MK7 6ZS, United Kingdom: tel. +44 (0)1908 653231; e-mail ces-gen@open.ac.uk

Alternatively, you may visit the Open University website at www.open.ac.uk where you can learn more about the wide range of courses and packs offered at all levels by The Open University.

To purchase this publication or other components of Open University courses, contact Open University Worldwide Ltd, The Open University, Walton Hall, Milton Keynes MK7 6AA, United Kingdom: tel. +44 (0)1908 858785; fax +44 (0)1908 858787; e-mail ouwenq@open.ac.uk; website www.ouw.co.uk

First published 2005 by Routledge, Taylor & Francis
2 Park Square, Milton Park, Abingdon OX14 4RN, United Kingdom

Edited, designed and typeset by The Open University.

Printed and bound in the United Kingdom by The Alden Group, Oxford.

ISBN 0-415-351-60X (hbk)

ISBN 0-415-351-618 (pbk) ✓

1.1

258590B/k221b1prelimsi1.1

Contents

Contributors

Tom Heller is a general practitioner in a deprived area of Sheffield. His practice is associated with the integration of complementary and alternative forms of practice alongside orthodox medical approaches. For the last 20 years he has also been a Senior Lecturer at The Open University School of Health and Social Welfare and involved in the production of a series of health-related courses.

Geraldine Lee-Treweek is a sociologist of health and illness and was a Lecturer in Health Studies at The Open University until autumn 2004. Her main field of specialism is complementary and unorthodox healing, in particular CAM therapeutic relationships, the experience of long-term users of CAM and the professionalisation of modalities. She also has long-standing interests in chronic illness and disability, trust and belief in contemporary society, social gerontology and the sociology of unexplained phenomena.

Jeanne Samson Katz is Director of Postgraduate Studies and a Senior Lecturer in the School of Health and Social Welfare at The Open University. She is a medical sociologist and has contributed to many courses in the health curriculum in the School since 1990. Much of her research has focused on the care of people dying in different settings, most recently in residential and nursing homes.

Julie Stone is Deputy Director of the Council for Healthcare Regulatory Excellence. She was previously a lecturer in health care ethics and law, teaching pre- and post-registration health care practitioners across a wide range of conventional and CAM professions. A lawyer by training, Julie has advised many CAM bodies on ethical and legal responsibilities and has contributed to policy initiatives in the CAM arena both nationally and internationally. Julie has written and lectured extensively on legal, ethical and regulatory aspects of complementary and alternative medicine. Her books include: *Complementary Medicine and the Law* (1996, Oxford University Press) with Joan Matthews; *An Ethical Framework for Complementary and Alternative Therapists* (2002, Routledge); and *Psychotherapy and the Law* (2004, Whurr) with Peter Jenkins and Vincent Keter.

Sue Spurr is a Course Manager at The Open University School of Health and Social Welfare, working on health-related courses. She is a qualified teacher of science and biology and is currently training to become a shiatsu practitioner.

Professor Mike Saks is Pro Vice Chancellor at the University of Lincoln. He was formerly Dean of the Faculty of Health and Community Studies at De Montfort University. He has published extensively on professionalisation, health care and complementary and alternative medicine and given many presentations at national and international conferences. His latest books include *Regulating the Health Professions, Complementary Medicine: Challenge* *and Change* and *Orthodox and Alternative Medicine: Professionalization, Politics and Health Care*. He has been a member and chair of numerous NHS committees and has served on a range of national groups on complementary and alternative medicine, including the NHS research and development capacity building committee for this area. He is a member of the Executive of the International Sociological Association Research Committee on Professional Groups and the editorial team for the new international journal *Knowledge, Work and Society*, as well as the current Chair of the Research Council for Complementary Medicine.

Sarah Cant is Senior Lecturer in Applied Social Sciences at Canterbury Christ Church University College. She has written extensively on the sociology of complementary medicine and is currently researching the use of and access to complementary medicine on the internet as well as continuing her interest in professionalisation.

Andrew Vickers is a research methodologist and statistician who has focused on complementary and alternative medicine for much of his career. He received his Bachelor's degree in the History and Philosophy of Science from the University of Cambridge and his doctorate in Clinical Medicine from the University of Oxford. He has been an investigator on numerous clinical trials and systematic reviews of complementary therapies, including a study of acupuncture for headache that is among the largest randomised trials of acupuncture ever conducted. He has also conducted considerable statistical and methodological research, with a particular emphasis on randomised trials with quality-of-life outcomes. Dr Vickers now works at Memorial Sloan-Kettering Cancer Center in New York where he has appointments in the Departments of Medicine, Biostatistics, Urology and Public Health (Weill Cornell Medical College). Dr Vickers' most recent methodological research has centred on medical prediction.

Acknowledgements

Grateful acknowledgement is made to the following sources for permission to reproduce material in this book.

Chapter 1

Figure
Figure 1.1: Reproduced by permission of CPPIH.

Photographs
p. 12: Nigel Stead, LSE; p. 16, left: The Wellcome Trust; p. 16, right: unknown source.

Chapter 2

Photographs
p. 40: The Wellcome Trust; p. 50: Anthea Sieveking/The Wellcome Trust.

Chapter 3

Photographs
pp. 61, 67 and 70: The Wellcome Trust; p. 73: Rex Features.

Chapter 5

Photographs
p. 112: Photographer Terry Di Paolo; p. 113: Hulton Archive; p. 120: Susan Tyler Hitchcock, www.mdx.ac.uk/www/study/ylamb.htm; p. 128: Bernhard/Fotex/Rex Features; p. 131: The Wellcome Trust.

Chapter 6

Photographs
p. 153: Sally and Richard Greenhill; p. 161: Science Photo Library.

Chapter 7

Photographs
p. 174: Wellcome Library, London; p. 191: Maximilian Stock Ltd/Science Photo Library.

Tables
Table 7.1: Thomas, K. J., Nicholl, J. P. and Coleman, P. (2001) 'Use and expenditure on complementary medicine in England: population based survey', *Complementary Therapies in Medicine*, Vol. 9, Harcourt Publishers Ltd; Table 7.2:

Ernst, E. and White, A. (2000) 'The BBC survey of complementary medicine use in the UK', *Complementary Therapies in Medicine*, Vol. 8, Harcourt Publishers Ltd.

Chapter 8

Photograph
p. 210: BSIP Keene/Science Photo Library.

Chapter 9

Photographs
p. 243: Courtesy of Hay House, Inc.; p. 250: The Wellcome Trust.

Chapter 10

Photographs
p. 272: St Christopher's Hospice; p. 276: Photograph courtesy of Marie Curie Cancer Centre; p. 281: From *Love, Medicine and Miracles* by Bernie S. Siegel, MD, Arrow Books; p. 282: Reprinted by permission of SLL/Sterling Lord Literistic, Inc. A/A/F Bernard Siegel.

Figures

Figure 10.1: Payne, S., Seymour, J. and Ingleton, C. (eds) (2004) *Palliative Care Nursing*, Open University Press; Figure 10.2: Barraclough, J. (ed.) (2001) *Integrated Cancer Care*. Copyright © Oxford University Press.

Chapter 11

Photographs
p. 295: Courtesy of Center for Adventist Research, James White Library, Andrews University; p. 298: Courtesy of Matt Utting; p. 301: Courtesy of J. D. Lasica; pp. 303 and 304: Science Photo Library.

Text
Box 11.11: R. Carroll (2003) 'It's green, prickly and sour, but this plant could cure obesity and save an ancient way of life', *The Guardian*, 4 January.

Chapter 12

Photographs
p. 336: Banana Stock/Alamy; p. 342: Courtesy of South Hams Tourism; p. 345: Copyright © The Guardian.

Chapter 13

Photographs
p. 356: Science Photo Library; p. 369: Material reproduced with kind permission of the Publisher, How To Books Ltd; p. 371: *Today's Therapist*, Issue 25, www.todaytherapist.com, www.chexpo.com.

Chapter 14

Photographs
p. 382: Sally and Richard Greenhill; p. 386: Wellcome Library London; p. 391: Alamy; p. 394: Dr Amita Raja, Homoeopathic Physician at the Royal London Homoeopathic Hospital (Complementary Medicine on the NHS); p. 397: Science Photo Library; p. 402: Photo courtesy of Mid Somerset Newspapers.

Figures
Figure 14.1: House of Lords Science and Technology Committee Sixth Report. © Crown copyright material is reproduced under Class Licence Number C01W0000065 with the permission of the Controller of HMSO and the Queen's Printer for Scotland.

Chapter 15

Photograph
p. 411: Science Photo Library.

Front cover

Photograph
Copyright © Getty Images

Introduction

The title *Perspectives on Complementary and Alternative Medicine* was chosen for this book to reflect the need for a critical overview of the subject areas that relate to the development of complementary and alternative medicine (CAM) as part of a dynamic process of change in contemporary society. The recent changes and developments in and the exponential growth of CAM are explored from a wide range of perspectives and covering several academic disciplines. This book represents a collaborative process among many academic disciplines and is designed to help you to understand and contextualise the phenomenon of contemporary CAM. Political, historical, ethical, geographical and economic perspectives are drawn on throughout this book in the search for understanding.

Sociologists such as Anthony Giddens (1991) claim that the key drivers leading to the growth of interest in CAM as part of a more general social change in 'late modernity' include: a more assertive consumer; a more accepting audience of a greater diversity of ideas and sets of knowledge; and an increase in the number and range of people having the confidence to set themselves up as 'new experts' in their field. A further significant force that is integral to understanding the development of CAM is the political and historical dimension. The history of CAM cannot be dissociated from that of orthodox medicine. Before the Medical Registration Act 1858, when state-supported biomedicine emerged and became protected as the dominant discipline, herbalists, healers and many others, including lay people known as 'wise women' or 'cunning men', competed with the same level of status as physicians, surgeons and apothecaries (Cant and Sharma, 1999). When orthodox medicine was established on a formal national basis in the mid-19th century, the realm of CAM came into being by exclusion (Saks, 1992).

Is there a single entity called 'complementary and alternative medicine'? Some commentators such as Ursula Sharma (1992) argue that CAM represents such a broad range of practices that have so little in common with one another that it is very difficult to talk of them as a whole. This book explores and examines many different definitions of CAM. A rationale is developed for considering CAM as a fluid description, which changes according to dynamic processes internal to both the CAM movement itself and its relationship with orthodox medical practice and other wider features of contemporary society.

In general terms, health-related behaviours are determined by a highly complex variety of influences. What motivates people to turn to CAM and what are they are seeking from CAM? A huge range of CAM therapies are available, with differing philosophies, claims and treatments. Most CAM remains in the private sector, unsupported by the National Health Service (NHS) and requiring some financial investment from the individuals seeking help. This financial constraint certainly prohibits many people from using CAM. An examination of how many people use CAM and of their sociodemographic profile highlights some of the current inequities associated with CAM use, but it also offers some insights into the reasons why people step outside the biomedical realm. Although users can access CAM for a variety of reasons and conditions, in the UK, patients tend to see their biomedical practitioner (usually a general practitioner or GP) before seeking care from a CAM practitioner, and they rarely abandon biomedical care completely (Sharma, 1992; Thomas et al., 1991).

Historical perspectives demonstrate that the politicised marginalisation of CAM in the UK reached a low point by the mid-20th century. Bakx (1991) describes this period as an 'eclipse' in which biomedicine became pre-eminent in the field of health and healing post-industrialisation, temporarily eclipsing other forms of health work. Consumers' and practitioners' interest in CAM grew dramatically since then, after the emergence of a strong counter-culture that led to a CAM renaissance. This development increased the political support for, and legitimacy of, several types of CAM therapy. The social and cultural process underpinning this shift stems from changing ideas about health and illness, and changing ideas about what doctors can and should deliver. People are taking a much more active and critical role as consumers of health care and are increasingly sceptical about the value of science (Giddens, 1991) and orthodox medicine in particular (Gabe et al., 1994). However, as Giddens (1991) suggests, these changes are not simply related to scepticism about biomedical knowledge: they also relate to lifestyle choices and the search for alternative experiences that CAM might offer.

This interest, in turn, prompted the growing incorporation of some forms of CAM into orthodox medicine. In many ways the report by the British Medical Association (BMA, 1993) can be considered a watershed in that it included the argument that an awareness of CAM should be part of basic education for students of medicine and other health professions. This does not mean that there is not considerable resistance to medicalisation and incorporation from within the ranks of CAM. In particular, for some groups of CAM practitioners, the growth of 'integrative medicine' represents an undermining of counter-cultural values, as more holistic paradigms based on challenging orthodox biomedical or 'scientific' theories may become displaced through proximity to the dominant biomedical systems.

This book explores the challenge for CAM practitioners in their attempt to gain legitimacy through acting ethically and responsibly. Ethical practice requires the application of appropriate knowledge, skills and attitudes, including the consideration of users' rights and values, being non-judgemental, developing listening skills and delivering culturally sensitive care. All of these attributes, in addition to the knowledge base, need to be acquired during the process of professional training and/or apprenticeships for

CAM therapists, as well as for those wishing to practise more orthodox forms of health care. They are every bit as important as practitioners' technical skills. To be a 'good' practitioner requires both technical skills and ethical awareness.

It is hard to define or describe the nature of the therapeutic relationship commonly found in CAM. In many ways it could be considered to reflect some of the key drivers of the CAM renaissance described above. In its most developed form, the relationship itself can be intrinsically beneficial and may become a catalyst for self-healing. However, expectations of the therapeutic relationship vary within and among cultures, locations, user groups and demographics. This book explores many of the problems associated with attempts to research and evaluate therapeutic relationships. The paradox remains that, although CAM is becoming increasingly popular and there are increasing numbers of personal testimonies to its effectiveness, firm 'scientific' proof that the interventions work remains elusive.

Complementary and alternative forms of health care are not the exclusive domain of contemporary British society. This book takes a wider look at traditional as well as folk forms of health care, with the aim of shedding light on current CAM practice in the West. This immediately exposes the fluid nature of CAM definitions and practice: some modalities and practices that were sited within folk practice, and were often transposed from diverse cultures, have developed into current CAM practice. Also, the redefinitions are not entirely one-way: some previously established orthodox medical practices have become marginalised and now are either abandoned or considered to be CAM. In a similar vein, certain traditional medical practices originating from developing countries have crossed the barrier and become accepted into orthodox western medical practice. This is particularly true of the use of certain herbal products. Examples are given in this book of the commercial exploitation of traditional herbal remedies. In some cases the indigenous peoples who first understood the healing properties of particular biologically available remedies cannot now afford the commercially developed products derived from 'their' locally grown products.

This book explores ways of finding out about the patterns of contemporary CAM use. Using expertise from a geographical knowledge base, this book demonstrates how the growth and spread of CAM use can be charted. CAM developments often reflect changes within secular society (Doel and Segrott, 2003), which is apparent from the types of people who are motivated to become CAM practitioners. For example, Andrews (2003) has researched the large numbers of nurses who have left the NHS, often because their ability to provide satisfactory standards of care within the formal system was constrained. The world of CAM, by contrast, has enabled them to provide individualised and often intensive care for people in need. All too often people in need of the services of a CAM practitioner have to find the money to pay for their attention. The complex 'cash nexus' within the world of CAM is explored in this book. Although CAM has become a large consumer industry, evidently many CAM practitioners continue to provide services at the level of a cottage industry. Often the small-scale practitioners and private therapists struggle to make a living from their new vocation. There may also be tensions between working as a CAM therapist and the business of running a small private enterprise. However, many large companies are not similarly constrained and there is evidence of considerable profitability in marketing CAM products and services to the wider public.

One way of avoiding the problems of market forces potentially contaminating the delivery of CAM services would be to incorporate more CAM within the NHS. This possibility is explored and some of the problems of, as well as the considerable potential for, this 'integrated' development are discussed. Although there are many examples of the successful integration of CAM developments in the NHS, several problems remain, and the continued development of integrated medicine is not supported by central government policy directives or by mainstream NHS funding.

The final part of this book explores some of the information sources that are available to help members of the general public access the changing world of CAM. Which therapies should they use for specific problems? How can they check whether the information sources are accurate and reliable? Here again the user is faced with a changing and potentially perplexing plethora of sources of information. The world of CAM cannot be simply delineated, and the multiple sources of available information reflect this diversity and rapidly changing and expanding milieu. However, in this part, as in the rest of the book, you will find ways to understand and interpret changing perspectives that can be used to further your understanding of this exciting subject area.

Tom Heller and Sue Spurr, The Open University, September 2004

References

Andrews, G. (2003) 'Nurses who left the British NHS for private complementary medical practice: why did they leave? Would they return?', *Journal of Advanced Nursing*, Vol. 41, No. 4, pp. 403–15.

Bakx, K. (1991) 'The "eclipse" of folk medicine in western society', *Sociology of Health and Illness*, Vol. 13, pp. 20–38.

British Medical Association (BMA) (1993) *Complementary Medicine: New Approaches to Good Practice*, London, BMA.

Cant, S. and Sharma, U. (1999) *A New Medical Pluralism? Alternative Medicine, Doctors, Patients and the State*, London, UCL Press.

Doel, M. and Segrott, J. (2003) 'Beyond belief? Consumer culture, complementary medicine, and the dis-ease of everyday life,' *Society and Space*, Vol. 21, pp. 739–59.

Gabe, J., Kelleher, D. and Williams, G. (eds) (1994) *Challenging Medicine*, London, Routledge.

Giddens, A. (1991) *Modernity and Self-Identity. Self and Society in the Late Modern Age*, Cambridge, Polity Press.

Saks, M. (1992) 'Introduction', in Saks, M. (ed.) *Alternative Medicine in Britain*, Oxford, Clarendon Press.

Sharma, U. (1992) *Complementary Medicine Today: Practitioners and Patients*, London, Routledge.

Thomas, K., Carr, J., Westlake, L. and Williams, B. (1991) 'Use of non orthodox and conventional health care in Great Britain', *British Medical Journal*, Vol. 302, 26 January, pp. 207-10.

Complementary and Alternative Medicine in Context

Edited by Jeanne Katz and Geraldine Lee-Treweek

Chapter 1 Changing perspectives

Geraldine Lee-Treweek

Contents

AIMS

- To show how complementary and alternative medicine is evolving as part of the process of social change in which there are competing sets of knowledge, diverse lifestyles, more choice for some members of society and a rise in consumerism.
- To contextualise complementary and alternative medicine in the western health care system in terms of changing patterns and challenges to the dominance of medical knowledge and ideology.

1.1 Introduction

Contemporary society is continuously changing and increasingly complex. Along with this change there is also greater choice about lifestyle and belief. At the same time, many sets of knowledge and ideas about the world coexist and compete for attention – different accounts of how things are. This is the case with choice and knowledge about health, illness and wellbeing. Complementary and alternative medicine (CAM) offers a vast array of choices in dealing with issues of health and wellbeing. This chapter invites you to consider CAM in a critical way and to see what it can offer to society. It outlines some of the debates and issues that highlight the social changes, which include popular interest in CAM.

The chapter begins by introducing CAM as a fascinating and fast-changing area of social life. It also discusses the concepts that are often seen as underpinning CAM and some of the assumptions people make about what it involves. It highlights the debates within CAM about how these forms of treatment and therapies should be defined and understood. In many ways the issue of what CAM is can be considered contentious and open to debate. You will be encouraged to engage with such debates and reach a view about how you understand such contentious issues.

This chapter goes on to contextualise CAM as part of much broader changes in modern western society. To understand CAM in contemporary society, the social trends and structures that allow it to flourish and grow must be considered. In particular, the chapter discusses where differing opinions, or world views, of health and healing come from and why increasing numbers of people want to use different types of therapy. It is also useful to consider why the number of people offering CAM in the UK has grown so much since the 1980s. These new 'experts' on health and wellbeing are highly visible in the media, on the high street and even in people's bathroom cabinets (in the complementary therapy products they buy to treat themselves). In the last 100 years, priorities in life and expectations of health have changed dramatically, as have people's ideas about appropriate ways of managing illness and lack of wellbeing. This chapter will involve drawing on your own experience to examine how you see your health and think about the impact of CAM on society.

The chapter title highlights **changing perspectives**. Change also incorporates a struggle between different paradigms as well as competition. There is competition between and among a variety of groups: between CAM and orthodox medicine, but just as likely between different types of CAM. Issues of power, knowledge and change permeate the contemporary study of CAM. Indeed, the diversity within CAM makes it such an interesting topic. As well as considering this issue, the focus is on various integrations and collaborations. That is to say, the emphasis here is on the way in which not only is CAM continually developing but also some people who, at first sight, might be expected to be negative towards it. In particular, not only are the medical profession and members of professions allied to medicine moving towards greater acceptance but also many medically qualified practitioners are now training in CAM as an adjunct to their orthodox skills (Zollman and Vickers, 1999).

1.2 Defining complementary and alternative medicine (CAM)

The term 'complementary and alternative medicine' (CAM) is used in a variety of places: pharmacies, local newspapers, *Yellow Pages*, television and radio, general practices, the high street, complementary health clinics, etc. As with many other terms, CAM has different meanings for different people. Most people have assumptions about what the term means and, from these assumptions, expectations about what CAM can offer in terms of treatment.

Sometimes such assumptions can lead people to overestimate or underestimate a particular CAM: viewing it with suspicion or open acceptance. To understand this subject you need to examine your own assumptions and consider how they might affect your views of CAM and whether you choose to use it.

'USERS', 'PATIENTS' AND 'CLIENTS': A NOTE ON TERMINOLOGY

In this chapter the term 'user' refers to people who use CAM. In many CAM disciplines you will hear different terms for the service user. For instance, you may read or hear the terms 'patient' or 'client' in leaflets about different forms of CAM, on websites, or when practitioners discuss their work. Here 'user' is the most common term. However, when a specific CAM is discussed, the term chosen will be the one most often used by practitioners in that field. In this way, the term used in this text will always be the most authentic to that particular CAM discipline.

ACTIVITY   WHAT ARE YOUR ASSUMPTIONS ABOUT CAM?

Allow 10 minutes

List five words you associate with CAM and what it is about. You may not have much personal experience of CAM, in which case list terms you have seen in the media or heard friends or family use.

Comment

There is a range of words and ideas you might associate with complementary and alternative medicine, including natural, mumbo jumbo, weird, relaxing, hippy, healthy, unscientific and traditional. Certainly a diversity of words spring to mind when thinking about CAM! Quite often they depend on people's personal experience of the area or the information gathered from friends, relatives and the media.

Commentators with a variety of perspectives on CAM have tried to identify what key concepts can be associated with it. For instance, Anthony Campbell, a consultant physician at the Royal London Homoeopathic Hospital, argues that there are four assumptions underpinning many CAMs (Campbell, 2002, pp. 3–12).

CAM as natural

Campbell (2002, p. 3) notes that the idea of particular forms of medicine or health care being natural is a fairly new concept that developed and gained strength during the 20th century. Nowadays the concept relates not just to the idea of particular remedies or treatments as being 'more natural' than pharmaceutical or orthodox ones but also to the growing social idea that the body heals naturally. The human body is seen as having a natural ability to repair itself and so CAM is there to help this process along.

CAM as traditional

CAM medicines are often claimed to have a long history of healing or links and connections with allegedly older ideas of medicine and health. Some forms of CAM, such as traditional Chinese medicine (TCM) demonstrate a heritage of healing going back thousands of years. Campbell (2002, p. 6) draws attention to how tradition and the appeal to the idea of tradition is often a key feature of many types of CAM. Thinking critically about the use of the term 'traditional' in relation to health practices raises important questions. Just because something is 'traditional', does that necessarily mean it is safe or effective? Are treatments from the past or with a long history better than newer treatments? The term 'traditional', while used to justify some types of CAM, does not really help to answer such questions.

CAM as holistic

There is a widespread view that different types of CAM (or **modalities**) try to understand illness in the context of the whole person (Campbell, 2002, p. 7). That is, a person is not just a physical body but can be seen as having several levels – mind, body and spirit – which need to be considered together to understand and treat illness and disease. Many CAM practitioners believe that consultations should include more time to discuss with an individual not only health and illness but also how they feel 'in themselves', their background, and their emotions and thoughts. Holistic treatment tries to tailor the whole treatment experience to suit the user as a unique person. Another way of understanding this is to consider the opposite of holism, which is reductionism. A reductionist approach sees illness and disease as being associated with a particular part of the body – in the cells of the body for instance – and deals with that problem without considering the needs of the whole person with the ailment. Modern orthodox medicine is often said to take a reductionist view of health and illness, treating only the diseased part and taking less interest in the individual as a whole. This way of viewing medicine, although undoubtedly true in some settings, is a generalisation that ignores the way in which many aspects of medicine are moving towards being more holistic and person-centred.

CAM as energy

CAM often refers in some way to the notion of energy. Campbell (2002, p. 11) maintains that the idea of people having a vital force or energy is shared by many CAMs. This often relates to energy flowing around the body in a particular pattern. Different therapies use different names for energy: you may hear the terms qi, chi, prana or life force, depending on the type of practitioner. Many CAM practitioners see at least part of their role as getting energy moving properly around the body, helping to remove blockage, or rebalancing problems in the energy field. Normal flowing energy is usually considered a prerequisite to health as, allegedly, the body can heal itself better if energy moves through it correctly.

Other ideas about the features of CAM

Campbell (2002) discusses what he views as the key assumptions of CAM. However, other people emphasise very different features or identify more differences than similarities between CAMs (Sharma, 1992). For instance, it could be argued that the way the practitioner treats the user varies across the different CAMs. Hypnotherapy involves using deep states of relaxation or trance to attempt to modify users' behaviour. The practitioner's role is to facilitate the trance state and, allegedly, to use suggestion to help the user attain their goal, such as to stop smoking or to be more confident. Here the practitioner often sees the user only two or three times. In other CAMs, such as massage, the user may return for treatments repeatedly. Clearly, the practitioner's role is different in such CAMs: they involve different styles of treatment – touching the body and talking. It is important to recognise that, as well as key similarities between CAMs, distinctions can also be drawn between different ones by focusing on aspects of treatment and approach.

Challenging assumptions

Given the assumptions people make about CAM, it is important to establish a set way of using the term in this book. It will become apparent that different groups, individual writers and organisations have a preference for (and tend to use) the terms 'alternative' or 'complementary'. For instance, 'alternative' implies separation or a complete difference from other types of medicine, whereas 'complementary' suggests working alongside or with other types of medicine. Some commentators, such as Sharma (1992), argue that CAM represents such a broad range of practices that have so little in common with one another that it is very difficult to talk of them as a whole. In this book CAM means forms of health care and treatment that are commonly regarded as non-conventional at present. This does not mean some CAMs will not be, and indeed are not being, integrated into more orthodox health settings and services. The definition and understanding of CAM used here focuses on how particular therapies or medicines are regarded by the majority of people.

non-conventional at present

definition of compl. and altern medicines

There are many non-conventional types of medicine. The most common ones are:

- **Osteopathy and chiropractic** – the 'hands-on' treatment and manipulation of the muscular and skeletal system.
- **Homoeopathy** – the treatment of illness with very small doses of medicines. The medicine used is chosen because it can cause the symptoms being treated if taken in larger doses.
- **Medical herbalism** – the use of herbal preparations to aid the individual.
- **Acupuncture** – the insertion of needles into the body to treat a range of problems.

These types of CAM are often collectively referred to as the 'Big Five' because of their popularity and high levels of usage (House of Lords Committee, 2000). However, there are many other types of CAM, which are introduced and explained briefly in Section 1.3.

It is important to note that a type of medicine or treatment considered to be a CAM today may become an accepted mainstream treatment tomorrow. In the field of CAM there is a high level of change, which is one reason why it is so interesting to study. There are changes in the public acceptance and use of CAM, and how the medical profession perceives it, in terms of regulation, in the types of training involved, and in the patterns of integration of CAM into conventional health care settings. Such change makes categorising CAM more challenging. It is worth noting here that people working in a particular CAM often find their work categorised by others – the media, groups within orthodox health care, other CAM organisations, etc. – in ways that run counter to how they see themselves. In Chapter 2 the difficulty of trying to categorise CAM is examined in more detail, along with the broader debates around using the terms 'alternative' or 'complementary'. Throughout this book it is important to remember that CAM is a highly contested field, in which there are often disputes and disagreements about what it is and its efficacy and role in contemporary society.

Why study CAM and why now?

Clearly, CAM is a contentious area. Its rapid change is enough to make it a fascinating area for scholarly investigation. However, some other issues also make it important to study this area.

- CAM is increasingly popular and more people use it today than in the recent past. Estimates suggest that in the UK between 6.6 per cent and 2 per cent of the population use CAM (Ong and Banks, 2003, p. 23). A study by Thomas et al. (2001) showed that people who consulted CAM practitioners for six of the most established CAMs rose from 8.5 per cent of the population of England in 1993 to 10.6 per cent by 1998. This may be an underestimate as it does not include the use of some 'less established' CAMs.

■ People are choosing to buy CAM products over the counter at a range of outlets – from high street retail stores to health food shops and over the internet. Statistics from Mintel (2003) show that £130 million was spent in the UK in 2002, the prediction being that the CAM market will be worth £200 million by 2008. This includes sales of such products as herbal remedies, homoeopathic preparations and aromatherapy oils.

■ The rise in public interest in CAM is mirrored by a rise in the interest of medicine, nursing and professions allied to medicine. In particular, orthodox health services now increasingly integrate CAM as part of their range of services (Zollman and Vickers, 1999).

ACTIVITY   THE CONSEQUENCES OF GREATER CAM USE

Allow 5 minutes

Think about the reasons why, and for whom, it might be important to know that people are increasingly using CAM for health and wellbeing.

Comment

The greater use of and interest in using CAM has consequences in terms of provision. CAM organisations need to know whether more training is necessary to meet public needs. As public interest grows, public pressure will also grow for health services to offer more CAM in hospitals, primary care services and other settings. Information about growing public demand will be needed for planning and organising such services. There are important issues around the safety of CAM and its efficacy (whether it works or produces the desired effect). People use CAM in their homes, as well as seeing practitioners, so it is important to know what they are self-treating and how they use the products, as well as being sure that the products work and are safe. Therefore, the different groups of people who might want information about the move towards the greater use of CAM include: health policy makers, hospital and primary care managers, doctors or members of the allied health professions and retail managers (who may like to know whether people want to buy aromatherapy oils in their stores, etc.).

CAM offers a range of services in the contemporary health marketplace. However, while there is more choice, there is also more need to ensure that people using CAM can make an informed choice, including the aspect of safety, about the services and products available. CAM can be seen as part of a wider move towards more choice in what can be bought, and indeed in what people want to buy, in contemporary society. It is important to understand the context in which CAM has become popular: the changes in general society that provide the context to the choices that CAM offers.

1.3 Living in a complex and diverse society

Many people, including social scientists, believe that UK society is complex and diverse (for example, Andersen and Taylor, 2003). Certainly, life experiences seem to have become increasingly diverse and often geographically wide ranging, including the following areas.

- **Where people live.** People are now more prepared (and indeed may have no choice) to move long distances for work, or for other commitments, and they may do this several times in their lives.
- **Where people work and what they do.** There is a trend towards regular occupational change: people do not generally stay in the same job for life and often retrain in a completely different field.
- **People's tastes, interests and lifestyles.** Today people are more likely than in the past to combine diverse and unusual pastimes and interests. These tastes are influenced by factors such as family background, places visited, television and other media.
- **People's choice of health care and products that enhance their wellbeing.** The range of people offering their services in the fields of health and wellbeing is diverse and there is a greater choice for users. This means there is a wider choice of health providers for individuals to choose from, as long as they can afford the treatment. Some people also buy over-the-counter health treatments, such as herbal remedies or aromatherapy oils, while simultaneously taking prescription medications from their GP and continuing to attend a National Health Service hospital.

Social trends indicate that people's lives in the UK have radically altered over the last 100 years, bringing a range of choice in many aspects of life. In other words, the mixing and matching of different ideas, activities and experiences is a feature of everyone's lives, to an extent, in a complex society.

ACTIVITY   HOW DOES DIVERSITY AFFECT YOUR LIFE?

Allow 15 minutes

Spend 15 minutes thinking about your life, interests and tastes. Write a list of your interests and tastes in food. Are there any apparent contradictions or examples of diversity in your list?

Comment

You may have noted that you combine many ideas to inform even your food tastes. For instance, because of access to both products and creative ideas about food, it is quite common for people to have Italian-inspired meals one day, curry the next, and vegetarian food the day after. The same applies to other aspects of life because, in contemporary society, so much is on offer that people can 'pick and mix' their approaches to any particular facet of their lives, which includes the choices made about health and illness.

The characteristics of a complex society

On a personal level, most people can identify with the 'pick and mix' approach to modern social life in their own lives. Social scientists have tried to go beyond these personal understandings to capture the key features of modern life and how people have become accustomed to diversity and change. To understand this it is necessary to outline the general patterns of change in recent history. The period after the industrial revolution in the 18th century is often referred to as 'modernity'. The industrial revolution seemed to bring endless possibilities for society, especially in the fields of science, medicine, technology and governance. At the same time, these areas of knowledge and understanding took a dominant and authoritative position in explaining and describing the world. So, taking science as an example of a key dominant set of knowledge, it can be seen that a scientific explanation is believed to be more legitimate in explaining events and phenomena than other types of knowledge. Lay knowledge, or the understandings and theories of the man or woman in the street, has generally been considered less useful than that of scientists, who test their knowledge with scientific methods. There is what can be termed 'a hierarchy of knowledge': that is, different knowledges are ranked, some being seen as having credibility and veracity and others being seen as less likely to be accurate or correct. Modernity can thus be viewed as a period in which certain sets of knowledge became well established as **the** way of understanding the world.

It may strike you that people do not trust science as much as they did. There are many examples of lay people refusing to accept or challenging the knowledge of science on the basis of their own knowledge, experiences or feelings. One example is parents who will not accept medical orthodoxy about immunisation (in particular the MMR – measles, mumps and rubella – vaccine) and openly challenge both scientific accounts and social policy by not having their children immunised (Heller et al., 2001). Commentators on social change in the West note that societies seem to have gone through another stage since modernity, which they call 'post-modernity' (Lyotard, 1984; Sarup, 1993). Whereas modernity was epitomised by the development of sets of knowledge which claimed to be the ways of understanding the world, in post-modernity this certainty is replaced with doubt and questions. The sets of knowledge that described the world became less powerful (Sarup, 1993). Several other key features are identified as part of post-modernity, including the following.

- A change towards a society driven by information technology, in which new forms of technology have changed both the nature of work and other aspects of life. At the same time, industries such as shipbuilding and steel production are in decline and new forms of work demand skills related to information technology.
- A mixing and matching of ideas that perhaps would not have been combined in the past.
- A growth in the area of consumer culture and consumption. The term 'consumption' relates to the goods and services individuals choose to buy and use.
- A 'pick and mix' approach to life. In particular, the tendency for people to engage in a wide range of leisure, work and social pursuits.

If modernity can be characterised by the development of sets of knowledge which sought to develop authority in explaining and describing the world, post-modernity can be characterised by the break-up of these large sets of knowledge (Lyotard, 1984). Put another way, in post-modernity people no longer tend to believe there is one authority on a topic. The 'professional' (doctor, lawyer, scientist, etc.) is no longer seen as having all the answers and always being right – an attitude that opens such types of knowledge to criticism and challenge.

The influence of Anthony Giddens

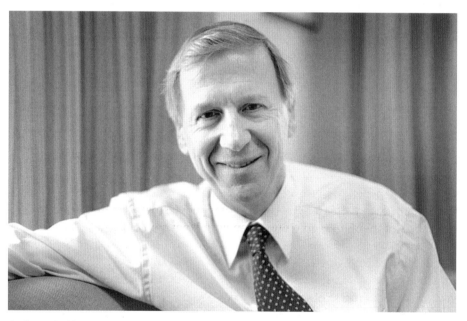

Anthony Giddens' highly influential work focused on describing and explaining social change in western societies

The ideas about social change of the eminent sociologist Anthony Giddens have been very influential in the social sciences and the humanities. He describes more recent modern life (within the last 30 years or so) as 'late modernity' (Giddens, 1990). He uses this term rather than 'post-modernity' because, he argues, if something is 'post' it suggests a complete change. He sees the processes of modernity and late modernity as merging together and so does not use the term 'post-modernism'. However, he writes about very similar changes in society to those suggested by his post-modernist contemporaries. Giddens (1990) adds other dimensions to the discussion of the features of present-day society that is of interest when discussing CAM:

■ The rise of new groups of people who present themselves as 'experts' on particular topics, such as how to be healthy or what to do when they are ill.
■ Despite disputes within academic discussion about terminology, there is general agreement that there has been a move away from believing in a set hierarchy of knowledge and a greater acceptance of a wider range of sets of knowledge, ideas and 'experts' within society.

Present-day society: changes in relationships, changes in ideas

In contemporary society in the UK there is a shift from fixed relationships and roles both at home and in the workplace towards what are termed more 'fluid' social relationships. For Giddens (1990) such changes demonstrate how roles in late modernity become more flexible or even reverse those seen before. For instance, traditional ideas of how men and women should relate to each other and behave in society are changing – both in terms of roles in the domestic sphere and in paid jobs and public roles. The idea of 'women's and men's jobs' is breaking down. This is borne out by the implementation of equal opportunity policies and practice, backed up by law. Social status is also less linked to traditional notions of social class. Whereas in the recent past a higher status went with a higher social class, status in contemporary society hinges on issues such as wealth, education, success in business and celebrity. In terms of personal identity, there is an array of influences around people which help develop a sense of self and a feeling of individuality. So for many people what they do for a living has become increasingly less important to their sense of themselves in comparison with what they believe, what activities they enjoy and who they want to be. New technologies such as the internet give people the opportunity to change identity further and 'play' with the idea of who they are. On the internet, attributes such as age, gender, social class, disability, ethnicity, illness and looks can be unimportant to the identity people use in chat rooms and discussion groups. Of course, this anonymity has its sinister side, such as the serious issues of paedophilia on the web and internet stalking. However, for the majority of internet users, the technology offers them new ways of thinking about and representing themselves to other people.

As well as the change in personal and public relationships and ways of thinking about themselves, many other aspects of people's lives have been mixed and matched. Factors such as living in a multicultural society, the ever-increasing opportunities for travel, and the new ideas offered by the media give people different perspectives on many issues and a wide range of concepts from which to make lifestyle choices. Restaurants often advertise 'fusion cooking', that is, a mixture of styles assembled in one dish. Similarly, living in a complex and diverse society can be characterised by the ability to indulge in 'fusion thinking', that is, bringing together a mixture of ideas. For example, although many people have some kind of spiritual belief, they often do not associate themselves with a particular institutionalised or recognised religion. There are many sources of information to inform a personal sense of spirituality, including formal religions, the media, the internet, music, books and magazines, films and other people. These information sources often provide ideas that go into the mix in developing people's personal approach to issues that matter to them. This is as true in the case of health and wellbeing as in other aspects of life and the proliferation of CAM gives ideas on which people can base their philosophies of health and wellbeing.

ACTIVITY   LOOKING AFTER YOUR HEALTH

Allow 1 hour

This activity will take about an hour and will start you thinking about the range of activities you do to maintain your own health and wellbeing. List all the health and wellbeing products you use in a week and write another list of all the activities related to health and wellbeing that you do in a week. Now try to write a sentence for each one identifying why you decided to use or do this.

Comment

You may have found this activity difficult. One reason could be the sheer number of activities that can be classified as related to health and wellbeing. Some are simple to audit in this way, for example taking antibiotics. However, others are more difficult to link to a cause. You may have started going to a gym because everyone else was or because you were given free membership initially.

You will have identified many other activities but your list should indicate that working at your health and wellbeing is a daily and a substantial task. Most people spend considerable time working on their own feelings about health and wellbeing but in different ways.

Lifestyle, consumption and consumer health

Along with mixing and matching ideas in personal philosophies and choices in life, there is a general trend towards diverse consumption. The term 'patterns of consumption' is commonly used to express the range of ways in which people choose to buy and use goods in contemporary society. When writing about the diverse types of consumption in society, commentators draw attention to the variety of goods and services people buy (Douglas and Isherwood, 1996). This term also highlights the diversity of places where these goods are grown or produced. Buying patterns have changed and in the UK the majority of people no longer buy the main produce or services they need from people they know, in their own communities, who have produced the goods themselves. There are some exceptions in small tight-knit communities or geographically remote ones.

In general, the 'geography of consumption' and buying from major stores links consumers with places all over the world. It is possible to buy clothes made in China, bananas from the Windward Islands and CDs from the internet. As with ideas about life, for most people consumption is now more eclectic and global. In the case of services, in a complex society buyers are unlikely to know the people who provide and sell them home-help services, holidays and double-glazed windows, or who offer complementary health services such as osteopathy or reflexology. It is impossible to know all the providers of goods and services, so people need to trust that such providers have the skills they claim. Alternatively, people rely on various forms of regulation and qualification that (it is hoped) demonstrate that those who offer services are suitably skilled (Lee-Treweek, 2002).

However, the idea of diverse consumption goes beyond what people buy to how they see themselves. Students often talk about themselves as consumers or customers of the educational system. Being a consumer is about embracing a set of values – being in control and buying what one needs and desires. In modern society, health care services, including complementary and alternative, is a growing area of consumption. Many commentators on complementary therapies argue that they offer a different kind of experience from being a patient in orthodox health services (Sharma, 1992; Stone, 2002; Lee-Treweek, 2002). For instance, in complementary therapy the individual seeking help drives the relationship; often self-refers; usually pays privately for the treatments; and, in theory, can choose to leave and select another therapist at will (Lee-Treweek, 2001). As the users of CAM seem to be more in control of their health care than in orthodox health care settings, they might prefer to see a CAM practitioner than go to orthodox health care practitioners. Also access to CAM is usually easy and people can select practitioners from *Yellow Pages* in the same way as they choose a plumber or caterer. In some types of CAM 'the patient' is often referred to as 'the client', a term which emphasises the individual as a consumer of a service who makes a choice about what they need.

Along with individuals' freedom of choice to seek help from complementary practitioners, there are risks attached to making the wrong choice, selecting the wrong care, or being treated by health 'experts' who are not fully qualified to help. This raises the important issues of safety and efficacy. It is important to bear in mind that when health care moves into the marketplace, there are both costs and benefits for the individual seeking treatment.

Consuming health

New patterns of consumption also extend to buying over-the-counter complementary health products, for example: herbal remedies for stress, homoeopathic medicines for allergies, and aromatherapy oils for massaging or bathing. There are also self-help hypnosis tapes, yoga classes and videos, and countless series of introductory books for home treatments. The rise in buying the services of complementary therapy practitioners is matched by this expansion in self-help (Mintel, 2003). Note that the consumption of orthodox health products has always been popular. You might have a home doctor book and/or many orthodox over-the-counter remedies in your bathroom cabinet. What is new about complementary therapy products is the amount being bought and the easy access to such products now compared with the recent past. For instance, in the 1980s outlets selling homoeopathic remedies or herbal supplements to the general public were limited to, for example, health food shops and specialist outlets.

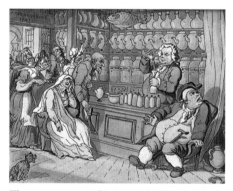 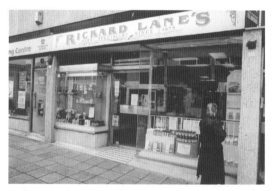

The resurgence of interest in CAM has led to much easier access to CAM products: (left) an 18th-century herbalist shop; (right) Rickard Lane's in Plymouth, a high street shop that sells health and CAM products and has specialised in providing herbal remedies since 1875

Now, most complementary therapy products can be bought on any high street in the UK. The boundary between the health care practitioner and the patient/client/user has become blurred as the public become more familiar with the ideas, products and potentials of complementary therapy and self-help. People often want to be their own therapist, to use oils at home, to learn how to massage and to use therapies to enhance their lives.

ACTIVITY   TREATING YOURSELF

Allow 30 minutes

This activity involves focusing on the reasons why people choose to self-treat with CAM. You do not have to use CAM yourself to do this activity – just use your imagination. Outline four reasons why people might choose to treat themselves or their families with complementary therapies rather than seeing a CAM practitioner.

Comment

You may have thought of the following issues.

1   Treating yourself with CAM can be cheaper than going to a practitioner.
2   Some CAMs are designed for self-treatment and are also relaxing to use in your own home.
3   You may distrust CAM practitioners.
4   You may use CAM along with orthodox treatments or to alleviate the symptoms of orthodox treatments.
5   For many people in the UK using CAM is part of their daily lifestyle and self-treatment is deeply embedded in their ideas about maintaining good health.

The rise of 'new experts' and new knowledge systems

While ordinary people are increasingly interested in gaining enough knowledge to treat themselves with complementary health care, there are plenty of people offering services as 'experts' in this field. This issue of individuals offering services to treat illness or increase wellbeing highlights an important feature of late modernity and health care: the diversification of knowledge and of 'new experts'. One feature of late modernity described by Giddens (1990) is the ever-increasing diversity of information and knowledge sources. At the same time, there is an apparent decline in the power of claims from orthodox sources of information. People are much more inclined to use a range of resources to understand areas such as health, illness and wellbeing. Interestingly, it is not only academics who have focused their attention on describing this process. William Bloom, a new age writer and holistic teacher from the CAM world, writes about the 'new buffet of information' in society (Bloom, 2001, p. vi). He goes on to argue that openness to different forms of knowledge has allowed individuals to explore new aspects of their health and wellbeing.

Giddens (1990) takes this idea further by identifying a general rise in the 'new experts' who create and then develop an area of expertise as their own. You might wonder who the 'old experts' are and whether it is easy to draw such boundaries. From Giddens' viewpoint, the 'old experts' are the purveyors of orthodox and mainstream knowledges: science, medicine and religion. In comparison, 'new experts' can spring up in the most unlikely places. All around, individuals and groups attempt to reconstruct their skills as specialised and more 'expert'. For instance, consider the change in terminology from 'hairdresser' to 'hair technician'. Health is no exception to these social changes and has spawned a range of people who profess to 'expertly' inform others how to live healthily, eat properly, detoxify their bodies or homes, make them think positively and change their lives. Hardly a week goes by without some new exercise fad, diet or idea. Daytime television is full of programmes that devote slots to complementary health care alternatives and to individuals – health gurus – who claim to have found the route to health. Many celebrities apparently have their own health gurus, if media coverage of their lives is to be believed. Invariably the new health experts have something to sell and therefore health in the diverse health marketplace generally comes at a price.

Are complementary therapists really 'new experts'?

You may wonder how useful the term 'new expert' is when discussing complementary therapists. Social science often provides concepts and terms to describe a broad sweep of changes. These are useful for getting an overview but they can be imprecise when applied to a particular area. Indeed, it may be necessary to modify Giddens' term to describe complementary and alternative therapists more accurately. There have always been people who treat disease and illness outside an orthodox medical framework in the UK: 'wise women' and 'cunning men' who worked for health in their communities, using a range of methods including, for example, herbs, bone-setting, charms, amulets and prayer (Chamberlain, 1982). It may be more useful to see the new experts of complementary medicine as having a remarkable resurgence in late modernity. This resurgence occurred after a period of, as Bakx (1991) calls it, 'eclipse'. Bakx refers to the way biomedicine became pre-eminent in the field of health and healing post-industrialisation, temporarily 'eclipsing' other forms of health work. Despite the recent resurgence of complementary therapy, biomedical thinking has maintained an authoritative position in a range of areas relating to health, illness, disease and the body. However, people still have to visit a general practitioner to access many health services and doctors are still considered by most people to be the best source of help for serious symptoms. To quote comedian Billy Connolly, if you are run over by a car in the street and break your leg, your spirits are unlikely to be lifted by someone who pushes through the gathering of onlookers saying, 'Let me through, I'm a qualified aromatherapist!' Most people have a sense of hierarchy in terms of who they want to treat them in an emergency.

Biomedicine has provided, and still does provide, the mainstay of formal health care services in the UK but there has been a diversification of other groups offering complementary health care. In particular, these groups can often provide services to patients whose conditions are not well served by orthodox health care or high-tech answers. People with musculo-skeletal pain, such as back and neck pain, are a good example of such a group. Although orthodoxy can provide physiotherapy services, pain clinics and analgesics, many people who have recurrent pain choose osteopathy, chiropractic or acupuncture treatment for their long-term care or management during flare-ups. People who treat themselves for back and neck pain may also choose meditation, herbal remedies and visualisation therapies, such as hypnosis or biofeedback. Although some of the skills offered by CAM are being integrated into a range of orthodox care and areas, it is fair to say that, at present, integration is most likely where chronic illness cannot be treated by orthodox means. Also some therapies have more chance of integration and collaboration with orthodox ones than others. However, in general, attitudes towards complementary medicine, in orthodox medicine, nursing and the allied health care professions are changing towards a more positive view of integration and recognition of different ways of thinking about and treating illness and disease (BMA, 1993), as Box 1.1 shows.

BOX 1.1 BIOMEDICINE AND KNOWLEDGE ABOUT HEALTH

After the industrial revolution in western society a narrow range of sets of knowledge became pre-eminent in describing and explaining both natural and social phenomena. In particular, science not only provided explanations but also developed specific methods for investigating and analysing aspects of the world. Biomedicine developed as a scientifically based form of knowledge, founded on laboratory research, clinical observation and a professional system of training, ethical standards and careful regulation. Through its close connections to the powerful knowledge of science, biomedicine could claim a monopoly over knowledge about the body, health and disease. Medicine developed with close connections to the state and soon became the authoritative voice on how disease and ill health should be managed and treated. These powers are still at work today. Medicine as a profession has statutory protection and a monopoly over many forms of health work. For instance, it is illegal to call oneself, or pretend to be, a medical doctor. Doctors also have powers of definition over individuals (in areas such as mental health, fitness to work, suitability for state benefits, or even whether a person is allowed to drive). However, it would be wrong to see modern medicine as pure biomedicine. Much has changed, not least the move towards primary care being pivotal to the provision of health and a restructuring of the relationship between doctors and patients towards greater equality. Modern medicine is difficult to assess as a whole because of the diversity of people, practices and ideologies within it.

Many commentators have argued that the traditional authority of medicine is being eroded as people turn to other sets of knowledge to understand, describe and treat their illnesses. At the same time, changing patterns of illness towards chronic conditions, combined with an increasing ageing population, mean that modern medicine sometimes cannot offer answers for commonly experienced symptoms and ills. According to this model, complementary health care is a threat to the traditional power of doctors. However, another way of looking at this recognises the overlap and integration of new knowledge with biomedical knowledge and practice. Integration and collaboration between traditional biomedicine and CAM is increasing and some 'orthodox' health care practitioners choose to train in CAM therapies or are well aware of what such therapies can offer. It is also very important to remember that running parallel to the rise and development of biomedicine, traditional and lay beliefs about health have continued and flourished in the UK.

You might have noted that, in discussing the changes towards widespread diversity in the health market, what is being described is a change in social relationships and not a judgement of that change. In other words, it is not presenting a particular position on whether new experts, and in particular the new experts that complementary therapies represent, are a good or a bad thing. Nor are biomedicine and orthodox health care services being held up as old-fashioned or inefficacious. The changes happening in many health settings mean that the future of health care most probably lies in an integrated model of care which recognises and values diversity. What can be said is that the general social trend towards individuals and groups setting up as health experts has real consequences for individuals' health choices, the state health services and private health services.

Recognising diverse traditions and heritages

Another issue about using the term 'new expert' is that it does not describe the background and development of many therapies. For instance, it is necessary to attend carefully to the differences between complementary therapies and medicines, as well as the apparent similarities. Herbalism and Chinese acupuncture are just two complementary therapies that are far from new. Their history goes back much further than modern biomedicine and they have, at different times, been the main form of medicine available in many cultures. Sometimes, as with TCM, practitioners have successfully been accepted in other cultures. TCM is used in a range of countries including Vietnam, India and the UK. Other therapies have only been developed in the last few decades: for instance, 'zone rebalancing' (an acupressure technique that purports to work with energy in the body in which pressure is applied to particular points). New therapies are being developed all the time, raising the problem of how CAM can be divided up, given the diversity of therapeutics and beliefs. This problem of definition and categorisation is called **taxonomy**, a theme you will meet again in Chapter 2.

The resurgence of interest in complementary medicine and therapy is perhaps most visible in the range of CAM practitioners in the marketplace advertising and selling their particular sets of knowledge on health and wellbeing. According to some statistics, one in five people have visited some kind of complementary practitioner in the past 12 months. However, behind the curtains of homes across the UK another resurgence is taking place. People are self-treating their ills with the wide range of proprietary complementary therapy products available: homoeopathic arnica for sprains and bruising; St John's Wort herbal tablets for mild depression; lavender aromatherapy oil for relaxation, and so on. Although it can be argued that there has always been self-treatment with CAM, the increased availability in a range of outlets and the growth in products mean that self-treatment is now more accessible for people. Also, people not only treat themselves: the range of aromatherapy and other CAM products for animals indicates a growing market. Most people use home versions of CAM while still believing in the efficacy of orthodox health care services. There is a trend towards mixing a range of health providers, both orthodox and complementary, so that seeing a GP one day to get painkillers for a bad back and attending an osteopath the next for some treatment is not considered incompatible – by either the service user or the practitioners involved. Indeed, the patient may be referred to the osteopath by the GP. There is increasing overlap and dialogue between old and new experts in health and many orthodox health practitioners are integrating complementary types of health knowledge into their work.

ACTIVITY   THE CONSEQUENCES OF NEW EXPERTS

Allow 20 minutes

Spend 20 minutes thinking about the growth of new experts in health. Note down three positive consequences and three negative consequences of having a diversity of health experts.

Comment

You may have noted some of the following positive consequences.

1   With more diversity, people have more choice.
2   With more experts, there is more access. It is easier to find someone to help you with your health problem.
3   With more experts, it is more likely that someone can help you with your particular problem or issue.

4   There is no need for your medical record to include problems you may be embarrassed about. For instance, you can take your emotional problems to an aromatherapist or a hypnotherapist privately, which is then not on your medical files.

Greater public acceptance of new experts has led to their integration into some aspects of orthodox health care, helping to broaden the options that orthodoxy can provide. For instance, many midwives have training in aromatherapy, acupuncture and massage: skills they can use alongside orthodox care to enhance the experience of women during maternity and childbirth.

You may have thought of the following negative consequences.

1   With the range of people available to help, it may be hard to choose which expert to go to. Choice is only good if you know what is on offer and can therefore make an informed choice.

2   It is not always easy to know whether an 'expert' is properly trained. New health occupations may not have formal training structures or adequate means for you to check the authenticity of a practitioner.

3   New experts may not uphold the ethical standards of other orthodox practitioners.

4   Orthodox health practitioners may not know enough about the range of new therapies on offer to be able to offer advice and support to patients who want to use them.

Choice in the range of treatments on offer may give people an array of ways to deal with their health problems. On the other hand, making informed choices and getting information about whether a treatment will help can become much harder. For professionals such as GPs there may be little time to update their knowledge on particular complementary therapies. Thus they cannot give informed advice to patients. As new sets of knowledge arise and people begin to use them, it can be difficult for orthodox health care practitioners to know about them all and be able to advise patients on what may help. Diversity of health knowledge can present practical problems to health workers who are often expected (unrealistically) to be knowledgeable about all the latest research. However, increasingly GPs will offer a CAM that they practise themselves or that they 'buy in' to their practice. Most often, the CAM available is one of the 'Big Five' therapies: osteopathy, chiropractic, medical herbalism, homoeopathy and acupuncture.

Giddens (1990) argues that the rise of interest in CAM can be considered as part of wider patterns of change in 'late modernity', because health consumers, patients or clients now have more choice, a subject addressed in the next section.

1.4   Pluralism and changing health needs

So far this chapter has described the changes that have occurred in the range of health services people can access and noted the rapid growth in CAM use. Plurality is a term used to describe the wide range of complementary forms of health care which are available to deal with people's ills (if individuals can afford them). There are many ways of addressing people's health needs. A range of issues confines these choices, including cost and the individual's or family's financial situation, access, knowledge of the availability of treatments, and people's ideas about their health and illness. However, another important issue is whether individuals see their health as 'worth' spending money and time on. In a sense, people prioritise health along with other aspects of their lives.

People may also prioritise **within** health. A good example of this is a person who goes to a pharmacy with a prescription which has several items on it. However, they choose to take only one of the items, thus 'saving' money, which they can spend on other 'essentials'. This kind of choice may seem absurd and yet it happens in pharmacies across the UK every day. Often the pharmacist is asked which medication is the most important or the most needed. When the choice is between clothes for the family, a meal or a prescription, many people will choose the clothes or a meal rather than prescription medications.

ACTIVITY   YOUR PRIORITIES

Allow 15 minutes

Think of as many of the important things in your life as you can. Present them as a list, as a doodle or in any other way that comes to mind. Now consider ranking them in order of priority. How will you begin to sort out which ones come first in your life? You could also consider whether this ranking would be the same if you had done this activity some years ago when your circumstances were maybe different from now.

Comment

Ranking priorities in your life is a completely subjective exercise. You may have put health and wellbeing at the top of your list, especially if you frequently have ill health or live with people who do. Alternatively, you may have ranked family, friendship or community ties as most important. It is interesting to consider how time and circumstances could change your list or ranking. For instance, whereas work may have been important to you at one time, starting a family tends to change this. If you imagine yourself in the future, becoming a carer for another person may also radically alter how you approach this task.

What people think they need and want also changes along with circumstances, yet the following comments are commonly made about CAM:

'I **need** a massage', 'I **must** get an appointment with the chiropractor', etc. It is interesting to think about need in relation to choice and the factors that constrain individual choice.

Maslow's hierarchy of need and changing desires

Abraham Maslow (1971) designed a model of need that is very influential in a variety of social science, business and arts disciplines. He argued that individual behaviour is determined by a person's strongest need at that particular moment. Maslow described five categories of need.

1 **Physiological needs:** these are the basic needs to sustain life – food, water, shelter, etc. They are associated with wealth in society, i.e. a basic level of money is required to sustain this need.

2 **Safety needs:** people need and desire to be safe from crime, disease, war and economic instability.

3 **Social needs:** people need to interact with others and to feel they 'fit in' and are accepted by other people.

4 **Esteem needs:** this is a diverse set of sub-needs and motives. Esteem is strongly related to the power and influence individuals have or their perception of their power and influence over other people.

5 **Self-actualisation needs:** these encompass people's need to realise their potential. This potential differs for everyone but it is about realising the full extent of their abilities in a variety of ways, e.g. studying and achieving through academic endeavour are ways of realising potential that can be satisfying and fulfil need.

This way of categorising need was developed further by several scholars. For instance, Bradshaw draws attention to the way in which professionals often define and compare the needs of groups for the purposes of providing health or social care services (Bradshaw, 1972). She also argues that the needs people feel or express can be very different from those identified by professionals. Defining and identifying needs can sometimes be a source of conflict between lay people and professional groups. More recently, researchers interested in consumption have used the term 'desire' to emphasise the way many people have wishes about acquiring or buying culturally valued products or services (Shove and Warde, 1998). The term 'desire' takes the focus away from need in the sense that Maslow used it. It relates more to the hopes people have in addition to their basic sustenance and survival. It is disputed whether the use of some CAMs is about desire, leisure and pleasure, rather than need. Certainly some CAMs are very pleasurable. However, about 60 per cent of people who use CAM have long-standing illnesses (Ong et al., 2002). Some people see CAM as central to coping with illness, pain and disability and prioritise its use above other needs.

In decisions about the public provision of CAM, for instance in the NHS, conflict can arise about what people need and want and what really works. Just as people have to make choices about using and prioritising their resources, so do public bodies. However, public pressure is now having more of an effect on how such bodies distribute and use resources.

Changing roles, changing policy

To talk about a 'health landscape', in which people can choose from a range of practitioners and consumers of health care, indicates another important change: in the relationship of patients to health providers. When considering CAM as part of the marketplace, the term 'consumer of health care' was introduced. Although this is not a new way of talking about health, some new policy initiatives are taking patient power much further than ever before. Patients' participation in health is a key tenet of New Labour's vision for publicly run health services. It is fairly unclear what patient participation will mean in reality but, certainly in theory, patients' views will be included in the decision-making process by involving individuals on panels and committees (see Figure 1.1).

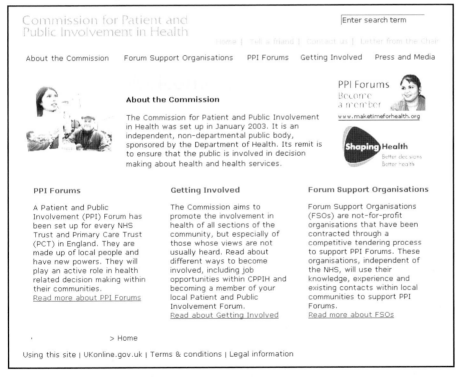

Figure 1.1   The PPI website offers information to lay people about possible ways of participating in health decisions and health policy planning
(Source: Commission for PPI in Health, 2004)

Introducing a consumer of complementary health care

Clearly, in theory individuals with health problems have a wide choice in a plural health market. This choice can give them opportunities for becoming healthy. However, it also has drawbacks in terms of how to make informed choices about using therapies. Time, money and access are important factors, not only in choosing where to get help for ill health but also in whether an individual can make a choice to use services such as CAM. Other factors at work, at home and in relation to roles and responsibilities can make it difficult to seek help and use some services. The following case study looks at the kind of circumstances that can lead a person to consider CAM.

LOUISE'S STORY

Louise is 35 and lives in Bristol. Until recently she enjoyed good health but over the past year she has experienced recurrent bouts of pain in her back. Initially she attributed this to picking up the children. As her partner is in sales and often works away from home she has to look after nine-month-old baby Lewis, three-year-old Cara and 13-year-old Daniel. Before the onset of her back problem the family went to a holiday cottage in Wales which turned out to be on two floors. Louise had to take the carrycot up and down the stairs and on several occasions twisted awkwardly while doing this. On her return she was bending to pick up some washing and her lower back 'locked'. She managed to lie down on the floor for 10 minutes before she could stretch herself out. She heard a 'click' and could move again without too much pain. Luckily, Cara was watching television in the same room, Lewis was asleep and Daniel was out playing football with friends. However, Louise was worried because, while she was incapacitated on the floor, she could not reach the children if anything happened.

At work in a local DIY superstore the bending and stretching involved in stacking the shelves became more difficult and her lower back continually ached, clicked and seemed to move. Working on the check-out involved using a broken chair, which did not help, and Louise often felt a tension in her back. She attributed some of this general tension to the threat of redundancies at the store and fear of how the family would cope if she lost her job. Louise decided to ask her friends and family what she should do. Two friends said they had both seen the same chiropractor for back pain and he sorted them out. His office was on the high street and it was easy to get appointments. An initial visit would cost £45, although subsequent treatments were £30.

Louise's mother suggested she took cod liver oil (to 'oil' her back) and ate more vegetables for vitamins. She also told Louise that her grandmother always suffered with her back and that it 'ran in the family'. Louise's partner said he thought painkillers would help and the problem might go away in time. Eventually events triggered Louise to seek help. After a two-week bout of low back pain, during which she was off work, Louise went to her GP. Initially she was examined, given painkillers and put on a waiting list for physiotherapy. A month later Louise was still in pain and waiting for physiotherapy. Fearing that she might lose her job if her problems went on much longer, she began to consider using CAM. In particular, she wanted to keep going to work and to cope with caring for the children.

ACTIVITY   OFFERING ADVICE TO LOUISE

Allow 15 minutes

Louise finds herself in a diverse CAM marketplace, being given advice from a range of sources, and trying to decide how to proceed with her health problem.

For this activity you will try to give Louise advice on what she could do next. The resources you can use include your own knowledge of 'bad backs' and any information you may have on CAM. If you are a practitioner in this field, you could imagine you are a lay person and think about what they might suggest for Louise.

Comment

You might have made the following suggestions to help Louise.

- Louise could find out exactly how long she has to wait for physiotherapy but, if she does want to go to a CAM practitioner, her doctor may be able to recommend a local osteopath or chiropractor.
- Research shows that people with back and neck problems need to keep active as much as possible and in all likelihood her back would get better on its own.
- Louise should be advised to speak to her Health and Safety Officer or union at work as using a broken chair is dangerous. As her back seems to go into spasm maybe massage would help.

It is easy to discuss Louise's situation without considering the context of her life, and specifically, the constraints that affect her ability to use CAM and make choices to help herself.

ACTIVITY   CONSTRAINTS ON USING CAM

Allow 20 minutes

Reread Louise's story.

1   Note down the key issues that may make her prone to back trouble.
2   List the factors that may make it more difficult for Louise to use CAM.

Comment

1   Several factors might predispose Louise to back problems or pain.
   - Louise has family responsibilities, which often involve much lifting and carrying.

- Her work also involves some lifting and sitting in a position that is uncomfortable on a broken chair. Although Health and Safety legislation should protect Louise from this, she seems to be unable to demand that her employers conform to the law.
- Given Louise's worries about her job, and often having to cope alone, stress may also be a factor affecting her overall health.

2   The factors that might make it more difficult for Louise to use CAM include:
- the cost of treatment and the family budget
- balancing work, family and time constraints to 'make time' for treatment
- Louise's knowledge of CAM and what treatment may be most effective
- how easy it is for her to access CAM near to her home.

Information about the family's financial situation is not provided; however, the cost of regular CAM treatment may prove prohibitive for Louise and her family.

Clearly, when deciding whether to use CAM, the daily constraints on people's lives have an important impact on the choice they make. When considering how Louise will choose which CAM to use, it is important to think about some of the common assumptions that may affect the advice she receives from those around her. The advice given to Louise by her family and friends will probably include all kinds of beliefs and ideas about the treatment she needs, orthodox or otherwise. A lack of knowledge about what the different CAMs actually involve could put Louise off attending or make it difficult for her to know which type of CAM would be the most helpful. Assumptions can influence people's ideas about CAMs but, in order to fully understand them, it is important to critically and carefully examine a variety of aspects of their use.

1.5   Conclusion

The processes of social change have led to a diversity of health knowledge in contemporary western society. One type of health knowledge – CAM – offers a vast and growing array of choices in dealing with health and wellbeing issues. However, along with choice, people also need information if they are to be fully informed consumers of these services. In a field of 200-plus modalities (Stone, 2002), in many cases understandings of CAM are led by assumptions that can result in overestimating or underestimating a particular CAM, and viewing it with suspicion or open acceptance. Your own assumptions are important in critically examining the issues raised in this book and the modern-day experience of being a user of CAM.

KEY POINTS

- The key features of CAM are very difficult to pin down. This is partly because of the wide variety of practices in CAM but also there are different views, among CAMs, about what the most important issues are.

- Holism, or treating and understanding the whole person, is often presented as a key feature of CAM. Reductionism, or treating the part of the individual that is ill with little reference to the whole person, is sometimes presented as a feature of contemporary orthodox medicine. There are good reasons to question this divide as orthodox medicine can be and sometimes is holistic in its approach and some CAMs may be less holistic than people's assumptions may at first suggest.

- The growth of interest in CAM is part of wider processes of change that are visible in society. Although there are debates about terminology, Anthony Giddens sees these changes as part of 'late modernity'.

- Important changes in contemporary society that have affected the use of CAM stem from the development of a consumer culture, a greater acceptance of diversity in ideas and sets of knowledge, and growth in the range of people offering their services as 'experts'.

- Although people have always used home remedies, herbal preparations, etc. as well as orthodox medicine, proprietary CAM products are more available and in a greater range than in the past.

- Priorities in life are constantly changing but in relation to health and wellbeing some people may prioritise the good feelings CAM treatments provide, while others may use them as a lifestyle choice.

References

Andersen, M. and Taylor, H. (2003) *Sociology: Understanding a Diverse Society*, Florence, International Thompson Publishing.

Bakx, K. (1991) 'The "eclipse" of folk medicine in western society', *Sociology of Health and Illness*, Vol. 13, pp. 20–38.

Bloom, W. (2001) *The Endorphin Effect*, London, Piatkus.

Bradshaw, J. (1972) 'The concept of social need', *New Society*, Vol. 19, pp. 640–3.

British Medical Association (BMA) (1993) *Complementary Medicine: New Approaches to Good Practice*, Oxford, Oxford University Press.

Campbell, A. (2002) 'Complementary and alternative medicine: some basic assumptions, in *Alternative Medicine, Should We Swallow It?*', pp. 1–14, London, Hodder & Stoughton.

Chamberlain, M. (1982) *Old Wives Tales*, London, Virago.

Douglas, M. and Isherwood, B. (1996) *The World of Goods: Towards an Anthropology of Consumption*, London, Routledge.

Giddens, A. (1990) *The Consequences of Modernity*, London, Polity.

Heller, T., Heller, R. and Pattison, S. (2001) 'Vaccination against mumps, measles and rubella: is there a case for deepening the debate?', *British Medical Journal*, Vol. 323, pp. 838–40.

House of Lords Committee (2000) *Complementary and Alternative Medicine*, London, The Stationery Office.

Lee-Treweek, G. (2001) 'I'm not ill, it's just this back: osteopathic treatment, responsibility and back problems', *Health*, Vol. 5, No. 1, pp. 31–49.

Lee-Treweek, G. (2002) 'Trust in complementary medicine: the case of cranial osteopathy', *Sociological Review*, Vol. 50, No. 1, pp. 48–69.

Lyotard, J. F. (1984) *The Postmodern Condition: A Report on Knowledge*, Manchester, Manchester University Press.

Maslow, A. (1971) *Motivation and Personality*, New York, Harper & Row.

Mintel (2003) *Complementary and Alternative Medicine in the UK*, London, Mintel.

Ong, C. and Banks, B. (2003) *Complementary and Alternative Medicine: The Consumer Perspective*, London, Prince of Wales's Foundation for Integrated Health.

Ong, C. K, Petersen, S., Stewart-Brown, S., Doll, H. and Bodeker, G. C. (2002) 'Use of complementary and alternative medical services in England: a population survey of four counties', *American Journal of Public Health*, Vol. 92, pp. 1653–6.

Sarup, M. (1993) *An Introductory Guide to Post-structuralism and Postmodernism* (2nd edition), London, Harvester-Wheatsheaf.

Sharma, U. (1992) *Complementary Medicine Today: Practitioners and Patients*, London, Routledge.

Shove, E. and Warde, A. (1998) *Inconspicuous Consumption: The Sociology of Consumption and the Environment*, Lancaster, Department of Sociology, Lancaster University. Available online at www.comp.lancs.ac.uk/sociology/papers/shove_warde_inconspicuous_consumption.pdf

Stone, J. (2002) *An Ethical Framework for Complementary and Alternative Therapists*, London, Routledge.

Thomas, K. J., Nicholl, J. P. and Coleman, P. (2001) 'Use and expenditure on complementary medicine in England: a population-based survey', *Complementary Therapies in Medicine*, Vol. 9, pp. 2–11.

Zollman, C. and Vickers, A. (1999) 'Complementary medicine and the doctor', *British Medical Journal*, Vol. 319, pp. 1558–61.

Chapter 2 Can complementary and alternative medicine be classified?

Julie Stone and Jeanne Katz

Contents

AIMS

- To demonstrate the diversity of terms used to describe CAM therapies.
- To illustrate the different ways to group different types of CAM according to factors such as level or type of regulations, ethical awareness and the nature of the treatment involved.
- To explore the impact on CAM of particular definitions and taxonomies.

2.1 Introduction

As Chapter 1 indicated, what may be viewed as complementary and alternative medicine (CAM) consists of at least 200 different types of therapy, ranging from the well known, such as acupuncture, to less well known sub-specialities, such as auriculotherapy (Chinese–French ear acupuncture). It is hard to ascertain the number of therapies in existence at any one time as new therapies or sub-specialisms are constantly emerging. The emergence of new therapies and the evolution of existing ones make the task of creating taxonomies (classifications) for CAM even more difficult.

First, consideration is needed of whether and why it may be important to rank or classify the different therapies.

This chapter extends the introduction to complementary and alternative medicine started in Chapter 1. As there, it will be more valuable to focus on the general issues in this chapter, than on details about the classification of individual therapies. The primary concern is the political charge to the terms that are used for CAM. Also, this chapter will help you explore why it is important for the different therapies that are believed to be outside the orthodox establishment to be classified. Finally, it is important to ask yourself repeatedly: do individual CAM practitioners practising the same therapy necessarily want to be seen as part of a homogeneous whole for that therapy?

ACTIVITY   MAKING A LIST OF CAM THERAPIES

Allow 30 minutes

List as many CAM therapies as you can think of (up to 20) and then consider the following questions.

1   Do you think there is a need to group these different therapies?

2   If your answer is 'yes', why do you think classifications are important?
     If your answer is 'no', can you justify your position?

3   Which people might need to classify CAM?

Comment

Your list probably includes some or all of the following CAM therapies (in no particular order).

Acupuncture	Ayurveda	Arabic medicine
Bach flower remedies	Shiatsu	Iridology
Crystal therapy	Osteopathy	Chiropractic
Spiritual healing	Aromatherapy	Reflexology
Reiki	Traditional Chinese medicine	Qi gong
Homoeopathy	Herbalism	Naturopathy
Massage	Therapeutic touch	T'ai chi

This activity raises some of the key issues about CAM and how its practice may be perceived as different from orthodox health care. In the same way that conventional health care can be divided into acute care or community care, and the practitioners can be called physicians, nurses and allied health professionals (physiotherapists, radiographers, etc.), you the reader or CAM practitioner may need a taxonomy to help you choose which therapy to recommend or use. Also, people other than practitioners may require classifications, for example users and purchasers of services, policy makers and regulators.

Individual CAM practitioners may not believe that classification is necessary, as they may be apolitical and not identify with other CAM practitioners beyond those practising the same therapy or belonging to the same organisation. Some practitioners may go further and discredit other therapies. However, consumer choices do not seem to be dictated by these groupings (Ong and Banks, 2003), so the reason why this is an issue needs to be considered further.

A primary reason for organising these different approaches (or **modalities**) into more manageable categories was to enable policy decisions to be made about research, regulation, risk assessment and patient access. However, the process of categorising CAM is complex and controversial. This is not surprising, given the lack of agreement about what CAM is or is not.

Many CAM practitioners recognise the need for some form of classification. In the absence of strong individual professional identity among many CAM modalities, it is hard for policy makers and health care purchasers to negotiate with, or work alongside, CAM. Other practitioners feel strongly that each CAM therapy should be considered on its own merits. For them, attempts to classify CAM are dangerous and could be used in ways that either marginalise lay practitioners or make it easier for certain therapies to be incorporated into orthodox medicine. This process of combining CAM therapies alongside conventional health care is known as **integrated medicine** in the UK or **integrative medicine** in the USA. Two main trends can be identified: first, the grouping together of therapies which either use similar therapeutic interventions (for example, product-based therapies) or have similar underlying philosophies (energy-based interventions); and second, classifying therapies according to their perceived level of risk of harm. This chapter considers the current forms of classification and suggests a different categorisation, based on the ethical issues arising from different therapies.

ACTIVITY   DESCRIBING CAM

Allow 30 minutes

This is a three-part activity, which builds on the activity 'What are your assumptions about CAM?' in Chapter 1.

1   Ask two people for their opinions about complementary and alternative medicine. Compile a list of all the terms they and you use to describe it.

2   Arrange these descriptions of CAM from the most positive to the most negative.

3   Reflect on both the positive and the negative terms. Write some notes on the context in which these terms are used. Do you think this reveals anything about the beliefs and values of the people using these terms?

Comment

This activity demonstrates how difficult it is to find terms that appropriately encapsulate the vast array of interventions that make up CAM. Some of the terms relate to the 'natural' or non-reductionist nature of CAM: seeing the whole person rather than their symptoms or the results of tests. Other terms include 'holistic' medicine, or 'médécin douce' in France ('sweet' or 'soft' medicine). However, you may have noted that many terms for CAM are pejorative: for example, voodoo medicine, witchcraft, quack medicine, New Age medicine, charlatanism, fringe medicine and marginal medicine. A unifying theme to these terms seems to be the notion that these approaches to health and healing are unscientific, or backward, especially in comparison with orthodox medicine. However, these pejorative terms may also reveal deeply held biases for the person using them. Some of these terms suggest an imperialist attitude towards healing practices from other cultures.

Some terms for CAM try to capture its inherent qualities, for example natural medicine, holistic therapies and traditional healing systems. An obvious criticism of these terms is that not all CAM practitioners are holistic (viewing the patient as a whole and part of their social network), in the same way that all conventionally trained doctors are not reductionist. Similarly, CAM may be more natural than orthodox medicine, but is this an appropriate term if the public mistakenly associate 'natural' with 'safe' and potentially expose themselves to harmful side effects as a result?

You might also have listed various terms that describe a range of practices within CAM, such as 'body work' or 'energy work'. These less value-laden terms are often the ones CAM practitioners themselves use to describe their work.

You probably also noted that CAM is often defined by what it is not, rather than what it is. For this group of terms, CAM is defined in opposition to conventional health care. The terms include 'alternative medicine', 'complementary medicine' and 'non-conventional medicine'. Do you think it is helpful to think of CAM and orthodox medicine in such binary (opposing) terms, especially when so many people now use an array of approaches as part of their personal health care?

Since this form of describing CAM is so common, the next section describes how these terms arose, and the impact they have on the public's perceptions of CAM.

2.2 Definitions of exclusion

Most descriptors of complementary and alternative medicine presuppose the dominance of the biomedical paradigm and describe CAM as being external to it. In other words, the dominant definition implies that these practices are 'complementary' or 'alternative' to orthodox medicine. Thus fringe, or marginal, medicine implies working at the edge of orthodox or 'allopathic' medicine.

For many years, what became known as 'the Harvard definition' of alternative medicine defined CAM as anything that was not taught in conventional medical schools in the UK or the USA. In a sense, this definition remains useful, if only for demonstrating how arbitrary the many different terms are. The medical school curriculum constantly responds to change and the medical education provided today is very different from in the past. As Prince Charles provocatively observed: 'today's unorthodoxy is probably going to be tomorrow's convention' (BMA, 1986, p. 1). Nowadays, the Harvard definition is particularly ironic, since many medical and nursing schools in the UK and USA offer students opportunities to learn about some aspects of CAM.

It is impossible to assess how much the use of negative terms has contributed to the marginalisation of CAM, both in the public's mind and in terms of health service provision. It is no coincidence that the most disparaging names for CAM often come from members of the medical profession even though the prevailing view of CAM has softened considerably: for example, see Morrell (2001) for a discussion of the pejorative use of the term 'quackery'. Many doctors in the UK now support the use of CAM. Some have even acquired their own training in it. This name-calling could be seen as orthodox medicine trying to preserve its professional monopoly on health (Stone and Matthews, 1996). At the very least, the use of these pejorative terms helped convey a general message that CAM is not to be trusted in the same way as conventional medicine and that CAM practitioners cannot be trusted in the way that doctors are. It may also have limited the realm of CAM in the public's mind to areas in which conventional medicine is least successful, for example treating chronic illness and allergies. This is misleading, as CAM can be used as a treatment for serious conditions (for example homoeopathy to treat acute asthma or acute infection, and acupuncture to treat addiction and help recovery from stroke).

In the USA, the National Center for Complementary and Alternative Medicine (NCCAM) is the Federal Government's leading agency for scientific research on complementary and alternative medicine:

> NCCAM's mission is to explore complementary and alternative healing practices in the context of rigorous science, to train CAM researchers, and to inform the public and health professionals about the results of CAM research studies.
>
> (NCCAM, 2004)

NCCAM offers the following definition of CAM.

> Complementary and alternative medicine ... is a group of diverse medical and health care systems, practices, and products that are not presently considered to be part of conventional medicine. While some scientific evidence exists regarding some CAM therapies, for most there are key

questions that are yet to be answered through well-designed scientific studies – questions such as whether they are safe and whether they work for the diseases or medical conditions for which they are used.

The list of what is considered to be CAM changes continually, as those therapies that are proven to be safe and effective become adopted into conventional health care and as new approaches to health care emerge.

(NCCAM, 2004)

The Cochrane Collaboration is an organisation which collects reviews on health-related issues in order to 'make the results of research assessing the effects of health care more easily available to those who want to make better decisions' (2003).

It gives another important definition of CAM as:

A broad domain of healing resources that encompasses all health systems and modalities, and practices and their accompanying theories and beliefs, other than those intrinsic to the politically dominant health systems of a particular society or culture in a given historical period.

(The Cochrane Collaboration, 2003)

Both definitions highlight the tendency to define CAM as that which is outside orthodox medicine. The Cochrane Collaboration's definition suggests that this can be considered principally a political issue. As in the Harvard definition, CAM is whatever orthodox medicine is not. However, the definition also hints that this is not fixed, because the dominant health system is a political and social construct, which changes from time to time and from culture to culture. When considered in conjunction with the NCCAM definition, it is possible to see that how other people describe CAM is not necessarily how CAM practitioners might define it. The definitions imply not only that orthodox medicine predominates but also that it has the power to incorporate a CAM modality into conventional medicine if and when it fits in with established biomedical criteria. This may partly explain why some CAM practitioners are wary of the medical profession's motives.

The differences between CAM and orthodox medicine are not limited to mere therapeutic concerns. Daniel Eskinazi challenges other popular definitions of CAM by calling the whole group 'alternative medicine':

I propose that **alternative medicine** be defined as a broad set of health care practices (i.e., already available to the public) that are not readily integrated into the dominant health care model, because they pose challenges to diverse societal beliefs and practices (cultural, economic, scientific, medical, and educational). This definition brings into focus factors that may play a major role in the a priori acceptance or rejection of various alternative health care practices by any society. Unlike criteria of current definitions, those of the proposed definition would not be expected to change significantly without significant societal changes.

(Eskinazi, 1998, p. 1622)

Stone (2002) notes that this definition is helpful in that it demonstrates the full extent to which CAM poses a threat to prevailing orthodoxies. In highlighting the various challenges alternative medicine poses, Eskinazi clarifies the point that acceptance or rejection by the medical profession is no longer the main or sole issue, because alternative healing systems are grounded in a wider range of concerns. This represents a significant shift in the debate, as in the past it was assumed that doctors, as the guardians of health, were best placed to comment on CAM. Eskinazi's definition recognises that the issues intrinsic to CAM philosophy go beyond what historically has been considered the concern of medicine, for example the impact of the environment on individual health, or the effects of social relationships on health, healing and coping.

The term 'traditional medicine' in itself is controversial. In the activity 'Describing CAM', you may have included 'non-traditional medicine' as a name for CAM. From what you have read so far, you will appreciate that when the term 'non-traditional' is used in this way, it implies that conventional medicine is traditional medicine. Unfortunately, the claim to ownership of this term is even stronger among therapies that have existed for hundreds or thousands of years. (Remember that western medicine in more or less its current form is only about 150 years old). About 20 per cent of the world's population have access to hi-tech western medicine. The remaining 80 per cent rely on traditional medicine (or TM). TM is used to describe indigenous healing practices falling outside western medicine, including traditional Chinese medicine (TCM), Indian ayurvedic medicine, Arabic unani medicine, and traditional Hawaiian healing.

As the World Health Organization notes (WHO, 2002), in countries where the dominant health care system is based on allopathic medicine, or where TM has not been incorporated into the national health care system, traditional medicine is often called 'complementary' or 'alternative' to conventional medicine. However, it is important to remember that in many societies TM is the only healing option and therefore it cannot be seen in that context as 'alternative'.

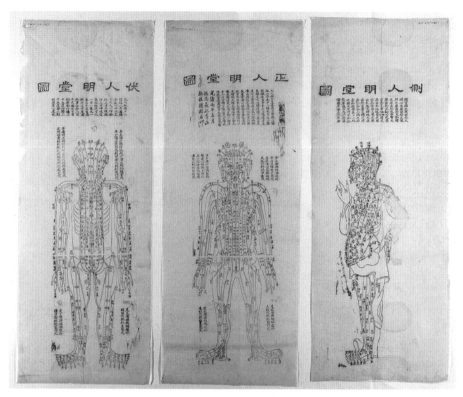

Traditional Chinese medicine has been the dominant health tradition in China for centuries. Its body of knowledge addresses a variety of conditions, using acupuncture as the main treatment

ACTIVITY   'COMPLEMENTARY' OR 'ALTERNATIVE'?

Allow 30 minutes

Reflect on the responses you had from the people you asked to describe complementary and alternative medicine.

1   Did they differentiate between 'complementary' and 'alternative' medicine?

2   Did they refer to 'traditional' medicine at all?

Comment

One person who did this activity noted that 'complementary' and 'alternative' are both unhelpful when considering the wider perspective of 'good' health care and suggested that they are only useful for the purpose of developing policy. By using these terms therapies will always be viewed as 'outside' or 'on the fringes of' conventional health care.

2.3   Is there a difference between 'complementary' and 'alternative' medicine?

The term 'complementary and alternative medicine' has been the main term used by both CAM practitioners and health providers in the UK and the USA since the early 1990s. So it is important to be clear what it means. Think about the differences between the two words 'complementary' and 'alternative'. Why are both terms used?

Although not all practitioners accept that the distinction between 'complementary' and 'alternative' is valid or meaningful, much of the literature makes a firm distinction between 'complementary' medicine on the one hand and 'alternative' medicine on the other. The BMA report (1993) states:

> It is worth briefly making the distinction between those therapies which are viewed as 'complementary' and those described as 'alternative'. 'Complementary' therapies are those which can work alongside and in conjunction with orthodox medical treatment. Within this category there is clearly a wide diversity of types of practice, which would include self-help therapies such as yoga; re-educational therapies such as the Alexander Technique; relatively non-invasive therapies such as healing and massage; and all interventive therapies such as acupuncture, osteopathy, and chiropractic. Practitioners such as osteopaths or chiropractors can, for example, treat the mechanical components of a musculo-skeletal problem whilst the patient is concurrently taking prescribed medications from their general practitioner, in the form of analgesics, non-steroidal anti-inflammatory drugs (NSAID), or muscle relaxants. In this role, the therapies are an additional and a complementary form of treatment. In the clinical practices of osteopathy and chiropractic, the basic training is largely grounded in the orthodox medical sciences and, as such, practitioners of these disciplines are able to have a close dialogue with their medical colleagues which is based upon a common language. Training modules for these practices increasingly place emphasis on working in conjunction and liaison with established health-care professionals.
>
> By contrast, 'alternative' therapies could be seen as those which are given in place of orthodox medical treatment. While clearly any non-conventional therapy could in some circumstances be used as an alternative form of treatment – for example, if a practitioner of any discipline suggested that the patient should not receive concurrent orthodox medical treatment – there are some therapies which, by their very nature, aim to **replace** orthodox medicine. Examples of such therapies might include herbal medicines, which are often given in place of orthodox medication, as an alternative to allopathic drugs.

(BMA, 1993, pp. 6–7)

In the USA, NCCAM makes a similar distinction to the BMA, differentiating between complementary and alternative medicine using the following definitions.

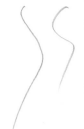

- **Complementary** medicine is used together with conventional medicine. An example of a complementary therapy is using aromatherapy to help lessen a patient's discomfort following surgery.

- **Alternative** medicine is used **in place** of conventional medicine. An example of an alternative therapy is using a special diet to treat cancer instead of undergoing surgery, radiation, or chemotherapy that has been recommended by a conventional doctor.

(NCCAM, 2004)

The House of Lords' report on complementary and alternative medicine in the UK draws the following distinction:

> CAM embraces those therapies that may either be provided alongside conventional medicine (complementary) or which may, in the view of their practitioners, act as a substitute for it. Alternative disciplines purport to provide diagnostic information as well as offering therapy.

(House of Lords, 2000)

A key element of alternative medicine is that it involves a diagnosis within a potentially different framework from a conventional diagnosis. For example, when an acupuncturist detects dampness in a patient's pulse, this bears no relation to an orthodox diagnosis. However, is this apparent differentiation based on diagnosis helpful, or is it politically inspired? Stone and Matthews (1996) argue that it is an unhelpful distinction, borne out of political considerations rather than reflecting the reality of the clinical encounter. The key distinction between 'alternative' and 'complementary' therapy is that the latter is considered to be an adjunct to conventional treatment. Complementary practitioners may work alongside a patient's medical practitioners and treat according to the medical diagnosis. Alternative practitioners work within a different diagnostic realm altogether and, as such, are perceived as more threatening to conventional medicine.

Stone and Matthews (1996) argue that all CAM practitioners diagnose within their own sphere of practice and belief systems, and make judgements based on their belief and knowledge to determine what treatment to offer. Any practitioner, at however basic a level, has to decide what the problem is and how to approach it. To draw a distinction based on whether the practitioner makes an official 'diagnosis' is unhelpful semantics, and seems to be a covert way of discussing the relative risks various therapies present. None the less, this distinction is still used by many people involved in CAM politics. Some CAM umbrella bodies have suggested that complementary practitioners should not make a 'medical diagnosis', as only medical doctors can do this. Stone and Matthews observe:

> Likewise, the [British Complementary Medicine Association's] code insists complementary practitioners may not make a 'medical diagnosis', this being something which only medical doctors can do (para. 1.14). The BCMA position is that new patients must be asked what medical advice they have received. If they have not seen a doctor they must be advised to do so (para. 1.11). Given, however, that a patient cannot be forced to consult an allopathic doctor, the BCMA cautions that this advice must be recorded for the practitioner's protection. Note that the code does not go on to say that practitioners must refuse to treat patients unless they have received a medical diagnosis.
>
> There are obvious political reasons why an organization dedicated to stressing that use of these therapies is complementary to orthodox medicine, should stress, as a matter of territorial boundaries, that therapists do not make a 'medical diagnosis'. There are also the strongest consumer protection grounds for emphasizing this point. Without a full medical training, it would be highly dangerous for complementary therapists to attempt to give a diagnosis in medical terms, which is highly likely to be wrong and may be a diagnosis upon which the patient relies to his or her detriment. Moreover, from a legal point of view, complementary practitioners would place themselves in an extremely vulnerable position were they to make medical diagnoses, on the basis of which the patients did not receive urgent medical treatment and suffered harm. (This is not to suggest that diagnosing is a precise science, or that doctors, even if consulted, always make an accurate diagnosis.)
>
> (Stone and Matthews, 1996, p. 197)

2.4   Integrated or integrative health care: the name of the future?

In the same way as the term 'complementary and alternative medicine' was commonly used in the 1990s, **'integrated'** (or **'integrative'** as it is called in the USA) medicine or health care is increasingly used to denote the incorporation of some CAMs or concepts of CAM alongside orthodox medicine.

Rees and Weil (2001, p. 119) describe integrated medicine as:

> practising medicine in a way that selectively incorporates elements of complementary and alternative medicine into comprehensive treatment plans alongside solidly orthodox methods of diagnosis and treatment.

This implies a far greater linkage of CAM with the world of evidence-based practice. Rees and Weil also point out that, inevitably, integrated health care must be different from CAM:

> Integrated medicine has a larger meaning and mission, its focus being on health and healing rather than disease and treatment. It views patients as whole people with minds and spirits as well as bodies and includes these dimensions into [sic] diagnosis and treatment. It also involves patients and doctors working to maintain health by paying attention to lifestyle factors such as diet, exercise, quality of rest and sleep, and the nature of relationships.
>
> (Rees and Weil, 2001, p. 119)

NCCAM's definition is particular, specific and exclusive:

> Integrative medicine, as defined by NCCAM, combines mainstream medical therapies and CAM therapies for which there is some high-quality scientific evidence of safety and effectiveness.
>
> (NCCAM, 2004)

The Prince of Wales's Foundation for Integrated Health defines integrated medicine in a more all-encompassing way, explicitly suggesting that integrated health is not simply CAM repackaged:

> Integrated medicine or healthcare is not another term for complementary medicine, nor does it represent an alternative to conventional care. An integrated approach is much wider. It focuses on health and healing, rather than just disease and treatment and seeks to bring together body, mind and spirit so that healthcare encompasses the whole person. Integrated healthcare sees each human being as an individual and starts by recognising that each one of us has many dimensions and lives in a unique social and environmental context. It acknowledges the high level of responsibility individuals have for their own health ...
>
> In such a partnership, conventional and complementary practitioners would work together. For example, a physician might prescribe medication for migraine, but look for underlying factors such as stress or diet that could cause or perpetuate the condition. An integrated therapeutic package agreed with the patient and with complementary practitioners could include acupuncture to reduce the frequency of attacks and induce relaxation, nutritional advice, a herbal remedy as a preventive measure and yoga, relaxation and other stress-management techniques to encourage natural healing processes.
>
> (The Prince of Wales's Foundation for Integrated Health, 2003, p. 9)

As with all new ways of working, the term 'integrated' or 'integrative' medicine makes several implicit assumptions with which CAM practitioners may or may not agree. The use of the term 'integrated medicine' indicates how far CAM has come in a relatively short time. In 1986 the BMA published a report called *Alternative Therapy*. This fostered negative stereotypes about CAM and fuelled the hostility between CAM practitioners and the medical professional in a most unhelpful way (this is elaborated on in Chapters 3 and 7). However, in 1993 the BMA's second report reversed some of its earlier conclusions, sounding cautiously positive:

> It is clear that there are many encouraging initiatives currently taking place in the field of non-conventional therapy, and it is to be hoped that good practice in each can be extrapolated for general use.
>
> (BMA, 1993, p. 3)

The BMA (1993) recommends that potential CAM clients should find out:

1   Whether the therapist is registered with a professional organisation.
2   Whether that body has a public register of members, a code of practice, effective disciplinary procedures and sanctions, and a complaints mechanism.
3   What qualifications the therapist has, and where they were obtained.
4   How long the therapist has been practising.
5   Whether the therapist is covered by any form of malpractice insurance.

The most interesting aspect of the report's recommendations is the focus on therapies being registered and the professional association having a code of practice, etc. These issues are discussed in Chapter 4.

In the past 20 years there has been a shift in orthodox medical practice away from a mechanistic, reductionist model towards a model that recognises the fact that behavioural and social influences are as important as biomedical factors.

ACTIVITY   COMPETING BELIEF SYSTEMS

Allow 15 minutes

Read the following excerpt by Julie Stone (2002, pp. 273-4) on integration.

> Although [in certain societies] models of integrated health care exist in which competing belief systems flourish and are equally valued, this tends to be where the alternative modality was highly valued in the culture prior to the emergence of western, hi-tech medicine. Elsewhere, the might of modernist medicine will prevail. Integration, at least in the USA and Europe, will almost certainly take the form of conventional medicine incorporating evidence based aspects of CAM and dismissing what remains as having no place in modern, effective health care systems. This prediction is made quite explicit by Stephen E. Straus, MD, Director of the US National Institutes of Health National Center for Complementary and Alternative Medicine. [He writes]:

As a result of rigorous scientific investigation, several therapeutic and preventive modalities currently deemed elements of complementary and alternative medicine will have proven effective. Therefore, by 2020, these interventions will have been incorporated into conventional medical education and practice, and the term 'complementary and alternative medicine' will be superseded by the concept of 'integrative medicine' ... Advances in neurobiology will elucidate mechanisms underlying ancient practices such as acupuncture and meditation, as well as the phenomenon of 'the placebo effect' ... Other modalities will have proven unsafe or ineffective, and an informed public will have rejected them. The field of integrative medicine will be seen as providing novel insights and tools for human health, and not as a source of intellectual and philosophical tension that insinuates itself between and among practitioners of the healing arts and their patients.

1   Do you share Stephen Straus's view of the future of CAM?
2   Do you think the public share the medical profession's concern about the scientific basis for CAM?

Comment

Picking up on a theme discussed earlier, many CAM practitioners fear that 'integrated/integrative health care' is a disguise for the incorporation of CAM by orthodox medicine. Other CAM practitioners are more optimistic (for example, the Prince of Wales's Foundation statement cited above). For them, the term 'integration' reflects broader transformations within medicine, away from a reductionist, mechanistic model and towards a 'wellness' model that takes account of the effects on health of environmental, socioeconomic and political as well as physiological and psychological factors. The philosophies underpinning CAM are certainly well placed to contribute to this gradual paradigm shift, but 'integrative health care' may mean something different to CAM practitioners' current understanding of the term. The influential report of the US National Research Council (2001) sees an integrative approach as incorporating research and practice in social, behavioural and biomedical sciences. According to this wider approach of integrative health care, CAM would certainly make a contribution, but a contribution alongside biomedical science.

2.5   Classifying different CAM therapies

As the nomenclature of CAM is constantly changing, so are the taxonomies to categorise the many therapies within CAM and TM. The sheer number of therapies has led to categorisation and subcategorisation. These groupings are commonly based on the type of intervention. For example, the US Chantilly report divides therapies into seven broad categories of holistic practice:

1   mind–body interventions

2   bioelectromagnetic applications in medicine

3   alternative systems of medical practice

4   manual healing methods

5   pharmacological and biological treatments not yet accepted by mainstream medicine

6   herbal medicines

7   treatments focusing on diet and nutrition in the prevention and treatment of chronic disease.
(Department of Health and Human Services, 1994)

NCCAM classified CAM therapies into five similar categories or domains (see Box 2.1).

BOX 2.1   THE MAJOR TYPES OF CAM

1 Alternative medical systems

Alternative medical systems are built upon complete systems of theory and practice. Often, these systems have evolved apart from and earlier than the conventional medical approach used in the United States. Examples of alternative medical systems that have developed in Western cultures include homeopathic medicine and naturopathic medicine. Examples of systems that have developed in non-Western cultures include traditional Chinese medicine and Ayurveda.

2 Mind-body interventions

Mind-body medicine uses a variety of techniques designed to enhance the mind's capacity to affect bodily function and symptoms. Some techniques that were considered CAM in the past have become mainstream (for example, patient support groups and cognitive-behavioral therapy). Other mind-body techniques are still considered CAM, including meditation, prayer, mental healing, and therapies that use creative outlets such as art, music, or dance.

3 Biologically based therapies

Biologically based therapies in CAM use substances found in nature, such as herbs, foods, and vitamins. Some examples include dietary supplements, herbal products, and the use of other so-called 'natural' but as yet scientifically unproven therapies (for example, using shark cartilage to treat cancer).

4 Manipulative and body-based methods

Manipulative and body-based methods in CAM are based on manipulation and/or movement of one or more parts of the body. Some examples include chiropractic or osteopathic manipulation, and massage.

5 Energy therapies

Energy therapies involve the use of energy fields. They are two types:

- **Biofield therapies** are intended to affect energy fields that purportedly surround and penetrate the human body. The existence of such fields has not yet been scientifically proven. Some forms of energy therapy manipulate biofields by applying pressure and/or manipulating the body by placing the hands in, or through, these fields. Examples include qi gong, Reiki, and Therapeutic Touch.

- **Bioelectromagnetic-based therapies** involve the unconventional use of electromagnetic fields, such as pulsed fields, magnetic fields, or alternating current or direct current fields.

(Source: NCCAM, 2004)

The House of Lords Select Committee Report

In 2000, the House of Lords Select Committee on Science and Technology published a highly influential report covering all aspects of CAM. They took evidence from a wide variety of sources, and their report is the most important policy document about CAM produced in the UK so far. As with any policy document about CAM, an early task for the Committee was to devise a form of classification that facilitated discussion about the different groups of practitioners and modalities falling within the report's remit. The Committee's categorisation is set out in Box 2.2.

BOX 2.2   THE HOUSE OF LORDS' CATEGORISATION OF CAM

In the opinion of the Committee, these therapies and disciplines fall into three broad groups:

- The first group embraces what may be called the principal disciplines, two of which, osteopathy and chiropractic, are already regulated in their professional activity and education by Acts of Parliament. The others are acupuncture, herbal medicine and homeopathy. Our evidence has indicated that each of these therapies claim to have an individual diagnostic approach and that these therapies are seen as the 'Big Five' by most of the CAM world.

- The second group contains therapies which are most often used to complement conventional medicine and do not purport to embrace diagnostic skills. It includes aromatherapy; the Alexander technique; body work therapies, including massage; counselling; stress therapy; hypnotherapy; reflexology and probably shiatsu; meditation and healing.

> ■ The third group embraces those other disciplines ... which purport to offer diagnostic information as well as treatment and which, in general, favour a philosophical approach and are indifferent to the scientific principles of conventional medicine, and through which various and disparate frameworks of disease causation and its management are proposed. These therapies can be split into two sub-groups. Group 3a includes long-established and traditional systems of healthcare such as Ayurvedic medicine and Traditional Chinese medicine. Group 3b covers other alternative disciplines which lack any credible evidence base such as crystal therapy, iridology, radionics, dowsing and kinesiology.
>
> (Source: House of Lords, 2000, para. 2.1)

The House of Lords' grouping stirred up considerable confusion and anger within the CAM field. Acupuncturists found the report particularly baffling, since they seemed to fall within both Group 1 and Group 3 (that is, simultaneously highly credible and unreliable because they also fall within the TCM category).

Group 1 seems to conflate related but distinct issues. The first issue is whether the therapy has been regulated, and the second whether the therapies in this group have an individual diagnostic approach. Assuming this means these therapies diagnose within an alternative diagnostic framework, the real interest in Group 1 therapies could be interpreted as their perceived level of safety and risk. However, the level of risk in these therapies is not equal. Homoeopathy has few side effects compared with, say, chiropractic, which can cause serious injury if practised by unskilled hands. Also, some people might question how alternative the diagnostic system within chiropractic and osteopathy is to a conventional musculoskeletal diagnosis. Group 1 therapies also bring together the so-called 'Big Five' (acupuncture, osteopathy, chiropractic, herbalism and homoeopathy). Retaining a group in the Big Five is short-sighted unless they are linked by useful criteria. A desire for statutory self-regulation is not limited to the Big Five, and other therapies are just as popular with patients.

Group 2 perpetuates the distinction between complementary and alternative therapies criticised by Stone (2002) but widely used in debates about what CAM is or is not. Moreover, many practitioners listed in this group would probably dispute that they do not diagnose and treat.

However, Group 3 gives most cause for concern by combining highly respected forms of traditional medicine that fall outside western medicine (Group 3a) with discredited therapies, which have no evidence of acceptability to the scientific community (Group 3b). Apart from merging therapies that have been in recorded existence for several thousand years in the same group with therapies that may have existed for only a few years, the conceptual basis for this group is also unclear.

2.6   Whole systems versus non-whole systems

The BMA (1993) points out that several of the CAM therapies are not claimed to be 'whole systems' of medicine in the same way as orthodox medicine. It prefers the term 'discrete clinical disciplines'. However, the 'complete system' approach of these therapies distinguishes this group most clearly from other complementary therapies and, accordingly, exercises a critical influence on such issues as organisation and education.

Furthermore, this group is usually identified as having the greatest potential to cause harm, as doctors believe that patients are less likely to seek the medical advice they might need if the therapy they pursue has an answer or an explanatory model for everything. It seems somewhat inappropriate to prejudge the issue of potential to cause harm in the absence of systematically collected data, showing that particular therapies do put patients at greater risk of harm. Moreover, policy makers need to consider the consumer freedom issues involved in patients voluntarily rejecting conventional medical advice and preferring to rely on a CAM practitioner.

The 'Big Five'

This classification by the House of Lords Committee concerns the professional organisation and the regulatory aspirations of the five therapies more than the inherent characteristics of acupuncture, homoeopathy, herbalism, osteopathy and chiropractic. Although they all might have claimed to be whole systems originally, there has been a shift, so that osteopathy and chiropractic are less vocal about their 'cure-all' claims and holistic approach. This may be to gain acceptance by the medical profession as a modality that could most easily be integrated with the dominant biomedical paradigm. For example, chiropractic is not necessarily seen as a CAM now that it is regulated but as part of the dominant biomedical model.

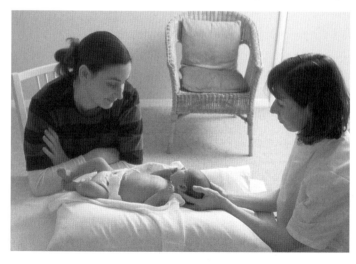

A baby having cranio-sacral osteopathy, which is meant to relieve the distress suffered at birth. This addresses a particular problem and does not purport to provide long-term care

However, as whole systems, each of the 'Big Five' therapies is considered riskier and therefore more in need of urgent regulation than other therapies. They are also among the most popular therapies in the UK.

Categorising CAM according to regulatory status or potential

Many professions in the UK are regulated by representative or formally constituted bodies. Regulated professionals include doctors, lawyers, accountants, architects, and so on. Regulation provides security for the profession, as well as the population at large, that standards are set and adhered to by practitioners. In a regulated profession, practitioners have to pass specific professional exams to demonstrate their fitness to practise and they are increasingly required to undergo revalidation procedures to ensure their continuing competence. The General Medical Council regulates the medical profession. For example, it has a professional conduct committee which assesses the fitness to practise of doctors who have been reported for unethical or unprofessional behaviour. It has the power to withdraw the registration of medical practitioners who are deemed unfit to practise, or to recommend or demand further training for practitioners who practise below the required standard.

In the UK, where only a few CAM therapies are statutorily regulated (or exhibit mature self-regulatory characteristics), there are concerns about classifying all types of CAM therapies under the same heading. Therapies with a long history of safe usage, whose mechanisms are known and which are based on an extensive body of knowledge (such as acupuncture or herbal medicine), may have little in common with untried, unresearched and unproven techniques (such as the less well known therapies of crystal therapy or aura cleansing).

None the less, therapies that seem to fall into a similar regulatory 'category' can be grouped together. For example, herbalism and homoeopathy most obviously sit within medicine-licensing provisions. Aromatherapy oils claiming specific therapeutic uses also seem to require product licensing, although oils that are marketed for general wellbeing purposes could also sit alongside beauty product regulation. The position of food supplements is also controversial. Should they be classified as foods or medicines? By classifying them as foods, they do not have to satisfy the requirements of quality, safety and efficacy that medicines do. However, if this regulatory avenue is ignored, the public is denied any knowledge about the intended or possible medical effects and side effects.

Classifying CAM therapies according to ethical issues

Stone (2002) categorises CAM disciplines by grouping therapies based on the ethical issues they raise. Whereas the other classifications have implicitly political overtones, Stone believes that a categorisation explicitly based on ethical issues takes account of the underlying concerns, such as inherent risk and capacity to cause harm. An appreciation of this classification requires an understanding of the scope of **ethics**. Here, ethical considerations include the following principles:

■ any form of treatment should have the capacity to benefit and not harm
■ treatment should usually be given on the basis of a voluntary, informed decision
■ appropriate mechanisms should be in place in case anything goes wrong.

Stone's classification divides therapies into the following six groups.

1 **Hands-on therapies** include chiropractic, osteopathy, shiatsu, massage, rolfing, reflexology, aromatherapy and therapeutic touch.

2 **Invasive therapies** include acupuncture, colonic irrigation, chelation therapy and any therapy using an invasive technique.

3 **Product-based therapies** include homoeopathy, herbalism (western and traditional Chinese herbal medicine), ayurveda, unani, aromatherapy, nutritional therapy and Bach flower remedies.

4 **Energy-based medicine** includes spiritual healing, intercessory prayer, crystal healing, radionics, channelling, reiki, therapeutic touch, acupuncture, shiatsu, ta'i chi and qi gong.

5 **Psychological intervention** includes hypnotherapy, counselling and psychotherapy.

6 **Self-help techniques** include yoga, biofeedback, meditation, visualisation, self-hypnosis, relaxation techniques, the Alexander technique, ta'i chi, qi gong and autogenic training.

Each group is based on a predominant ethical concern. For example, hands-on therapies are linked by respect for bodily sovereignty and the extent to which lawyers and ethicists regard the slightest 'unwanted touching' as infringement of a patient's autonomy. In hands-on therapies, autonomy and boundary issues are thus paramount, as touching the patient inappropriately could be construed as abusive, and lead to professional disciplinary proceedings.

Product-based therapies are linked by their capacity to cause harm as well as good. Thus there is a need for quality control and for practitioners to give the patient adequate information about the product so they can make an informed choice about its use. The linking of product-based therapies also highlights regulatory issues, including the evidence base which is required before specific medicinal claims can be made about CAM products.

Self-help techniques are linked from an ethical perspective by the extent to which patients are expected to take responsibility for themselves and the consequent sharing of responsibility for outcomes.

Stone acknowledges that this grouping may require further refinement. None the less, her classification is intended to bring the specific concerns about groups of therapies to the forefront rather than to blur the issues with spurious distinctions such as whether CAM practitioners truly 'diagnose'.

The position outside the English-speaking world

The classification of CAM is very different outside the UK, especially in parts of the world where the influence or availability of orthodox medicine is limited. Eighty per cent of the world's population rely on traditional forms of healing, so the status of non-conventional medicine is radically different because it is often the only medicine people can access.

The World Health Organization identified four major organisational relationships characterising the provision of orthodox and traditional medicine (Stephan, 1983). The four systems are described in Box 2.3.

BOX 2.3 DIFFERENT SYSTEMS OF CAM

1 The **monopolistic system** in which orthodox medical practitioners have the exclusive right to practise medicine. All other forms of healing are illegal, although enforcement of this monopoly varies from country to country. In France, for example, osteopathy is unlawful unless practised by a medical practitioner.

2 The **tolerant system** in which orthodox medicine has exclusivity within the official health services, but non-conventional medicine is still legally available outside that sector. This system most closely resembles the organisational relationship between orthodox and unorthodox medicine in the UK.

3 The **parallel system** in which practitioners of both orthodox and unorthodox medicine are officially recognised. While both services are available to patients, the organisational systems controlling the two divisions of medicine remain separate.

4 The **integrated system** in which the two systems of medicine are merged into one both for the purposes of medical education and when made available through the health services. For non-conventional therapies to be incorporated into health care systems in the West, there will have to be a shift to a more flexible system in which such therapies can be legalised or formally recognised by the state. For example, in India, ayurvedic medicine and homoeopathy are practised alongside western orthodox medicine.

(Source: adapted from Stephan, 1983)

Although there has been a significant growth of CAM throughout the European Union (EU) since the 1970s, there is no European-wide classification system covering complementary and alternative medicine

(Fisher and Ward, 1994). In general, each Member State determines whether a professional activity should be regulated or not. The EU position is explained by Fisher and Ward:

> In most member states of the European Union, including Belgium, France, Spain, Italy, and Greece, the practice of medicine, except by statutorily recognised health professionals, is illegal. This is also technically the situation in the Netherlands, but the Dutch government has stated that it will not prosecute non-medically qualified practitioners unless there has been malpractice. A comprehensive reform of the law governing medical practice in the Netherlands is under way. This will create a system of statutorily regulated registers and protected titles. In Denmark non-medically qualified practitioners may practise but the scope of their activities is restricted by law.
>
> Germany has the unique Heilpraktiker (health practitioner) system. Originally introduced in 1939, it licenses practitioners who are not members of recognised health professions to practise provided they have passed an examination in basic medical knowledge and are registered. The system is administered by the Lander (provincial governments), and standards vary considerably between regions. Heilpraktikers are specifically prohibited from practising obstetrics, dentistry, and venereology.
>
> (Fisher and Ward, 1994)

The peculiarities of national legal systems give rise to national idiosyncrasies. For example, reflexology is popular in Denmark (39 per cent of complementary medicine users), which reflects the legal situation: in 1981 the Danish High Court ruled that acupuncture is a form of surgery since it pierces the skin (Fisher and Ward, 1994).

Towards classification?

In the absence of a single overarching body for CAM in the UK, part of the problem with any model of classification is the difficulty in establishing what the different groups in CAM believe or want in relation to classification or regulation. There is a distinct lack of cohesion even between different schools of the same CAM. For many years there was considerable in-fighting among these groups, although this has receded recently; acupuncture is an example of the partial rationalisation of disparate groups. The issues of classification continue to concern some practitioners. Political aspirations or regulatory needs are taking precedence over what practitioners may believe are their main priorities: the therapeutic potential of the CAM or consumer choice.

For orthodox medical practitioners, the earlier tendency to condemn CAM has become politically unwise because of the dramatic surge in its popularity. While the UK government attempts to centralise health care and assure the public that efforts are being made to improve its quality (partly through evidence-based medicine), the private sector, which includes CAM, is still largely unregulated. Also, there is still the problem of CAM practice leading to indirect harm: for example, doctors' allegations that CAM practitioners suggest their patients should throw away their antibiotics. The BMA's report on acupuncture conveys the view that, with increasing numbers of people using CAM, there is the potential for more harm, and that orthodox medical practitioners will have to pick up the pieces and deal with the ensuing medical problems (BMA, 2002).

2.7   Conclusion

Several points emerged from this chapter. First, attempts to categorise CAM rarely concern the nature of the therapeutic intervention. Rather, the literature implies that the classification of CAM is inherently political, often reinforcing the polarised distinction between orthodox and non-orthodox medicine. In fact, most of this chapter focused on the terms that other people use for CAM practitioners, rather than the classifications CAM practitioners use. The respective names given to CAM historically represent its ongoing successes or failures vis-à-vis the dominant biomedical paradigm. The term 'integrated/integrative' is very significant because it represents the ultimate political realisation that CAM will not go away, so 'good' CAM practices (that is, those that have been proved to work and have an acceptable risk:benefit ratio) will become part of 'good' medicine. Much of the language used about integration may give CAM practitioners cause for concern that integration ultimately means incorporation. As the House of Lords' attempt shows, it is not easy to categorise CAM. You might think categorising CAM would be easier if the parties involved were honest about their motivations. Until then, several unsatisfactory terms will remain in use, most of which are unhelpful to patients, practitioners and policy makers alike.

KEY POINTS

- Classifications are necessary to organise hundreds of therapeutic modalities into categories that are more useful to consumers and other stakeholders.
- Classifications of CAM are more political than therapeutic, and are often disputed by CAM practitioners themselves.
- Previous definitions of exclusion helped maintain the marginal status of CAM, although this position is now changing.
- The term 'traditional medicine' is particularly contentious and claimed by both conventional medicine and indigenous healing systems.
- Classifications inform and are shaped by regulatory processes.
- Outside the UK there is very little consistency in classifications of CAM.

References

British Medical Association (BMA) (1986) *Alternative Therapy*, London, BMA.

British Medical Association (BMA) (1993) *Complementary Medicine: New Approaches to Good Practice*, Oxford, Oxford University Press.

British Medical Association (BMA) (2002) *Acupuncture: Efficacy, Safety and Practice*, London, Harwood Academic Publishers.

The Cochrane Collaboration (2003) [online], www.cochrane.org/Cochrane/revabstr/mainindex.htm [accessed 26 February 2004].

Department of Health and Human Services, Public Health Service, National Institutes of Health, Office of Alternative Medicine (1994) 'Alternative medicine: expanding medical horizons: a report to the National Institutes of Health on alternative medical systems and practices in the United States', *Proceedings of the Workshop on Alternative Medicine*, 14–16 September 1992, Chantilly, Virginia, HHS publication no. NIH 94066.

Eskinazi, D. (1998) 'Factors that shape alternative medicine', *Journal of the American Medical Association*, Vol. 280, No. 18, pp. 1621–3.

Fisher, P. and Ward, A. (1994) 'Complementary medicine in Europe', *British Medical Journal*, Vol. 309, pp. 107–11.

House of Lords (2000) *Complementary and Alternative Medicine*, London, The Stationery Office. Available online: www.parliament.the-stationery-office.co.uk/pa/ld199900/ldselect/ldsctech/123/12301.htm [accessed 1 June 2004].

Morrell, P. (2001) *On Quacks and Quackery* [online], bmj.com/cgi/eletters/311/7021/1712#11705 [accessed 4 January 2001].

National Center for Complementary and Alternative Medicine (NCCAM) (2004) 'What is complementary and alternative medicine (CAM)?' [online], www.nccam.nih.gov/health/whatiscam [accessed 25 February 2004].

National Research Council (2001) *New Horizons in Health: An Integrative Approach*, Washington, DC, The National Academies Press.

Ong, C. and Banks, B. (2003) *Complementary and Alternative Medicine: The Consumer Perspective*, The Prince of Wales's Foundation for Integrated Health, London.

The Prince of Wales's Foundation for Integrated Health (2003) *Setting the Agenda for the Future: A Consultation Document*, London, The Prince of Wales's Foundation.

Rees, L. and Weil, A. (2001) 'Integrated medicine imbues orthodox medicine with the values of complementary medicine', *British Medical Journal*, Vol. 322, pp. 119–20.

Stephan, J. (1983) 'Patterns of legislation concerning traditional medicine', in Bannerman, R.H.O., Burton, J. and Ch'en, W. C. (eds) *Traditional Medicine and Health Care Coverage*, Geneva, World Health Organization.

Stone, J. (2002) *An Ethical Framework for Complementary and Alternative Therapists*, London, Routledge.

Stone, J. and Matthews, J. (1996) *Complementary Medicine and the Law*, Oxford, Oxford University Press.

Straus, S. (1999) '2020 Vision: NIH heads foresee the future', *Journal of the American Medical Association*, Vol. 282, No. 24, 22–29 December.

WHO (2002) *Traditional Medicine Strategy 2002–2005* [online], www.who.int/ medicines/library/trm/trm_strat_eng.pdf [accessed 1 June 2004].

Chapter 3 Political and historical perspectives

Mike Saks

Contents

AIMS

- To demonstrate the processes of social change that have led to the diversity of health knowledge in contemporary western society.
- To illustrate and explain how the history and changing fortune of biomedicine is intertwined with the fall and the current resurgence of CAM today.

3.1 Introduction: The politics of complementary and alternative health care

This chapter outlines the historical development of complementary and alternative approaches to health in the UK. It traces the position of complementary and alternative medicine (CAM) in the health field over several centuries, spanning from practitioner-based therapies to self-help. This is done with reference to the development of orthodox medicine, since CAM cannot be fully understood in isolation. Such developments are explained in terms of political factors, which have been more important formative influences than technical changes in the health field. Politics here means the formal and informal use of power by groups in society to shape the development of CAM and health care more generally. It is assumed that this was shaped more by conflict than by consensus. Therefore, this chapter focuses on several interconnected levels of the exercise of power from interest-based skirmishes between the occupational groups concerned in this area to the involvement of the state and commercial interests. Indeed, as Chapters 1 and 2 showed, the definition of CAM itself is a matter of political debate.

Defining complementary medicine

As noted in Chapter 2, CAM is popularly seen as covering a variety of therapies, from aromatherapy and reflexology to acupuncture and homoeopathy. There have been various attempts to define such practices, based on the intrinsic nature of the therapies themselves. These include such claims as they are uniquely holistic, traditional or natural. However, such blanket definitions do not stand up to scrutiny (for example, see Saks, 1992). In terms of holism, while some complementary and alternative approaches, such as traditional Chinese medicine (TCM) and ayurvedic medicine (which originates from India), are based on generic views of health derived from philosophies linking mind and body to the wider environment, many are not. Practices such as osteopathy, while designed as a whole therapy that can treat a range of health problems, often have very mechanistic methods, in this case focusing primarily on back pain. Similarly, although some forms of CAM such as herbalism have strong traditional origins, others are more recent. Homoeopathy, for instance, only emerged in the 19th century, while biofeedback is barely 50 years old. Biofeedback is a form of therapy that uses technology to detect tiny changes in the body. Users of this therapy are taught by a practitioner to respond to feedback from the machines to help control their heart rate, relax particular muscle groups, etc. The aim is to enable users to identify problems in their bodies and to learn to respond in a way that helps them take control of the symptoms. This therapy, therefore, is completely based on the fairly recent development of appropriate technology to allow the monitoring of bodily processes. Notwithstanding the use of plants such as lavender and rosemary in aromatherapy, what could be less natural than inserting steel needles into a person's body for therapeutic purposes, as in acupuncture?

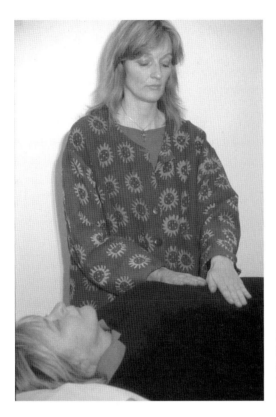

Not all CAMs have a long history. Reiki is a Japanese hands-on healing system that was developed in the late 19th century and did not arrive in the UK until the 1980s

Complementary and alternative health care

As highlighted in Chapter 2, CAM therapies are very diverse. However, they do have one feature in common: their political marginality (Saks, 1994). This is because, while CAM practitioners in the UK can practise under the Common Law and are consulted widely by the public, their therapies have not been well supported by the state through such mechanisms as research funding or inclusion in the mainstream medical educational and training curriculum. In this respect, CAM is very different from orthodox medicine. In the past orthodox medicine centred mainly on drugs and surgery, which attracted support and drew financial backing from the state. While the current biomedical orthodoxy can be distinguished by its underlying conception of the body as a symptom-bearing organism, in which the patient is viewed as a cluster of cells, the main difference lies in its legitimation by the state. However, as we shall see, such political differentiation did not fully arise until the mid-19th century.

3.2   Health care pluralism in the pre-industrial era

Health care has historically been a concern in many different cultures. It was an even more central concern for people in earlier times when life expectancy was much shorter and freedom from illness was far less common than in developed countries today. Traditionally, such health care was very simple and based mainly on self-administered treatments, for example, plant remedies and religious rituals. In early societies, medicine men and women – including shamans and witch doctors – were also important, as much for their ability to explain misfortune as to treat its consequences. Their interventions were typically centred on beliefs about the displeasure of the spirits and/or the gods of nature and had limited resonance with the ideology of 'science' that underpins orthodox medicine (Cule, 1997).

Early forms of health care

What is now regarded as orthodox medicine was influenced by the work of Galen (AD 129–201) and Avicenna (AD 980–1037), who wrote on subjects such as anatomy, physiology and prescribing in early Roman and Arabian medicine respectively (Duffin, 1999). Their work had a less substantial impact in some historical periods, particularly in medieval times in Britain, when religious dogma heavily influenced health care, and before the Renaissance, when medicine began to develop more strongly through universities (Cule, 1997).

Neither CAM nor orthodox medicine existed in pre-industrial Britain in the early 16th to mid-19th centuries because there was no clearly supported dominant practice. This did not happen until orthodox medicine formally emerged on a national basis with the Medical Registration Act 1858. Before then there was a relatively undifferentiated and diverse field of people who claimed to be able to heal in various ways: almost anyone could claim to be able to treat illness. In this field, herbalists, healers and others – including lay people living in the community called 'wise women' or 'cunning men' – competed in an open market with the emerging groups of physicians, surgeons and apothecaries (Cant and Sharma, 1999).

Although physicians, surgeons and apothecaries progressively formed associations with limited powers to license people to practise from the 16th century onwards, they did not establish a widespread unified legal monopoly of the practice of medicine until much later. On the contrary, even the small group of high status physicians who won the limited power to oversee medical practice in and around the City of London as early as 1518 coexisted with a range of different types of health practitioner. This was in an age when self-help was also widespread (Saks, 2003). However, neither self-help nor the developing medical practice appeared to be very effective in resolving the many illnesses the population was exposed to at this time (see Box 3.1).

BOX 3.1   ILLNESS AND ITS TREATMENT IN PRE-INDUSTRIAL BRITAIN

The illnesses to which the public were exposed are well illustrated by the diaries kept by the Reverend Ralph Josselin which these describe the illnesses suffered and feared by his family over the period from, 1643 to 1683. Their experiences are not necessarily typical, but they indicate the type of conditions that arose and the responses made. During the period when he kept a diary, Josselin reported 148 cases of his wife being unwell, half of which were linked to pregnancy and childbirth. She had at least five miscarriages and five of his ten children died before him. She also suffered from a variety of ailments such as agues, eye disorders, measles, rickets, skin conditions, smallpox and worms. Ralph Josselin himself reported 317 episodes of illness ranging from many long-lasting colds, coughs, double vision and depression to the, perhaps fatal, pain, swelling and ulceration of his leg in later life, which never healed. At the same time the family also feared, but fortunately did not contract, the plague which was the most deadly disease of the day and generally viewed as incurable.

A variety of actions were taken to counter the conditions they directly encountered. This included praying to God to enhance the prospects of successful childbirth and to overcome illness. Ralph Josselin himself occasionally took medicine for his colds and had evacuations to improve his condition, based on the humoral theory of the day. Interestingly, he suggests that only in a tiny minority of cases was there consultation with healers, including physicians, surgeons and apothecaries, as well as practitioners such as bonesetters and midwives. Like many members of the public, Josselin and his wife were fairly knowledgeable about the medical issues of the day and were not averse to examining and treating themselves and their family using a range of approaches from leeches to herbal remedies, such as syrup of roses and violet cake. They also sought friends' advice to improve their experience of health and illness.

(Source: adapted from Beier, 1985)

ACTIVITY   ILLNESS AND TREATMENT IN THE JOSSELIN FAMILY

Allow 25 minutes

Read Box 3.1 again carefully. Reverend Josselin's diary gives an interesting insight into the ailments and means of alleviating them in the 17th century. After reading it, answer the following questions.

1   What key issues strike you about the ailments that the Josselin family suffered?

2   What kind of strategies did the family use to treat and prevent illness?

Comment

1   The Josselins suffered a range of ailments, including both chronic and acute illnesses, and parasitic and skin disorders. They were lucky to escape the plague. The children were particularly vulnerable, five being lost. The Reverend's wife also lost five babies to miscarriage and suffered considerable ill health during pregnancy and childbirth.

2   The strategies used by the family to prevent and cope with illness were invoking supernatural or spiritual help, self-treatment of remedies tried and tested over time, and seeking lay help and advice from other members of the community. They also made limited use of healers of various sorts but mainly used their own and friends' knowledge to deal with the many ailments they encountered daily. Note that the range of healers used included physicians and bonesetters (people who claimed to be able to set broken or fractured bones, sometimes through physical manipulation but also through magic or prayer.). The Josselins, therefore, had access to many different healers. It seems fair to say that people at this time experienced almost constant ill health or discomfort.

In the 16th and 17th centuries health care in Britain was largely practically based, often using plants and minerals. Other forms of health care in a more religiously oriented era were overlain with conceptions of witchcraft. Lay women and men healers were often accused of causing and removing disease with charms, for example by wearing amulets. At this time there was also a great belief in the King's touch to cure ailments of the head, neck and eyes, which originated in the divine nature of kingship (Larner, 1992). Among the public, self-help was even more popular than today, with entrenched beliefs in the importance of a balanced constitution, coupled with a strong ethos of neighbourliness and religious duty in maintaining health in a period when the plague and other hazards posed great challenges (Porter, 1995).

During this time, women were important players, both as healers, in dealing with everything from childbirth to life-threatening illnesses, and in their health care role in the home (Oakley, 1992). They were sometimes attacked by disparagers who criticised them for their lack of knowledge and wisdom and the damage they caused to health. However, this hostility was related to the dominant theological view of women and the fact that they posed a competitive threat to other practitioners. In fact, at this time, women were generally seen by communities as fulfilling a positive role. In the 16th and 17th centuries, healing was viewed as part of women's normal duties, whether in the family or outside in the wider community. They were typically regarded as capable of dealing with everything from domestic medicine, fractures and burns to infections and surgery. However, as the 18th century approached, this role was challenged by the Church, physicians and the witchcraft laws (Chamberlain, 1981).

Health care in the 18th century

In the 18th century in the UK a far more explicitly entrepreneurial context emerged as the industrial revolution and capitalism took root, and there were high sickness rates and growing consumer demand. In this period, which has been described as the **great age of quackery** (Maple, 1992), it was still difficult to distinguish between different types of healing practitioner who competed in the market for custom. There were often parallels in the theories and language they used, as well as in their training and social standing. Such practitioners provided a mixture of therapies, from the hucksters who published testimonials in newspapers to sell patent medicines with secret formulae, to physicians and surgeons who delivered aggressive and barbaric therapies to a paying clientele, based on cupping, bleeding and blistering (Porter, 2001). Despite the unpleasantness, and often lack of efficacy, of these types of treatment, they are often called **heroic medicine**. Although many of the healers' activities at this time had less than positive effects on health, some of their interventions helped on a day-to-day basis, such as remedies for ruptures and toothache (Barry, 1987). The self-help culture also continued in parallel, with a strong commitment to prevention, as illustrated by the popularity of vegetarianism at this time. However, there was more influence than before from the market in the self-help sector, with panaceas such as Ward's pills being peddled for all manner of illnesses, alongside the intensified sale of domestic health guides such as *Culpepper's Herbal* (Porter, 1995).

However, the more-or-less open, pluralistic health care field, in which doctors worked alongside complementary and alternative practitioners, progressively evaporated with the development of medical orthodoxy in the first half of the 19th century. Lobbies to create a unified medical profession grew at this time with the emergence of the scientific ideologies of the Enlightenment. Also, apothecaries and surgeons were increasingly allied with physicians to augment their position. The market for their services grew as the new middle classes, created by the industrial revolution, demanded health care. The establishment of the Provincial Medical and Surgical Association, the forerunner of the British Medical Association (BMA), was central to the campaign to win a medical monopoly. This brought the three branches of medicine together, as Parliament was petitioned from the early 1830s onwards for an exclusive register underwritten by the state, giving distinctive privileges to insiders (Waddington, 1984).

Authors such as Wallis and Morley (1976) take what is called a **functionalist perspective** on the rise of orthodox medicine because they see it as meeting the functional needs of the wider society. They argue that the decline of health care pluralism is related to the development of the ability of the medical profession to organise and provide effective treatment in the face of growing public demand. However, despite the technological developments at this time, medicine was still not that effective and could be very risky for patients. Medical care was often based on dangerous heroic interventions, at a time before anaesthetics and hygienic antiseptic and aseptic practices were introduced. Medicine also offered little hope of a cure for many conditions: indeed, voluntary hospitals, which were emerging at this time, were popularly seen among the working class as 'gateways to death' (Saks, 1994).

The state of medicine in the first half of the 19th century

Despite the developments in scientific medicine, hospitals offered little hope to ordinary people and could pose terrible risks to their health. What could be termed the medical profession's 'public image problem' perhaps helps to explain why the Medical Registration Act, which was eventually passed in 1858, had such a difficult ride, only finally being supported after 17 bills (Waddington, 1984). Researchers on this subject suggest that the main reason for the success of medicine in the UK was political (Johnson, 1972; Berlant, 1975; Navarro, 1978; Witz, 1992). This was because of the campaign of the Provincial Medical and Surgical Association which:

- built on the increasing solidarity of medical practitioners, as physicians, surgeons and apothecaries joined to form a political force
- exploited the growth of, and changes in, users and consumers of health care (in particular, the industrial revolution created new wealthy groups of people who could afford to use doctors)
- drew on allegiances with the middle and upper classes through the links with the elite clientele they served
- complemented liberal ideologies of the day by focusing on and promoting definitions of health centred on practitioner–patient relationships
- reinforced the gender-based biases of the time, because medicine was initially established as an exclusively male profession
- provided a legitimate group of workers to police the labour force, through the certification of illness and other means, thus reinforcing the interests of the dominant and wealthy capitalist class.

Another key strategy of the lobby for medical professionalisation for the newly defined area of CAM was to attack rival health groups. The emerging medical profession disparaged competing practitioners in medical journals such as the *Provincial Medical and Surgical Journal* and *The Lancet*. This helped to distinguish doctors from other health care groups by discrediting the latter. These included people practising therapies such as homoeopathy that were popular among the richest sections of society at a time when many medical practitioners were comparatively impoverished (Nicholls, 1988). Even practitioners within the incipient medical profession who were associated with deviant therapies were not immune from attack – as highlighted by the case of Professor John Elliotson in Box 3.2.

BOX 3.2   PROFESSOR JOHN ELLIOTSON

Professor John Elliotson was one of the most eminent medical practitioners in the first half of the 19th century in Britain. He held the posts of both Professor of Medicine at the University of London and President of the Royal Medical and Chirurgical Society. However, he had interests in therapies that were increasingly defined as deviant in the developing medical profession: most notably, in acupuncture and mesmerism. The latter caused his downfall. Mesmerism is often seen as the forerunner of modern clinical hypnotherapy although its founder, Anton Mesmer, was eclectic in his use of different methods for healing. Mesmer's views on health and illness were underpinned by the idea of energy running through and around people. He argued that sometimes the fluidity of such energy was blocked and he worked with people to help them recover. His work is often termed 'animal mesmerism', but Mesmer is most famous for using trance as one of his healing methods – and thus the link with modern hypnotherapy. Mesmerism became a disreputable popular cultural phenomenon in the Victorian period. Attempts to incorporate it within medicine were seen as a major impediment to professionalisation that was held to require the highest standards of 'scientific' respectability.

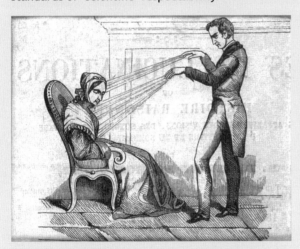

Trance was one of the main methods of medical mesmerists in the 19th century. Images such as this, in which the recipient is depicted as completely under the control of the mesmerist, reinforced public and medical fears about this form of therapy

The editor of *The Lancet*, Thomas Wakley, Elliotson's former friend, denounced his experiments with mesmerism as trickery, going beyond the pale of a civilised society. As a consequence of this and other attacks from within medicine, Elliotson was forced to resign his chair at University College Hospital in London in 1839 after he refused to stop giving public demonstrations of mesmerism. The medical students at University College debated whether or not to support him in his dispute with the Council of the University but, given the potential damage to their own careers and the College itself as a result of the association with mesmerism, even they did not reach a majority in support of Elliotson and his fate was sealed.

(Source: adapted from Parssinen, 1979)

3.3 The development of medical orthodoxy and marginality

When orthodox medicine was established on a formal, national basis in the mid-19th century, the realm of CAM came into being (Saks, 1992). The professionalisation of medicine resulted in legal support, among other effects, for forming a register held by the General Medical Council (GMC) and engaging in self-regulation, including control over medical education. In addition, this successful professionalisation granted exclusive rights over state medical practice. By extension, the effect was to marginalise other forms of health care outside the orthodox medical fold. Although CAM therapists could still practise under the Common Law, they were put at a substantial legal disadvantage by not being on the medical register. The Medical Registration Act 1858 also more generally diminished the legitimacy of unorthodox therapies (Saks, 1994).

As noted in the literature (for instance Saks, 1995), the dominant position of orthodox medicine was subsequently reinforced leading up to the mid-20th century by the following events.

- The increasing unity of the professional elite, consisting of the leaders of the Royal Colleges and the British Medical Association, and the development of a medical–ministry alliance, in which the government typically deferred to the opinion of the leaders of the medical profession on matters of health policy.
- The rise of biomedicine under this leadership, which provided greater ideological coherence to the practice of orthodox medicine as its philosophies increasingly underpinned medical theory, education and research.
- Positive technical developments in medicine, such as the discovery of X-rays, the introduction of aspirin and penicillin, and refinements in surgery.
- The introduction of the National Insurance Act 1911 and the NHS Act 1946 greatly increased the scope of state-funded practice and gave orthodox health care practitioners a key market advantage as they had a monopoly over state medicine.
- The emergence in the first half of the 20th century of subordinated professionals allied to medicine, such as midwives, nurses and physiotherapists, and limited professions such as dentists and opticians, which extended the scope of the medical monopoly.

Researchers such as Jewson (1976) note that there were stages in the development of orthodox medical practice, as described in Box 3.3.

BOX 3.3 STAGES IN THE DEVELOPMENT OF ORTHODOX MEDICINE

Medicine went through three stages from the 18th to the late 19th century:

1 **Bedside medicine** – where the individual paying client largely set the agenda in dialogue with the practitioner.

2 **Hospital medicine** – in which the emphasis was on doctors classifying rather than curing diseases.

3 **Laboratory medicine** – where the patient was objectified and conceived as clusters of cells.

These stages in the development of medicine can be seen to enhance its coherence around biomedicine by the first half of the 20th century. However, the price paid was the disempowerment of patients. Their conditions were depersonalised with the rise of laboratory medicine. They could henceforth be diagnosed through blood and other bodily samples by technicians many miles away, even without seeing a doctor. However, this is where CAM practitioners often now claim the higher ground as they usually adopt more holistic approaches, in that they place a stronger emphasis on face-to-face, interpersonal contact with the client. They also argue that this is what users of health services want now, rather than depersonalisation.

(Source: adapted from Jewson, 1976)

As orthodox medicine became increasingly firmly established, these changes further marginalised CAM – especially since its practice was largely confined to the private pay-for-service sector. Moreover, under the law, its practitioners could not certify statutory documents and were excluded from the right to recover medical charges (Waddington, 1984). In addition, legislation was passed in the first half of the 20th century limiting the claims that non-medically qualified practitioners could make about treating conditions such as cancer and epilepsy. These practitioners were also adversely affected by decisions made through the medical–ministry alliance that developed as a result of government deference to the biomedical paradigm. This is illustrated by the rejection of attempts to establish an independent register for specific CAM therapies, through the establishment of a Herbalists' Council in the 1920s and state registration for osteopaths in the 1930s (Larkin, 1995).

Meanwhile, the medical profession adopted codes of ethics that restricted collaboration with non-medically qualified CAM practitioners. As a result, offenders could be struck off, which happened early in the 20th century to an anaesthetist to Sir Herbert Barker, the celebrated bonesetter (Box 3.4).

BOX 3.4   SIR HERBERT BARKER: AN EXAMPLE OF EXCLUSION

Sir Herbert Barker was one of the most celebrated bonesetters. He discovered the art of manipulating bones when – with no formal training – he put back into alignment a passenger's dislocated elbow while on a cruise liner to Canada in the 1880s. After an apprenticeship with a bonesetter, he set up in practice in London. Here he successfully challenged the medical profession in public, through articles in the press, and by apparently curing seven out of the eight patients sent to him by doctors who had said nothing more could be done for them. In 1922, after a long career in which he had the backing of some of the more eminent physicians and surgeons of his day, Barker was given a knighthood in recognition of his services to patients.

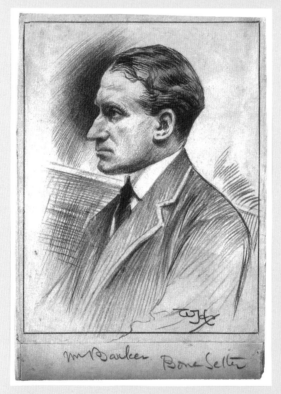

Sir Herbert Barker challenged notions of what doctors of his day were supposed to do. His use of bonesetting set him apart as a threat to developing medical monopoly

Despite his popularity, Barker was once successfully sued by a patient who received only derisory damages. However, the GMC struck off his anaesthetist, Axham, who had helped him with the procedure in question. Even after Barker's knighthood, the GMC refused to restore Axham to the register, despite the fact that the King's physician publicly supported his case. This case exemplifies the way in which orthodox medicine sought to exclude those within the profession acting in support of its most threatening CAM rivals.

(Source: adapted from Inglis, 1980)

The codes of ethics helped protect the profession and its privileged status from doctors associated with CAM, who risked legitimating its occupational rivals. An intensified attack was also launched on CAM therapists and their remedies through journals, for example the *British Medical Journal*. Groups such as hydropaths – who used spa and other water-based therapies – were frequently portrayed as irrational quacks seeking to rob customers of their money. This attack was extended to members of the public who used the wide range of preparations sold through the patent medicine industry, including healing balms and elixirs. It also included medical practitioners who used methods and treatments that other doctors considered were outside orthodox practice. They were often subject to informal control by colleagues, such as entry restrictions, ostracism and career blocking (Saks, 1996).

Of course, CAM therapists fought back – not least through the columns of their own journals and other publications – but they did not occupy strong political ground. So it is not surprising that the number of CAM practitioners dropped sharply from a position where they greatly exceeded medically qualified practitioners in the mid-19th century to much lower levels by the mid-20th century (Saks, 1995). This downward spiral is confirmed in the listings of such therapists in the *Report as to the Practice of Medicine and Surgery by Unqualified Persons in the United Kingdom* (HMSO, 1910). At the same time, the BMA was involved in a campaign that strengthened the regulation of secret remedies produced by the manufacturers of patent medicines, including CAM therapies. Rather startlingly, these included morphine-based preparations for children who were teething and the use of caustic substances such as zinc chloride to treat cancer, which may not have had the most positive effect on the patients' health (Vaughan, 1992).

However, despite the potential public health hazards of some CAMs, both developments could generally be considered as in the interests of the leaders of the medical profession, given the threat of competition to the income, status and power of its members (Saks, 2003). The few rival practitioners who survived remained wide ranging, from empirics operating with no explicit theoretical framework to those with theories that conflicted with orthodox biomedicine, such as homoeopaths, who believed that the more dilute the remedy, the greater its potency. However, the fate of such groups changed significantly as the second half of the 20th century unfolded.

Allow 1 hour

For this activity you need to gather some information from people you know. List at least five lay ideas you know about illness or keeping healthy. These might be termed 'old wives' tales' but, despite this, they are often important in people's lives. To get you started, one example is 'To prevent piles don't sit on cold surfaces.' Then ask your family or friends to tell you of any other 'old wives' tales' about health that they know and note down whether they still use them.

Comment

You probably gathered a range of examples, from ideas about going out in the cold without a coat on or with wet hair, to sitting in a draught, or what happens if you eat certain foods. You may also have found a wealth of remedies, such as mustard baths for your feet if you have a cold, or drinking stout to 'build you up' after an illness. You may have found variations in remedies and ideas between different cultures. Even geographical locations can mean a remedy from Yorkshire is seen as bad for you in Dorset. This shows that remedies and folk ideas about health and illness are still prevalent today. Indeed, this chapter illustrates that such ideas have always existed. The growth and prevalence of biomedicine and orthodox medical care has not stopped people having personal remedies and ideas about health and illness.

3.4   The resurgence of complementary and alternative medicine

A major formative influence on health care in the UK after the lull of the mid-20th century was the emergence from the mid-1960s to the mid-1970s of a counter-culture. In this context a counter-culture is a sub-culture set up to oppose the dominant medical culture. In the 1950s and early 1960s there was little sign of the developments to come, in particular the dramatic growth in public interest in CAM. For example, a report by the BMA in the 1950s rejected the claim that spiritual healing had any effect, other than that based on suggestion; while osteopaths were rejected as a supplementary profession to medicine as the 1960s approached (Inglis, 1980, p. 103). The medical elite, therefore, maintained its external controls on CAM, while simultaneously keeping in check any deviance from the biomedical model by practitioners operating within the ranks of medical orthodoxy (Saks, 2003).

However, by the mid-1960s a strong medical counter-culture emerged, which was linked to the critique by Dubos in 1959 of scientific progress based on the search for technocratic solutions to problems. This was associated with a desire for alternative lifestyles in many areas: from fashions to taking hallucinogenic drugs. At this time, interest grew in Eastern philosophies, including mysticism (Saks, 2000). This trend was associated with a challenge to professional experts, from which medicine was by no means exempt. It is highlighted by the work of writers such as Illich (1976), who believed that modern medicine had reached a watershed where it had become counterproductive, despite the pharmacological revolution and developments in cutting-edge areas such as heart transplants.

The counter-culture of the 1960s and 1970s

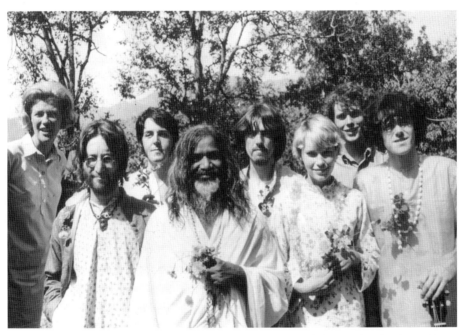

In the 1960s the public attitude changed towards traditional forms of authority and accepted ways of living. Famous people, such as The Beatles and their friends, led the way in questioning 'objective' knowledge and whether there were alternative ways of living

The counter-cultural critique was a strike against 'modernity', as defined by such features as rational progress, objective knowledge and the pivotal role of the professional expert within orthodox medicine. (You met these arguments in Chapter 1.) In this sense, it can be seen to represent the themes of fragmentation and choice that underpin the notion of 'post-modernity' (Saks, 1998). Although there are debates about whether 'modernity' has been supplanted (Giddens, 1991), the counter-culture of the 1960s and 1970s can be linked to escalating public demand for CAM therapies. As noted in the literature (for example, Saks, 1992), by the 1980s:

■ more than one in seven of the population were visiting unorthodox practitioners
■ the number of CAM therapists had correspondingly increased to 30,000
■ about 75 per cent of the population wanted established forms of alternative medicine to be available on the National Health Service.

None the less, these trends – reinforced by up to one in three members of the public using some form of CAM therapy (Fulder, 1996) – raise the question of why the upsurge of consumer interest in such therapies was so significant in this period. Certainly there was increasing awareness of the limits to biomedicine in terms of safety – as illustrated by the case of thalidomide – and the restrictions on the ability of medical orthodoxy to deal with conditions such as chronic illness. The frustration at the depersonalisation and disempowerment of the patient within orthodox biomedicine was also tangible, especially with increasing specialisation, which tends to fragment care by splitting the conceptualisation of the mind and body into many unconnected parts (Saks, 2003).

The attractions of CAM?

People's increased wish to be more active participants in their health care, with greater personal control, is apparent in many alternative therapies. However, care is needed when considering how far there has been a growth in consumer interest in CAM because of a large-scale conversion to 'new age' thinking as a result of the counter-culture (Coward, 1989). Survey evidence suggests that much of this growth in practice was simply linked to the pragmatic desire of patients to try such therapies for conditions where orthodox medicine had been unsuccessful. In such cases, return visits to orthodox health practitioners, rather than an exodus to CAM on a first-resort basis, usually followed the next episode of illness (Thomas et al., 1991).

Whatever caused the rise in public interest in CAM, by the 1980s there was still much medical opposition to such therapies. Although the GMC moved to relax prescriptive ethical codes on referrals to CAM practitioners, the informal stigma associated with CAM continued in medical circles – to the extent that careers were jeopardised by adverse local and national publicity. This negativity was accentuated further by ongoing publications in medical journals that disparaged CAM practitioners and their therapies, variously condemning them for their irrationalism and lack of safety (Saks, 1995). This raised a major debate about whether this stance was designed to protect the public, given all the developments in medicine at this time – from cataract surgery to hip replacements (Le Fanu, 1999) – and the hazards linked to CAM, such as punctured lungs from acupuncture and the high toxicity of some herbal remedies (Ernst et al., 2001). More cynical authors claim this was a political smokescreen, masking the interests of the profession to protect its income, status and power – and, at a wider level, the financial interests of large multinational companies in preserving their markets in pharmaceuticals and other medical supplies (for example, Gould, 1985).

The negative attitude towards CAM was perhaps most fully epitomised by the report on alternative therapy produced by the BMA (1986), which was referred to in Chapter 2. This focused on extolling scientific medical progress, while associating CAM therapies with superstition and witchcraft. This is reflected, for example, in the disparaging view taken of 'religious cults', and the claim that there is no rational basis for the link between increasing dilution and the rising potency of homoeopathic remedies. The report suggested that there were fundamental obstacles to progress in relation to the medical establishment, along with the continuing relatively low levels of state research funding of CAM and its ongoing marginality in the undergraduate medical curriculum. However, this situation changed with the publication of a further report by the BMA (1993) on what had been rebadged 'complementary' rather than 'alternative' medicine, in which CAM was looked on more favourably. This signalled the start of the medical incorporation of some forms of CAM therapy.

3.5   The medical incorporation of complementary and alternative health care

The report by the BMA (1993) was in many ways a watershed. It included the argument that an awareness of CAM should be part of the basic education for students of medicine and other health professions. It also advocated better communication between non-medical CAM practitioners and doctors, and that there should be more research into CAM. The main reasons for this change of heart seem to relate not so much to changes in the CAM field as to increased political pressures on medical orthodoxy. These arose from the following events (Saks, 2003).

- The further growth in consumer demand for treatment by CAM therapists.
- The associated increase in the number of CAM practitioners, which was now some 60,000.
- The large increase in CAM self-help, as shown by the sale of over-the-counter health foods and remedies.
- The growing number of medical practitioners using CAM, 16 per cent of GPs now practising one or more alternative therapies themselves.
- The development of CAM political lobbies, as exemplified by the work of Prince Charles and the All-Party Parliamentary Group for Complementary and Alternative Medicine.

■ Increasing government support for CAM, as witnessed in the early 1990s by the approval given to the National Health Service in subcontracting out such therapies.

These pressures meant that a more positive response to CAM was politically in the interests of the medical establishment. A point had been reached where it was more beneficial for the medical profession to incorporate CAM on its own terms than to reject it: particularly as this also opened up new territory for the profession to colonise, especially in private practice where most CAM practitioners operate.

The medical practice of CAM

The medical control of CAM therapies was central to ensuring that orthodox medicine maintained and/or increased its income, status and power. This helps to explain why the BMA's report (1993) emphasised that doctors should be in control of CAM through medical referral and that CAM practitioners should establish a more medicalised curriculum – including disciplines such as anatomy and physiology. It also accounts for the tendency of doctors themselves to practise CAM in a limited manner. Thus, acupuncture is used in medicine mainly to help treat pain and substance misuse. It is justified by theories about the release of endorphins rather than classical Chinese philosophies (Saks, 1997). The position of the medical profession was reinforced by developments in the pharmaceutical industry that began to see growing consumer interest in CAM not as a threat to its core business but as an opportunity to capture new markets in supermarkets, pharmacies and other outlets.

This is not to suggest that in some cases CAM therapies do not continue to be delivered through practitioners and self-help channels in a non-medicalised way. Indeed, there is considerable resistance to medicalisation in some areas of CAM. In particular, for some groups and CAM practitioners, counter-cultural values are seen as being undermined as more holistic paradigms based on challenging theories are gradually being displaced (Sharma, 1995). However, the drift towards medical incorporation has been clearly manifested by the fact that CAM therapies such as aromatherapy and reflexology are now widely practised in pain clinics and hospices: over 40 per cent of general practices now offer one or more types of CAM (Thomas et al., 1995). Osteopathy and chiropractic have gained further credibility and won the right to create statutory professional registers in the 1990s (Saks, 2002). The growth in legitimacy of therapies such as acupuncture, chiropractic, herbalism, homoeopathy and osteopathy was subsequently underlined by the report on CAM of the House of Lords Select Committee (2000). As noted in Chapter 2, a main recommendation of this report was the division of CAM therapies into three categories: the principal disciplines of osteopathy, chiropractic and acupuncture; complements to conventional medicine such as aromatherapy, massage and reflexology; and other disciplines including traditional systems such as ayurvedic and traditional Chinese medicine and those without evidence of efficacy. Category 1 medicines were seen as having the strongest evidence base. It was felt that the public should have access to such medicines where there was sufficient evidence to support their efficacy through NHS doctors.

ACTIVITY INTEGRATION OF CAM INTO ORTHODOX SETTINGS

Allow 20 minutes

For this activity you need to gather some information to decide whether CAM is increasingly being integrated into orthodox settings. You could collect information from the following sources.

- Current references to CAM (for example, ones you have read in newspapers, heard on the radio or seen on television).
- Your general knowledge of CAM provision in your local hospital or health centre.
- Information from friends and relatives about their use of CAM in an orthodox setting.

Note down your responses to the following questions.

1 How far does the information you gathered suggest that CAMs have been medically incorporated?

2 Are any particular CAM therapies incorporated more than others?

Comment

1 You may have noticed a proliferation of CAMs in a variety of 'orthodox' settings and provided by a range of different individuals. For instance, your GP or other staff at the practice may offer herbalism or homoeopathy. Aromatherapy and counselling are often available and provided by practitioners from outside the general practice staff group. You may know of friends or family who have received CAM in hospital. It is also clear from reading newspapers and magazines that advice given in question-and-answer pages often suggests speaking to orthodox health professionals about trying CAM. You could ask whether CAM is more positively portrayed now than in the past.

2 You may have noted that certain CAMs are more likely to be offered in orthodox settings. In particular, the 'Big Five' tend to be offered more. This is not surprising given how the House of Lords report gave more credibility and support to these five CAMs by grouping them together as 'principal disciplines'.

3.6　Conclusion

Having discussed political perspectives on the historical development of CAM in the UK at a variety of levels, it is helpful to conclude by briefly placing such development in its international context. Note that there are both similarities and differences between British and other societies. This is illustrated by the contemporary resurgence of CAM, both in the USA and across Western Europe (Eisenberg et al., 1998; Fisher and Ward, 1994), even if there are variations – such as in the pace, level and form of medical incorporation – in the countries concerned. In this respect, the UK is very much the exception rather than the rule, in permitting people without medical training in most types of CAM to treat clients under the Common Law. In most of continental Europe, medical dominance has been more explicit and only doctors have been allowed to practise CAM therapies such as acupuncture (Huggon and Trench, 1992).

In other western societies there are also cultural differences in the CAM therapies that have attracted most popular interest and support, which have in turn played into the agenda of health politics. These range from reflexology in Denmark and spiritual healing in the Netherlands to chiropractic and naturopathy or health in Canada (Saks, 2001). Looking beyond the West, and in terms of the political definition of CAM and medical orthodoxy outlined at the start of this chapter, some practices currently seen as CAM in the UK are far more mainstream. This certainly applies to therapies such as herbalism in China and homoeopathy in India (Saks, 1997). This distinction, together with the current understanding of the history and politics of CAM in the UK, underlines the point already made in Chapter 2 – and famously by Prince Charles – that, in any particular country, the orthodoxy of one age can readily become the unorthodoxy of another, and vice versa.

KEY POINTS

- The recognition of political forces is integral to understanding the historical development of CAM.

- The history of CAM cannot be dissociated from that of orthodox medicine.

- Although there is debate about definitions, CAM can helpfully be defined in terms of its political marginalisation.

- In these terms, CAM is a broad concept, including a great diversity of practices.

- In the UK, health care developed from a highly pluralistic field in which there was little differentiation between the standing of practitioners.

- CAM became marginalised from the mid-19th century onwards, when state-supported biomedicine emerged.

- The politicised marginalisation of CAM in the UK reached a low point by the mid-20th century.

- Consumers' and practitioners' interest in CAM have grown dramatically since then, after the emergence of a strong counter-culture.

- This increased the political support for, and legitimacy of, several types of CAM therapy.

- In turn, this interest prompted the growing incorporation of some forms of CAM into orthodox medicine.

- There are parallels – and contrasts – in the definition and position of CAM in different societies, which are linked to politics and history.

References

Barry, J. (1987) 'Publicity and the public good: presenting medicine in eighteenth century Bristol', in Bynum, W. F. and Porter, R. (eds) *Medical Fringe and Medical Orthodoxy 1750–1850*, London, Croom Helm.

Beier, L. M. (1985) 'In sickness and in health: a seventeenth century family's experience', in Porter, R. (ed.) *Patients and Practitioners: Lay Perceptions of Medicine in Pre-industrial Society*, Cambridge, Cambridge University Press.

Berlant, J. L. (1975) *Profession and Monopoly: A Study of Medicine in the United States and Great Britain*, Berkeley, University of California Press.

British Medical Association (BMA) (1986) *Report of the Board of Science and Education on Alternative Therapy*, London, BMA.

British Medical Association (BMA) (1993) *Complementary Medicine: New Approaches to Good Practice*, London, BMA.

Cant, S. and Sharma, U. (1999) *A New Medical Pluralism? Alternative Medicine, Doctors, Patients and the State*, London, UCL Press.

Chamberlain, M. (1981) *Old Wives' Tales: Their History, Remedies and Spells*, London, Virago.

Coward, R. (1989) *The Whole Truth: The Myth of Alternative Medicine*, London, Faber & Faber.

Cule, J. (1997) 'The history of medicine: from its ancient origins to the modern world', in Porter, R. (eds) *Medicine: A History of Healing*, London, Ivy Press.

Dubos, R. (1959) *Mirage of Health: Utopias, Progress and Biological Chance*, New York, Harper.

Duffin, J. (1999) *History of Medicine*, Toronto, University of Toronto Press.

Eisenberg, D., Davis, R., Ettner, S., Appel, S., Wilkey, S., Rompay, M. and Kessler, R. (1998) 'Trends in alternative medicine use in the United States, 1990–1997', *Journal of the American Medical Association*, Vol. 280, pp. 1569–75.

Ernst, E., Pittler, M., Stevinson, C. and White, A. (eds) (2001) *The Desktop Guide to Complementary and Alternative Medicine: An Evidence-Based Approach*, London, Mosby.

Fisher, P. and Ward, A. (1994) 'Complementary medicine in Europe', *British Medical Journal*, Vol. 309, pp. 107–11.

Fulder, S. (1996) *The Handbook of Alternative and Complementary Medicine* (3rd edition), Oxford, Oxford University Press.

Giddens, A. (1991) *The Consequences of Modernity*, Cambridge, Polity Press.

Gould, D. (1985) *The Medical Mafia*, London, Sphere.

HMSO (1910) *Report as to the Practice of Medicine and Surgery by Unqualified Persons in the United Kingdom*, London, HMSO.

House of Lords Select Committee on Science and Technology (2000) *Report on Complementary and Alternative Medicine*, London, The Stationery Office.

Huggon, T. and Trench, A. (1992) 'Brussels post-1992: protector or persecutor?', in Saks, M. (ed.) *Alternative Medicine in Britain*, Oxford, Clarendon Press.

Illich, I. (1976) *Limits to Medicine*, Harmondsworth, Penguin.

Inglis, B. (1980) *Natural Medicine*, Glasgow, Fontana.

Jewson, N. (1976) 'The disappearance of the sick-man from medical cosmology 1770–1870', *Sociology*, Vol. 10, pp. 225–44.

Johnson, T. (1972) *Professions and Power*, London, Macmillan.

Larkin, G. (1995) 'State control and the health professions in the United Kingdom: historical perspectives', in Johnson, T., Larkin, G. and Saks, M. (eds) *Health Professions and the State in Europe*, London, Routledge.

Larner, C. (1992) 'Healing in pre-industrial Britain', in Saks, M. (ed.) *Alternative Medicine in Britain*, Oxford, Clarendon Press.

Le Fanu, J. (1999) *The Rise and Fall of Modern Medicine*, London, Abacus.

Maple, E. (1992) 'The great age of quackery', in Saks, M. (ed.) *Alternative Medicine in Britain*, Oxford, Clarendon Press.

Navarro, V. (1978) *Class Struggle, the State and Medicine: An Historical and Contemporary Analysis of the Medical Sector in Great Britain*, London, Martin Robertson.

Nicholls, P. (1988) *Homoeopathy and the Medical Profession*, London, Croom Helm.

Oakley, A. (1992) 'The wisewoman and the doctor', in Saks, M. (ed.) *Alternative Medicine in Britain*, Oxford, Clarendon Press.

Parssinen, T. (1979) 'Professional deviants and the history of medicine: medical mesmerists in Victorian Britain', in Wallis, R. (ed.) *On the Margins of Science: The Social Construction of Rejected Knowledge*, Sociological Review, Monograph, Vol. 27, Keele, University of Keele.

Porter, R. (1995) *Disease, Medicine and Society, 1550–1860* (2nd edition), Cambridge, Cambridge University Press.

Porter, R. (2001) *Quacks: Fakers and Charlatans in English Medicine*, Manchester, Manchester University Press.

Saks, M. (1992) 'Introduction', in Saks, M. (ed.) *Alternative Medicine in Britain*, Oxford, Clarendon Press.

Saks, M. (1994) 'The alternatives to medicine', in Gabe, J., Kelleher, D. and Williams, G. (eds) *Challenging Medicine*, London, Routledge.

Saks, M. (1995) *Professions and the Public Interest: Professional Power, Altruism and Alternative Medicine*, London, Routledge.

Saks, M. (1996) 'From quackery to complementary medicine: the shifting boundaries between orthodox and unorthodox medical knowledge', in Cant, S. and Sharma, U. (eds) *Complementary and Alternative Medicines: Knowledge in Practice*, London, Free Association Books.

Saks, M. (1997) 'East meets West: The emergence of a holistic tradition', in Porter, R. (ed.) *Medicine: A History of Healing*, London, The Ivy Press.

Saks, M. (1998) 'Medicine and complementary medicine: challenge and change', in Scambler, G. and Higgs, P. (eds) *Modernity, Medicine and Health*, London, Routledge.

Saks, M. (2000) 'Medicine and the counter culture', in Cooter, R. and Pickstone, J. (eds) *Medicine in the Twentieth Century*, Amsterdam, Harwood Academic Publishers.

Saks, M. (2001) 'Alternative medicine and the health care division of labour: present trends and future prospects', *Current Sociology*, Vol. 49, pp. 119–34.

Saks, M. (2002) 'Professionalization, regulation and alternative medicine', in Saks, M. and Allsop, J. (eds) *Regulating the Health Professions*, London, Sage.

Saks, M. (2003) *Orthodox and Alternative Medicine: Politics, Professionalization and Health Care*, London, Sage.

Sharma, U. (1995) *Complementary Medicine Today: Practitioners and Patients* (revised edition), London, Routledge.

Thomas, K., Carr, J., Westlake, L. and Williams, B. (1991) 'Use of non-orthodox and conventional health care in Great Britain', *British Medical Journal*, Vol. 302, pp. 207–10.

Thomas, K., Fall, M., Parry, G. and Nicholl, J. (1995) *National Survey of Access to Complementary Health Care via General Practice: Report to the Department of Health*, Sheffield, University of Sheffield.

Vaughan, P. (1992) '"Secret remedies" in the late nineteenth and early twentieth centuries', in Saks, M. (ed.) *Alternative Medicine in Britain*, Oxford, Clarendon Press.

Waddington, I. (1984) *The Medical Profession in the Industrial Revolution*, London, Gill & Macmillan.

Wallis, R. and Morley, P. (1976) 'Introduction', in Wallis, R. and Morley, P. (eds) *Marginal Medicine*, London, Peter Owen.

Witz, A. (1992) *Professions and Patriarchy*, London, Routledge.

Chapter 4 Ethics in complementary and alternative medicine

Julie Stone

Contents

AIMS

- To understand the main ethical concepts in delivering health care.
- To demonstrate a sound understanding of the roles of professional bodies in regulating CAM practitioners.

4.1 Introduction

This chapter considers what it means to practise ethically; why ethics is so central to the health care relationship; and the responsibilities of practitioners, professional bodies, users and those making health care decisions for other people (for example, parents and carers of users who are unable to make their own decisions). This chapter also explores the unique ethical issues raised by complementary and alternative medicine (CAM) and the extent to which ethical obligations and legal requirements overlap.

4.2 Ethics and health care relationships

Allow 30 minutes

Write down a few sentences about what you think 'acting ethically' means.

Comment

Most people understand 'being ethical' as having something to do with people acting in 'the right way'. 'Acting ethically' embraces ideas about what people ought to do or what they should do, which presupposes there are rules of conduct or behaviour by which people expressly or implicitly agree to be bound. In this sense, acting ethically is similar to acting legally: following a set of rules that determine how people ought to behave. However, whereas the law lays down hard-and-fast rules, ethics presumes that people have a degree of choice about the decisions they make: they can choose to act either ethically or unethically. The notion of choosing to do 'the right thing' is important because society largely holds people accountable for the actions they take. So when a person's actions are judged, the pertinent questions are why did they act in the way they did, what were their motivations, and what did they hope the consequences of their actions would be? To be held accountable, people have to understand what they are doing. So, a child would not necessarily be called to account for doing something wrong, on the basis that they are considered to lack the capacity to understand the fundamental difference between right and wrong.

The term 'ethics' is often used interchangeably with 'morality', although people sometimes draw a distinction between them on the basis that morality is personal to each individual or to a particular group, for example Christian morality. There is probably a more relevant distinction between individual ethics and professional ethics. Each profession has a set of rules and obligations that are central to how professionals acting within that sphere of practice must behave. Many of the requirements of professional practice reflect the expected obligations of the ordinary citizen, including:

- a duty to tell the truth
- a duty to act honestly and fairly
- a duty to respect people's wishes, and not to treat people as a means to an end, but as individuals with rights
- a duty not to harm people.

Another way of thinking about ethics is to concentrate on people's rights, both in everyday life and specifically as health service users. As individuals, people have a right:

- not to be harmed
- not to be lied to

- not to be touched without their permission
- to be treated fairly and justly.

The obligations of a health professional embrace all of these rights. Ethics is important in health care for several reasons, but primarily because failing to act ethically can harm someone. Also, the unique vulnerability associated with being a patient leads people to trust that health practitioners will act ethically, by putting their best interests first. This includes taking their wishes into account, and not doing anything without their express permission (for example, by obtaining informed consent). Health care ethics concerns both professionals' duties and users' rights. Ethics in health care tends to concentrate on the following four key principles (Beauchamp and Childress, 1994).

1 **The principle of respect for autonomy** – giving competent adults the information they need to make their own decisions, based on their own values and their personal assessment of risk factors, free from coercion or undue influence.

2 **The principle of beneficence** – benefiting or acting in the patient's best interests.

3 **The principle of non-maleficence** – not deliberately causing the patient harm, or making sure that the benefits outweigh the harm if harm is unavoidable.

4 **The principle of respect for justice** – treating all patients equally and providing mechanisms for when care goes wrong.

While these four principles underpin the range of duties that health professionals owe their patients, they do not provide an exact blueprint for how a practitioner ought to act in every given situation. However, they do provide a good starting point for making decisions, so that a practitioner faced with an ethically contentious choice does not make a decision solely on personal preference (for example, a doctor refusing to agree to a woman's abortion because of their personal opposition to it).

Sometimes these four ethical principles clash. For example, a doctor might be reluctant to tell patients they are dying, believing this will cause distress. In the past, doctors could override patients' autonomy by withholding that information from them in what they perceived were the patients' best interests. These might include keeping hope alive and encouraging the dying person to take the prescribed medication. Nowadays, such an action would be regarded as unacceptably 'paternalistic'.

'Paternalism' has a distinct meaning in health care ethics. It describes the actions of a health care practitioner who overrides or does not seek the wishes of a competent person (that is, someone who has sufficient autonomy to make their own decisions), believing that they are better able to decide what is in the patient's best interests. A paternalistic action is always well intentioned but is ethically unacceptable because it usurps people's rights to make their own decisions, based on their own values and beliefs. Since the 1970s, there has been a cultural shift towards respecting rights and promoting self-determination. This means it is now considered more preferable for people to make their own choices on the basis of all the relevant facts than for other people to make decisions for them. This example also demonstrates that ethics is not static but reflects what is considered ethically appropriate by a society at different points in time, and that different cultures may have differing views on what is ethical. This explains why euthanasia can be lawful in the Netherlands but not in the UK: in the Netherlands, the emphasis is on respecting people's autonomy, whereas in the UK, the emphasis is on not causing harm.

Historically, health care ethics tended to concentrate on the responsibilities owed by the practitioner to an individual person. However, the true scope of health care ethics is considerably wider. Practitioners have duties not just to the individual in front of them but to all of their clients. They may even have duties to the public in general. For example, a practitioner who treats someone for a sexually transmitted disease has a duty to act in that person's best interests, but may also have a duty to that person's sexual partner, who could be a client. The practitioner may have a duty to warn third parties, who may not be clients, that they are at risk. Practitioners have ethical duties not just to service users but also to their profession and their employers. Users have ethical responsibilities as well as rights. These include doing what they can to maintain their own health; not drawing inappropriately on health services (for example going to the accident and emergency department with a routine or trivial complaint); and providing all necessary relevant information to a practitioner to facilitate an accurate diagnosis.

In the next activity you will reflect on your experiences as a user of health services and consider some of the ethical issues that arise in everyday health encounters.

ACTIVITY   ETHICS IN HEALTH CARE

Allow 25 minutes

Reflect on your last health care consultation (for example, a routine check-up with your GP or practice nurse, a visit to the dentist, a hospital appointment or a consultation with a CAM practitioner).

1   Did any aspects of the encounter give rise to ethical issues? Focus on the positive as well as the negative aspects.

2   Try to consider as broadly as possible, for example, whether the receptionist was polite to you, whether you felt confident to discuss personal information, whether the practitioner seemed genuinely interested in your problem or whether your appointment was on time.

Comment

Ethics permeates every aspect of the health care encounter. Healing relationships are, at their heart, based on trust. When people are ill, they need to believe that everyone involved in providing their health care is acting appropriately and treating them in their best interests (for example, giving them the treatment that is best for their condition, not simply the cheapest or the quickest to administer). Acting ethically involves health carers respecting users' rights and supporting their choices (for example, giving them as much information as they want about the range of treatments available and the alternatives to treatment); being good at what they do (keeping up to date with and undertaking continuing professional development); refraining from actively harming users (by following approved and appropriate practices); and treating people in a fair and consistent manner (for example, not having 'favourite' users with whom they spend twice as long as they do with 'difficult' users).

In the activity at the start of Section 4.2, it was probably easier to think about instances of unethical practice than examples of ethical practice. The following list identifies some of the areas you may have considered as giving rise to ethical issues.

- When you made your appointment did you feel that the initial contact with the receptionist or the professional was handled sensitively? Was the information you provided managed in a sensitive way, with respect for your privacy?
- When you arrived for your appointment did the receptionist (if one was present) give you the chance to say why you were there (if relevant) and privacy in which to give your personal details?
- Did the practitioner respect your autonomy, by asking you what you think is wrong and what you want to do about it, by gaining your consent to treatment, by respecting your personal health information as being confidential, by not discussing your details with anyone who does not need to know (other than to benefit your health), and by ensuring that written notes or computer records about you are kept safely?
- Did the practitioner act in your best interests, by obtaining an adequate history from which to form a diagnosis and consider the right treatment plan, by providing treatment that should bring about the desired outcome with a minimum of side effects, and by keeping up to date with professional developments?
- Did the practitioner act detrimentally towards you in any way: for example, being rude or dismissive, suggesting an inappropriate treatment, or charging you excessively for their services?
- As far as you could tell, did the practitioner treat you fairly: for example, was the appointment on time, or were you or other people kept waiting? If your appointment was much later than the arranged time, were you given an explanation or apology? Did you feel that you could complain if there was anything you were unhappy about?

The above list shows that most interactions in health and social care have ethical dimensions, even if you did not necessarily consider them as 'ethical' issues. Most ethical issues concern the ordinary, everyday relationships between practitioners and users, although the media tend to focus on the more dramatic life-and-death issues, often presenting them in a highly polarised way. Almost all interactions have an ethical aspect, which spans encounters from what might appear to be simple questionnaires sent to people at home, through all the interactions they have with the service providers, including the treatment. There are ethics about how people are referred to a practitioner, and the treatment prescribed to them. As previously mentioned, users also have ethical responsibilities, for example telling their doctor they are also receiving treatment from a CAM practitioner, which might have a bearing on the doctor's recommended treatment and vice versa.

4.3 Why ethical behaviour is central to the health care relationship

The health care relationship is basically a relationship of trust. This implies that practitioners are motivated by the users' best interests; will not exploit the therapeutic relationship to satisfy their own ends; will behave in an appropriate manner that is conducive to the healing process; and will refrain from behaviour that could harm users, including being physically or psychologically unfit to treat them. The examples in Box 4.1 give a clearer idea of what this means.

BOX 4.1   EXAMPLES OF ETHICAL SITUATIONS

- A patient may reveal extremely personal information to a practice nurse during a family planning consultation, even though the patient knows little about the practitioner.

- A dental patient who is paying for private dental treatment needs to trust that they will not be subjected to unnecessary and painful procedures simply to increase the dentist's earnings.

- An osteopathic patient needs to feel confident that she has been asked to undress down to her underwear only for the purposes of her treatment, and not for the practitioner's personal gratification.

- A surgical patient takes it on trust that the surgeon's skills are up to date, and that they know about all the available options that might obviate the need for surgery.

All of these examples demonstrate that people would be uncomfortable in trusting or confiding in a practitioner unless they can believe the practitioner is worthy of respect and can be relied on not to abuse their trust. Ethical behaviour is central to the health care relationship because of the inherent power disequilibrium between user and practitioner. This is based largely on the relative disparity in knowledge between health carers and the people they treat. Health professionals are consulted precisely because they have skills that lay people do not have.

People increasingly expect to be informed and involved in all aspects of decision making about their medical treatment, which is acknowledged in the development of the 'expert patient' (Department of Health, 2001). At the same time, many people are much more knowledgeable about health-related matters than in the past. This is hardly surprising given the attention health issues receive in the media. The internet has also helped to narrow the knowledge gap between doctors and users. In addition, television series such as *Casualty*, *ER*, *Holby City* and *Peak Practice* have made people more familiar with medical terminology and seeing health carers working through fictionalised ethical dilemmas. They also see documentaries about, for example, the ethics of assisted reproduction, separating conjoined twins and end-of-life decisions.

In contrast, many people know relatively little about CAM unless they have had personal experience. When people consult a complementary practitioner for the first time, they may not know what the therapy involves or what outcomes to expect realistically. For example, although people are increasingly aware of being asked to give their consent to conventional medical procedures, they would not necessarily expect a chiropractor to ask them to sign a consent form. They might also be unaware of the level of information they need before they can give valid consent to their first acupuncture session. In these situations, and from an ethical standpoint, it is even more important for the practitioner to openly discuss the form of treatment being offered, what it entails, and what it could achieve in the given situation, as well as to discuss alternative treatment strategies.

Another obvious inequality between practitioners and users is that most people who are 'ill' (loosely defined) may be frightened, in pain and vulnerable, and need to be able to rely on the practitioner. Health givers, in contrast, should be in robust psychological and physical health and in no sense reliant or dependent on the user. When people are ill, they usually look for a health practitioner who has the skill and expertise to make them better, and who may, conceivably, impose their own professional judgement when appropriate. The autonomy of people who are ill is already compromised. They may be unable to work, or their mobility may be restricted, limiting their ability to get about as they would like. They may be in too much pain or discomfort to continue with their normal business. Depending on the severity of the diagnosis, they could be anxious and possibly depressed. All of these factors compromise autonomy. To regain their health and full autonomy, many people are prepared to depend on advice and allow themselves to be cared for by others. People who are used to managing their own affairs can

by choosing not to be kept informed about changes in their condition, or the results of tests, preferring to rely on the practitioner's clinical judgement.

In the present climate, users may feel they are weak if they fail to take an active role in their healing and that somehow it is wrong to depend on their practitioner. This is unfortunate because, as discussed earlier, some users prefer to be wholly passive or to surrender some of their autonomy in order to be cared for. Clearly, a balance has to be struck between users' autonomy and their desire for dependence at a time of already diminished autonomy.

Law imposes more stringent requirements than ethics

All health care practitioners, including those in CAM, must work within the laws of the country where they practise. Although the law does not always reflect what is considered ethical – indeed, ethical duties may be thought of as higher than legal duties – in most jurisdictions it ensures that practitioners are subject, at the very least, to minimal requirements vis-à-vis respect for users' dignity, user information, confidentiality, and maintaining professional boundaries.

However, the state has a crucial role in governing decisions about a range of ethical issues, such as what is permissible for *in vitro* fertilisation (IVF) and human embryology research. These matters are not decided solely by the medical establishment. Often, when there is very strong public opinion, the government introduces legislation to control health care practices (for example, prohibiting trade in human organs, or commercial surrogacy arrangements).

What can be agreed about ethics?

Even though every person has an idea about what acting ethically means, when faced with an ethically contentious problem, or when it is not clear what will bring about the best outcome, 'good' people will act in diverse, and often opposing, ways, while maintaining they are 'doing the right thing'. While ordinary individuals also have ethical responsibilities to one another (for example, to tell the truth), the duties owed by professionals to their users go beyond everyday ethical responsibilities. For the reasons outlined above, users are in a uniquely vulnerable position when they are ill, which demands a higher standard of ethical propriety.

- **Professional ethics** is about how responsible practitioners ought to act when faced with ethically contentious choices.
- **Practical ethics** is about practitioners acting in an ethically appropriate way and being accountable for their actions.

It is worth reflecting on the idea that ordinary people are also accountable for their actions, in that they are held responsible for the outcome of their actions. A good example of this is acting within the law. When people seriously infringe the rules of society and break the law, they can be subjected to legal sanctions, such as a fine or even imprisonment. Mostly, though, people's decision to act ethically or not has little immediate comeback for them. It may affect how others think of them, but ordinary people are unlikely to be censured for acting unethically.

Health professionals are much more accountable for their actions because ethical duties form the foundation of their relationships with users. Infringements of those duties have serious consequences: for example, eroding the trust between users and practitioners. Accordingly, health professionals must be more accountable for their actions, because they have implicitly agreed to be bound by the rules and codes of their profession.

Accountability takes many forms, and practitioners are potentially answerable to their personal conscience, their professional body, an employment tribunal, or even a court of law. Being a practitioner is not easy. The freedom of health professionals to make choices goes hand in hand with being responsible for their consequences. The next activity shows how difficult these choices can be.

ACTIVITY   ETHICAL DILEMMAS

Allow 1 hour

Consider the following three ethical dilemmas, which are drawn from real-life CAM practice. Each dilemma raises one or more of the ethical issues discussed so far in this chapter. (To recap, they are respect for autonomy, a duty to benefit, a duty not to harm, respect for justice, and the concept of paternalism.) For each case, write a short paragraph saying what you would do if you were the practitioner. You do not need any technical knowledge to answer this. As you do this activity, try to take into account the aspects of good ethical practice that were discussed in the activity 'Acting ethically' (at the start of Section 4.2).

1   A chiropractor knows from past experience that if she explains to a user what the technique known as a high velocity thrust feels like before she applies it, the user will probably become tense and stiff. This would make it harder to do and possibly even dangerous for the user. Although the chiropractor was taught to explain in detail, she now acts first and explains later.

2   A homoeopath treating a 14-year-old girl for recurrent urinary tract infection is concerned that the girl is being abused by her stepfather but is unsure whether this concern should be disclosed and, if so, to whom. The homoeopath asks the girl if she will agree to let him talk to her mother, but she adamantly refuses. What should the homoeopath do?

3   A reflexologist suspects that the person he is treating has bowel cancer, but thinks the person's spirits will be damaged by disclosing bad news, so he keeps his opinion to himself. Although he is not a doctor, he is certain from his own one-year training that the user has cancer.

Comment

1   In this scenario the main ethical issue is **paternalism.** The chiropractor is trying to act in the user's best interests (**the duty of beneficence**) and not

cause the user harm (**the duty of non-maleficence**). This is why the chiropractor withholds the information about applying a high velocity thrust. However, by withholding this information the chiropractor is overriding the user's autonomy in not giving full information about what is being done (or, in this case, about to be done) to their body. Note that the chiropractor has been taught to give detailed explanations. Providing adequate information is essential if a practitioner is to gain a user's consent to treatment. Note, also, that the chiropractor's motivation for withholding the information is well intentioned but none the less ethically objectionable, since it removes the user's decision-making ability (in this case, to say they would rather not be given a high velocity thrust).

2   This case concerns both **respect for autonomy** and **the duty of beneficence**. The question is whether the homoeopath should **respect** the teenager's **confidentiality** as she insists. You may think that, if the teenager is old enough to consult the homoeopath and apparently give her consent to treatment, she is also old enough for her confidences to be respected. **Respect for confidentiality** is an aspect of **respect for autonomy**. A person being able to control who knows what about them is fundamental to their being in charge of their life. In UK law, a teenage or young person can consent to treatment as soon as they are sufficiently mature to understand fully what the treatment involves. However, at the same time, the homoeopath has a **duty to benefit the user** and a **duty to protect from harm**, which might be construed as a duty to report suspected abuse to the relevant authority. This case is an example of where ethical principles conflict. One solution might be for the homoeopath to persuade the young person to tell her mother. Certainly, the homoeopath ought to inform her whether he intends to disclose her personal information against her wishes. Remember, a paternalistic decision to go over the young person's head may be misguided. The homoeopath may not know all the facts and the decision to disclose these concerns could have unforeseen and bad consequences.

3   This case is also about **paternalism** and raises additional questions about the reflexologist's competence, an issue that goes to the heart of **the duty of beneficence** and **the duty of non-maleficence**. The reflexologist is acting paternalistically in withholding a suspicion that the user has bowel cancer. To withhold a potentially serious diagnosis from someone is a clear **breach of their autonomy**, even if it is aimed at protecting them from distress. It assumes that the practitioner knows better than the user: in this case, that the user would rather not know they have cancer, than know and be able to make decisions accordingly. Nowadays, in conventional medicine, withholding a serious diagnosis is almost always seen as unwarranted paternalism. In addition, in this case the reflexologist may be inadequately trained to diagnose bowel cancer (especially on the basis of one year of training). Unless the reflexologist has the necessary training to diagnose cancer, he is exceeding his limit of competence. To give a user an unsubstantiated diagnosis is a clear example of causing the user harm, and breaching **the duty of non-maleficence**.

So, knowing what to do or taking the 'correct' course of action is not always straightforward. In each situation, practitioners have to weigh up conflicting ethical issues and make an ethical deliberation, deciding what is the best course of action, allowing for all the circumstances. Practitioners are accountable for the decisions reached, and so have to be able to justify why they acted in this way. In each scenario, the problem is an ethical dilemma and not a technical problem. Being a 'moral agent' (someone who makes ethical decisions) requires the practitioner to consider the interests and rights of all relevant parties, any applicable laws, professional duties or regulations that might apply, and the likely outcome or consequences of choosing one course of action over another. The examples highlight that sometimes all the available options are problematic, in which case the best solution is to follow the course of action that will result in the least harm.

However, it is important to bear in mind that ethical dilemmas have cross-cultural dimensions. The comments on the three scenarios in the activity 'Ethical dilemmas' reflect western values. These stress individual autonomy and the rights of individuals to determine their own fates. The prevailing cultural preference in the UK and the USA is to respect an individual's right to self-determination. Accordingly, when health professionals override a patient's autonomy, it is seen negatively. However, not all cultures in the UK stress the rights of the individual in the same way. Some groups think of the family or even the community as the relevant decision-making unit. Here, ethical values may be interpreted differently, and a greater weight may be given to acting beneficently than to respecting the person's autonomy.

The principles underlying ethical practice

Box 4.2 describes four principles that are central to an understanding of acting ethically.

BOX 4.2   THE PRINCIPLES OF ACTING ETHICALLY

Principle one

Ethics is not solely about rare dramatic conflicts. It concerns all aspects of the therapeutic encounter, including the practitioner's competence, boundaries between the practitioner and patient, the patient's right to make decisions based on informed choices, respect for the patient's culture and values, and confidentiality. The fact that CAM rarely involves life or death decisions does not mean that there are fewer ethical issues in CAM therapeutic relationships [than in conventional health care relationships]. Any interaction with a patient (including a potential patient or a former patient) can give rise to ethical tensions.

Principle two

Ethical awareness is an ongoing process requiring active deliberation. Therapists can learn, through a process of reflection, how to apply a range of ethical theories to assist their decision-making and, indeed, have a moral duty to do so. Even though there may be no 'right answer' to a given dilemma, therapists have a moral responsibility to consider their options in the light of existing ethical theories, and to be sure that their decisions are ethically defensible and will stand up to external scrutiny. Since practitioners make most of their ethical decisions behind closed doors, practitioners must regulate their own conduct.

Principle three

Acting ethically requires a practitioner to be aware of all relevant professional codes and to know about any particular laws governing his or her sphere of practice, since these are additional mechanisms for regulating the individual therapist's conduct. The rules contained in codes of ethics represent standards of conduct which society expects professionals to follow. These may impose more onerous duties on health professionals than those which apply to ordinary members of the public, but to be a professional is a privilege, which confers both rights and responsibilities. The shortcomings of both ethical codes and law as a means of regulating the professional relationship make it all the more important that practitioners are aware of their ethical responsibilities, and become habituated to making good moral choices.

Principle four

Health care ethics involves benefiting patients and not causing them harm. Acting ethically requires practitioners to be aware of professional developments and research underpinning their therapy to ensure competence. It will rarely be ethical for practitioners to work in complete isolation from their professional colleagues and with little regard for developments in their field. In order to provide patients with a range of options, therapists should be aware of developments in health and social care generally.

(Source: Stone, 2002, pp. 37-8)

So far this chapter has considered some of the principles underpinning the ethical decisions of individual practitioners. This is important because most health care encounters are between an individual practitioner and an individual user. Clearly, there also needs to be consensus within a profession about what constitutes acceptable professional standards. If not, individual practitioners could take arbitrary and inconsistent decisions, with different practitioners adopting very different notions of what they consider ethical. Stone (2002) highlights that individual practitioners must act within the norms of their profession, as well as work within the law. This is important if the ethical principle **respect for justice** is to be met. The next section shows how professional bodies set relevant professional standards, and provide mechanisms for what happens when things go wrong.

4.4   Ethical practice and accountability: the role and function of professional bodies

The UK's medical profession is regulated by the General Medical Council (GMC). One of the main ways in which the GMC, and other regulatory bodies, influences its members is through its **code of ethics**. This sets out broad principles, rather than detailed guidance, for how practitioners should behave in specific circumstances. This is necessary because a practitioner retains individual accountability and ultimate responsibility for decisions taken during professional practice. Not all breaches of an ethical code result in disciplinary action being taken against the practitioner. However, the most fundamental breaches can lead to a disciplinary hearing, in which the professional conduct committee can remove the practitioner's licence to practise. In this way, a code of ethics can be a deterrent: that is, practitioners follow its principles because otherwise they could be 'struck off'.

A code of ethics is only one way of encouraging and promoting ethical practice. The functions of a regulatory body go much further than disseminating codes of ethics. Regulatory bodies need to set and enforce educational standards, keep a register of members, and have in place processes for practitioners whose performance is below par and rehabilitative procedures for those whose performance is marred by ill health. Many of these broader aspects of ethical practice can only be co-ordinated at a collective level if they are to protect users adequately, which is the key function of professional self-regulation. Box 4.3 summarises some of the main responsibilities of regulatory bodies.

BOX 4.3   FUNCTIONS OF REGULATORY BODIES

- Determine educational requirements for safe and competent practice at pre- and post-registration levels.
- Encourage research and professional development.
- Set standards through codes of ethics and codes of practice.
- Maintain and make available a register of members so that the public can distinguish regulated practitioners from unregulated practitioners.
- Maintain professional disciplinary procedures so that unethical practitioners can be held accountable for their actions.
- Have a complaints mechanism so that users' grievances can be heard and any appropriate reparation made.
- Install mechanisms for dealing with practitioners who are unfit to practise through ill health.
- Provide information to members of the profession, including information about the standards of care they should expect.
- Provide information to members of the public and promote user self-awareness.

Professionals have a special ethical responsibility to other people. Being a professional involves **rights** (respect from others and considerable freedom over what to do and how to do it) but also **responsibilities** (to act in the user's best interests at all times, and to surrender personal values if they conflict with providing optimum care). However, health professionals work mostly in an unsupervised context because another advantage of working in a professional capacity is relative autonomy over their work. This means it is extremely important for individual practitioners to be motivated and taught how to act responsibly and professionally in their dealings with service users. Equally, 'good' professionals may hold very different moral views. What then is the role of professional ethics and how does it relate to personal morality?

In essence, professional ethics refers to the ethos, rules and principles underpinning professional practice. In joining a professional body and assuming a professional title, a practitioner expressly agrees to be bound by the rules of that profession. Professional codes of ethics set down many general rules about how practitioners are expected to behave. This is an important aspect of professional self-regulation because it means there is a recognised standard against which professional practice can be measured, and an explicit statement about the level of commitment and behaviour the public is entitled to expect. A code of ethics represents the ethos of any given profession. Stone (2002) describes a code of ethics as a synthesis of minimal legal requirements and statements of ethical ideals, backed up with professional statements that represent the shared political and economic ideals of that particular group.

Currently, the only CAM professions that are statutorily regulated in the UK are osteopathy and chiropractic. Each profession has established a body with very similar functions to the GMC. As with the GMC, the General Osteopathic Council and the General Chiropractic Council have the right to remove or suspend practitioners from their registers. However, the usefulness of any regulatory body depends on the extent to which it is willing to exercise its range of regulatory powers. A professional body which is consistently soft on its members, and allows little scope for lay input, will fall short of its duty to protect the public.

4.5 Ethical practice and accountability: individual practitioners' responsibilities

The dynamics and working practices of many CAM practitioners mean the therapeutic encounters are rarely supervised and no one looks over the practitioner's shoulder. This places the responsibility to act ethically squarely with the individual practitioner. A European study of the practice of CAM states:

> Ethical issues are just as pertinent for conventional and unconventional medicine, alike. The labelling of a therapy as natural does not provide an excuse for practitioners to set aside standards of behaviour and ethical practice that are expected of all who care for the well being of individuals.
>
> (Research Council for Complementary Medicine, 1999)

Acting ethically means far more than following a code of ethics. Practitioners have individual ethical responsibilities towards their clients, and collective ethical responsibilities to foster and promote the ideals of the profession. This includes taking responsibility for the conduct of other practitioners, and exposing examples of misconduct or poor practice.

The centrality of consent

In the last 30 years there has been a strong move away from paternalism towards an emphasis on users' rights and involvement in the decision-making process. Nowadays, few users would accept treatment without knowing what it was or a health carer who withholds information about other treatment options. The importance of involving the user is exemplified by the need for practitioners to gain **informed consent**. This need to gain consent is enshrined in law, as well as being a central aspect of most professional codes of ethics. Competent users must be given a thorough explanation of what will be done, the risks involved in going ahead or not going ahead with the proposed treatment, and information about alternatives to the treatment. Therefore, the practitioner should have effective communication skills, because the information needs to be conveyed so that the user understands it. When giving consent, the user's decision must be voluntary and not subject to coercion. Failure to obtain consent is considered an extremely grave matter. If consent has not been obtained, and the user is harmed, they can sue the practitioner for medical negligence (for gaining inadequate consent). If the user has not been given any information or has been treated against their express wishes, they can sue the practitioner for battery (for not gaining consent at all). In addition, failure to gain consent can lead to disciplinary proceedings and the removal of the practitioner's right to practise.

So far, very few users have sued CAM practitioners, which is often attributed to CAM being more 'patient-centred'. It is debatable what this means in terms of information exchange. CAM practitioners have the same duty to obtain consent to treatment as other health professionals (Stone, 2002).

Acting ethically: tools for analysis

Do the usual principles underpinning conventional health care ethics provide an adequate or acceptable framework for the discussion of ethics in the CAM relationship? Most bioethics teaching in medical schools in the UK and USA draws on the principles-based approach to considering ethical dilemmas. To recap, the four principles are:

- respect for autonomy
- the duty to benefit (beneficence)
- the duty not to harm (non-maleficence)
- respect for justice.

As well as principles, practitioners need to be aware of the three types of ethical theory. Ethical theories are ways of judging whether an action is right or wrong. Two of the main theories were touched on earlier in this chapter: they are **duty-based ethics** and **consequence-based ethics**. The third theory is **virtue ethics**. Some ethicists believe that the practitioner's moral character is the most important basis for making good ethical decisions. According to this theory the focus is less on the facts of the particular scenario and more on the moral qualities required of the ethical practitioner. Virtuous practitioners, they argue, are inclined to make right decisions.

The ethical theories are described in Box 4.4.

BOX 4.4   THE THREE ETHICAL THEORIES

1 Duty-based ethics

The duty-based theorist (or 'deontologist') believes that an action is ethically right to the extent that it conforms with rules or duties. This theory prioritises certain duties, most notably, the duty to respect people's autonomy by treating people not as a means to an end but as an end in themselves. Within this theory, when a duty is considered to be important, it must be applied in all situations, regardless of the outcome. If, for example, a practitioner has a duty to respect confidentiality, this duty must be applied absolutely, in all situations. A duty-based theorist would not consider it acceptable to breach confidentiality even where this is necessary to protect the life or wellbeing of a third party. In health care ethics, the professional duties set out in a code of ethics are considered to be an important source of duties which the practitioner must comply with. For the duty-based theorist, the four principles become 'duties' which the practitioner has to apply absolutely.

2 Outcome-based ethics

An outcome (or 'consequence') based theorist believes that an action is ethical to the extent that it brings about a good rather than a bad outcome. Put another way, an action is good to the extent that it maximises happiness and minimises suffering. You may have heard this theory described as the theory of 'the greatest good for the greatest number, at the cost of the least suffering'. Unlike a duty-based theorist, an outcome theorist may sometimes override duties to an individual, if doing so would create a greater good. The outcome theorist is not compelled to apply a duty in the same way in every situation, if this would cause harm (for example, an outcome theorist might decide that it is ethically acceptable to breach the confidentiality of a sex offender who has threatened to attack a third party if breaching confidentiality will protect that person from harm). For the outcome-based theorist, the four principles provide a starting-point for moral deliberation, but a principle can be waived if its application would cause more harm than good. Since the outcome theorist judges an action to be right or wrong on the basis of anticipated risks or benefits, it is important to ascertain all relevant facts in advance.

3 Virtue ethics

Virtues are habituated character traits that predispose people to act in accordance with worthy goals and the role expected of them. Virtues include candour, fidelity, compassion, discernment and integrity. Virtues are an important component of ethical decision making:

> Principles do not provide precise or specific guidelines for every conceivable set of circumstances. Principles require judgment, which in turn depends on character, moral discernment, and a person's sense of responsibility and accountability. Often what counts most in the moral life is not consistent adherence to principles and rules, but reliable character, moral good sense, and emotional responsiveness.

(Source: adapted from Beauchamp and Childress, 1994)

It is hard to quantify the extent to which any of these theories are applied in real-life situations. Generally, health practitioners are not expected to justify the basis for every decision they make. Motives are not usually questioned unless something has gone wrong. For this reason, it may not necessarily be known whether a decision was made because of the practitioner's assessment of risks and benefits (outcome-based decision making), or because of the practitioner's perceived sense of duty towards the parties involved (duty-based theory), or because of what sort of person the practitioner is (virtue-based decision making). Medical decision making is no different from the ethical decisions that ordinary people make in everyday life. Sometimes ethical decisions are made through gut instinct, although if scrutinised in greater detail, even gut instinct involves a complex interplay of ethical decision making. Few people would be happy if the basis of their decision making was questioned, and most people are defensive when asked to justify why they behaved in a certain way. Trainee practitioners may believe they will know intuitively what to do in an ethically contentious situation. This may make health care students reticent about being taught how to make ethical decisions formally. Some practitioners may regard any instruction in professional ethics as an affront to their own personal sense of morality and a slur on their sense of propriety. This is misguided, since the obligations health professionals owe to their users go beyond normal moral obligations. Whereas everyday life usually requires nothing more than common decency, the health care relationship requires practitioners to consider their users' best interests at all times. This involves respecting the wishes about treatment of users who can participate in the decision-making process and acting in the best interests of users who cannot give consent for themselves.

Difficulties in applying conventional bioethics to the CAM relationship

> Much of the literature in bioethics views the doctor/patient relationship as the paradigmatic example of a health care encounter. Various assumptions are made about the roles of 'good' doctors and 'good' patients, gender, dominant cultural values, patient expectations and a shared (western) understanding of health and disease. These assumptions may not be shared by many CAM practitioners or, indeed, CAM patients. Can the language and constructs of bioethics be invoked in analysing CAM relationships? Bioethics is grounded in, and a product of, the dominant biomedical paradigm. Western values and western preoccupation with the rights of the individual underpin traditional discussions of what it means to be an ethical health practitioner.
>
> (Stone, 2002, pp. ix–x)

In view of Stone's words, it may not make sense to apply conventional medical ethics to such diverse CAM practices as traditional Chinese medicine or shamanistic healing. If this is done uncritically, several problems emerge, including the following.

■ There is no reason to assume that the autonomy-focused ethics of western, liberal democracies should automatically provide the theoretical underpinnings for CAM, much of which is grounded in different, non-rational, non-scientific cosmologies.

■ The dynamics of the CAM therapeutic relationship may mean users are far more willing to trust their CAM practitioner than their conventional doctor and are less inclined to take a hostile, litigious approach if the therapy is unsuccessful. This requires an ethical framework that goes beyond the confines of most duty-based, professional codes of ethics and embraces the notion of **mutual trust and mutual responsibility**, in which users are active participants in their own healing process.

■ Much of the current debate about ethics concerns the use of hi-tech, orthodox medicine. The low-tech or relatively low-cost nature of CAM interventions raises fewer of these issues, although the therapeutic relationship may generate as many, if not more, ethical issues than the typical doctor–patient relationship.

- Many aspects of CAM treatment are not evidence-based, so it may be very difficult to provide information, for example about known side effects, to users and to provide that information in the percentage terms preferred by law.
- Not all users of CAM are ill. The ethics of preventive medicine and wellness maintenance may require a separate ethical approach. In conventional ethics, the duties of the practitioner derive specifically from the fact that the patient is ill and their autonomy and decision-making ability may be compromised. This may not be the case when the user seeks treatment to prevent ill health and to maximise their autonomy.

4.6 Key ethical issues for CAM practitioners

Although CAM practitioners' duties may vary in nature from other health professionals' duties, the types of ethical concern remain broadly similar. The rest of this chapter considers the key ethical areas underpinning standards of best practice in CAM. Although CAM practice varies dramatically in scope, all the issues listed in Box 4.5 are central to ethical practice. Each one is considered further below.

BOX 4.5   KEY ETHICAL ISSUES

- Competence
- Research
- Negotiation of contracts with users
- Respect for autonomy and consent
- Consent for children receiving CAM
- Respect confidentiality
- Maintain professional boundaries
- Professional etiquette and whistleblowing
- An effective complaints mechanism

Competence

Practitioners must have a sufficient level of competence to benefit users. The proliferation of training bodies, and the diversity of qualifications available, make it harder to know what represents an appropriate standard of pre-registration training or continuing professional development (CPD). Bringing a therapy under a single regulatory body makes it easier to set national educational standards in which diversity can be maintained, but a basic level of competence to practise is ensured. A subsidiary factor is the extent to which CAM practitioners need to be aware of orthodox medicine, and vice versa. Given the extent to which users are increasingly integrating different therapeutic modalities in seeking health care, all practitioners need to understand the possible interactions between different treatments.

Research

Every therapy needs to have a sound theory underpinning it. Without it, a therapy cannot grow and mature. Research may extend and improve the knowledge base for a given therapy but not all practitioners are willing or able to participate in useful, well designed research. The issues are related to the ethical principles of benefiting (beneficence) and not harming (non-maleficence). Without evidence to support the claims that are being made, how can practitioners be sure that they are doing good rather than doing harm? What is at issue are ethical questions that go to the heart of knowledge, and how competing knowledge systems are assessed. Several CAM therapies still adhere to the teachings of their founder. Their knowledge base is passed down through the generations, remaining true to original principles. Such therapies have not made the transition to a knowledge base that can be externally validated and modified in the light of new findings. It remains to be seen whether public support for such therapies will continue in these increasingly evidence-based times.

Negotiation of contracts with users

To benefit users, the user and the practitioner must work towards common goals that have been explicitly discussed. It is especially important for the user to understand the limits of what the therapy can deliver and not be under any delusions about the likely extent of recovery. What should CAM practitioners tell users about the therapy and about themselves? Practitioners cannot assume that users know what their therapy entails. A useful starting point might be to give users an introduction to the therapy itself. The practitioner's responsibilities might also include:

- to agree a fee per session (the first session can be more expensive because it takes much longer than future appointments)
- to discuss how many sessions to have before progress is reviewed
- to indicate how long therapy is likely to continue
- to give users a copy of the notes at the end of the treatment so they can use them in the future when pursuing other or further therapies.

If the user is expected to contribute materially to the success of the therapy by exercising self-responsibility and following the practitioner's recommendations about diet and exercise, this should be made clear to them at the start of the therapy.

The user's responsibilities include:

- to attend appointments
- to follow reasonable advice given by the practitioner
- to show courtesy and respect for the practitioner as an individual
- to pay promptly for all therapy sessions (including cancelled sessions if this was agreed).

Respect for autonomy and consent

Many practitioners claim that the patient-centred nature of their therapy means they automatically respect the user's autonomy. On closer inspection, CAM practitioners' commitment to respecting the users' wishes and values may be less patient-centred than they would like users to believe. Some CAM practitioners may fail to acknowledge users' rights, particularly in the area of risk disclosure and gaining consent to treat, or even touch, the user. Some CAM practitioners mistakenly believe that the mere fact the user has consulted them counts as implied consent and that it is not necessary to seek any further consent. Many health professionals (both conventional and CAM) also mistakenly think that the primary function of obtaining consent is to stop them from being sued. Some CAM practitioners assume that, because hardly any practitioners are sued, their users do not need to give express consent, even to invasive and potentially dangerous procedures.

As a matter of ethics and law, consent requirements include giving users adequate information, ensuring that they are competent to consent, and making sure the decision is voluntary. Ernst (1996) argues that, if the practitioner does not have evidence about risks and side effects, it is not possible to gain consent. Certainly, not all therapies have the sort of scientific evidence necessary to give a meaningful risk:benefit ratio. Then again, many of the procedures that users consent to in conventional medicine are only just starting to be evaluated scientifically.

Stone (2002) argues that a better interpretation of the information requirement is to provide as much information as the user feels is necessary to make an informed decision. This fits in with the consent process being fundamentally about enhancing and facilitating a user's autonomy, including the absolute right of competent people to make decisions for themselves that others would regard as foolhardy. It is, arguably, a user's right as an autonomous agent to deliberately choose a therapeutic modality that has not been scientifically validated to give risk:benefit ratios with any precision or to identify the full range of possible side effects. By moving outside a more empirically researched, reductionist framework, users must accept that the risks and benefits will be expressed within the paradigmatic framework of that therapy only.

4.7 Conclusion

This chapter has shown that CAM practice raises a variety of ethical issues. Although ethical considerations have different dimensions when applied to CAM, this chapter demonstrated that ethical issues – such as consent, competence, boundaries and effective communication – remain central to good practice. CAM practitioners, like all other responsible health care workers, must be taught and encouraged to recognise the ethical dimensions of their work. All practitioners must be accountable for their own actions. Non-affiliated practitioners may escape accountability to a professional body, but they remain accountable to their users and to their own ethical standards. Professional codes of ethics are only a partial basis for ethical practice, but they may prove to be too vague for use in specific situations. As well as having ethical responsibilities, all practitioners must work within the law. They must be up to date with the law on informed consent, confidentiality and data protection, as well as provisions affecting their specific sphere of practice. Practitioners need to understand both the legal and the ethical implications of their duty of care and to remember that the privileges of being a professional depend on honouring and upholding the values and ethics of the profession.

KEY POINTS

- Ethics is as important to the CAM relationship as it is to health care relationships within orthodox medical practice.
- Western bioethics prioritises respect for autonomy over the duty of beneficence. This is demonstrated by the requirement to obtain explicit consent. Respect for autonomy is important to CAM practitioners and users, although the duty of beneficence also underpins CAM relationships.
- The professional relationship is a relationship of trust, which confers rights and responsibilities. Autonomous practitioners are accountable to their users, themselves, their professional body, their employers and society.
- Codes of ethics and conduct give basic guidance on what counts as ethical practice, but they must be supplemented by professional judgement.
- Sometimes ethical responsibilities for health care workers, including CAM practitioners, are more stringent than legal requirements.

References

Beauchamp, T. and Childress, J. (1994) *Principles of Biomedical Ethics* (4th edition), Oxford, Oxford University Press.

Cant, S. and Sharma, U. (eds) (1996) *Complementary and Alternative Medicines: Knowledge in Practice*, London, Free Association Books Ltd.

Department of Health (2001) *The Expert Patient: A New Approach to Chronic Disease Management for the 21st Century*, London, DoH.

Ernst, E. (1996) 'The ethics of complementary medicine', *Journal of Medical Ethics*, Vol. 22, pp. 197–8.

House of Lords (2000) *Complementary and Alternative Medicine*, London, The Stationery Office. Available online: www.parliament.the-stationery-office.co.uk/pa/ld199900/ldselect/ldsctech/123/12301.htm [accessed 4 December 2003].

POPAN (2003) *Response to Sexual Offences Bill (HL) 2003* [online], www.popan.org.uk/policy/lb01.htm [accessed 4 December 2003].

Research Council for Complementary Medicine (1999) *Final Report of the European Commission Sponsored COST Project on Unconventional Medicine* [online], www.rccm.org.uk/static/Report_COST.aspx [accessed 4 December 2003].

Stone, J. (2002) *An Ethical Framework for Complementary and Alternative Therapists*, London, Routledge.

Chapter 5 Complementary and alternative medicine and mental health

Tom Heller

Contents

AIMS

- To understand some of the diverse ways in which complementary and alternative therapies are used by people with mental distress.
- To discuss and review how the themes introduced in Chapters 1 to 4 are exemplified by the way in which complementary and alternative health approaches are used in the mental health field.

5.1   Introduction

In this chapter the focus switches to the health of people who use complementary and alternative approaches for their own mental health and possible mental distress. This chapter also uses mental health issues to explore the subject areas covered in Chapters 1 to 4, specifically the **context** in which people may use complementary and alternative medicine (CAM) to impact on their mental health, and various political, historical and ethical issues.

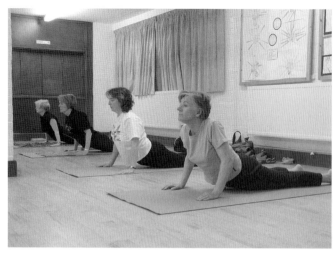

Many people use complementary or alternative therapies as a way of maintaining their own mental equilibrium

Conceptualising mental health issues

Mental health, and indeed mental 'illness' or 'distress', is a contested area, as illustrated by the range of ways in which various interest groups consider and may attempt to influence or change mental processes. Although the biomedical approach seems to be the dominant force in contemporary western society, many 'alternative' concepts are becoming increasingly accepted.

Indeed, in the world of complementary and alternative health there are many, diverse ways in which users and advocates conceptualise and attempt to tackle mental distress. It is difficult to characterise any single philosophical approach that underpins all CAM modalities. For example, some energy practitioners (such as reiki practitioners or spiritual healers) are not necessarily interested in the notion of mental illness and tend to work with the energy imbalances they believe they could find, rather than with any formal medical diagnosis. The reason for this lack of interest revolves around philosophical beliefs that place issues of energy over and above formal labels. Energy practitioners may not recognise labels such as 'mentally ill' and 'mentally well'. Instead they believe that everyone is somewhere on a spectrum at different stages of their lives and, therefore, medical diagnoses and categories do not make sense. In the diverse world of complementary and alternative medicine many people who have experienced severe, and maybe even life-challenging, bouts of mental distress have found a CAM approach that has helped them. For example, Rosalind Caplin recovered from severe anorexia:

> I decided to see a homeopath. I continued the homeopathic treatment for many years, finding my energy and vitality gradually increasing, as did my self-confidence. My experiences with the homeopath were similar to that of my counsellor – time and space to talk, respect and acknowledgement. My label was not considered in the remedy – which was given on the basis of

my overall personal makeup, my emotional, physical and energy states at the time. I was treated as an individual – a response far removed from the psychiatric one, which still considered me to be abnormal.

(Caplin, 1996, p. 145)

It is important not to imply a false dichotomy between current orthodox forms of mental health practice and holistic or complementary and alternative approaches. Indeed, the practice of mental health workers in the National Health Service (NHS) has been characterised by their increasing ability to adapt and incorporate some of the wider concepts of mental health that feature strongly in the CAM movement. Current 'conventional' or 'orthodox' forms of mental health work may, in fact, be more 'holistic' than they are sometimes stereotypically portrayed, especially when treating 'common' forms of mental distress. Anxiety and various manifestations of low mood may be considered more amenable to holistic approaches than the more severe forms of mental distress, such as bipolar disorders or psychotic illnesses such as 'schizophrenia'.

Many service users make comments about the detached, impersonal approach common in psychiatry. They believe psychiatrists are narrowly preoccupied with medical interpretations of emotional distress (see Box 5.1). Drugs and electroconvulsive therapy (ECT) signify the influence of technology and the medical model in psychiatry – an influence mediated through the dominance of clinical neuroscience in psychiatrists' training.

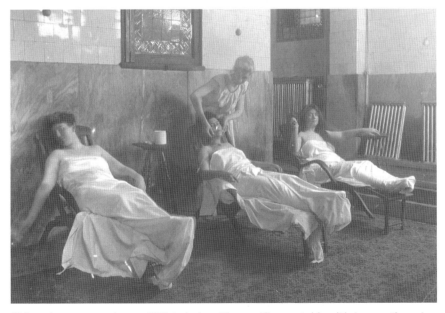

Although some people use CAM to help with specific mental health issues, there is a long history of its use to relieve general stress or prevent illness, including mental illness. In this photograph (taken in 1904) a group of women are given a face massage

> ## BOX 5.1 WHAT PEOPLE THINK ABOUT MODERN PSYCHIATRY
>
> There is evidence that many people who have mental health issues to confront are unhappy with the medical profession. MIND's survey *Experiencing Psychiatry* (Rogers et al., 1993) found deep dissatisfaction with psychiatry and the medical model. Only 12 per cent of over 500 service users who responded to the survey found psychiatrists helpful. Psychiatrists were reported to be the least helpful group by more than 21 per cent of respondents. There is also evidence that many people are turning away from medicine to use alternative and complementary therapies (Thomas et al., 2003). Many users value a wide variety of non-technological interventions, particularly creative and spiritual approaches, in coping with emotional distress. There is a clue to the reason for the dissatisfaction with medicine in the following quotations from the MIND survey.
>
> > I felt that I was treated too much as an object rather than a person.
>
> > They have a set diagnosis which they work to and treat with ECT and drugs. They do not search out the reasons for your illness with you so the illness just repeats again and again.
>
> > (Rogers et al., 1993, p. 50)

The stereotypical depiction of psychiatric intervention has become rather like mending an old car: something has gone wrong in the brain and this has affected the thought processes of the 'patient', who starts to 'suffer' uncomfortable thoughts, which then might be 'acted out' in 'disturbed' behaviour. Sometimes this sort of approach is seen to create a split between the mind and the body. In mental health disorders the biomedical model seems to see the mind as not functioning well, but the physical body remaining largely unaffected. More holistic approaches challenge this model. Often CAM is used by people who have not developed a specific mental health 'problem', but who want to find ways of improving mental health and general functioning. This preventive and self-reflexive aspect is the key to many of the paradigms of mental health that have been developed in complementary and alternative health approaches. Often these approaches challenge the notion of a split between the mind and the physical body.

CAM therapies can often offer a link between a person's physical ailments and their mental and emotional world:

> We can, for example, help clients improve the inner workings of their bodies by showing them how to handle their emotions. The teaching of such skills as *qi-gong*, acupressure and massage is not only good for the clients' physical health; it introduces an element of fun and variety in our intervention.
>
> (Chan et al., 2001, p. 273)

In effect, CAM can offer an integrated approach to what is now popularly known as 'mind, body and spirit'.

ACTIVITY   MENTAL STRESS AND DISTRESS

Allow 30 minutes

Think for a few minutes about a time when you were aware of your own mental health or were under some form of stress that affected your mood or thought processes. It does not have to be a serious condition: maybe a time when you could think about your mood.

- What was the situation?
- How did you feel at that time?
- What helped you return to more usual ways of thinking and behaving?

Comment

The following accounts of people who did this activity describe a wide spectrum of emotions and a remarkable range of ways of coping.

Angie remembered a time when one of her daughters became ill. This seems to have triggered her own low mood. She felt that everything was too much trouble and she could never concentrate on what was previously important for her. She did not function well at work and her line manager suggested getting professional help. Angie saw her own GP who persuaded her to see the practice counsellor. These sessions did not seem particularly helpful and Angie decided not to bother with them after a while. She eventually started to feel better after going to an aromatherapist for regular sessions.

Paul was very tearful and unhappy when he became unemployed. He felt that all his self-esteem and social contacts had been connected with his work and that these were all in jeopardy. He found it increasingly difficult to communicate with his wife and family. He saw his GP who prescribed some anti-depressant medication. The tablets made him feel sleepy and had various other side-effects, so he stopped taking them. He said his mood improved rapidly when he started going to the local gym. The exercise made him feel better about himself. He eventually got a job through a contact he made at the gym. He looks back on that time when he had such a low mood almost as though it had happened to someone else.

These accounts show that there is a wide range of stressors (factors that might cause mental distress) and an equally wide range of resources and ways people use to overcome their low mood.

Many people use CAM to alleviate what might be considered mild mental health problems – for example, stress or anxiety – and many CAMs are explicitly promoted on that basis. There is a more detailed examination of the ways in which various complementary and alternative therapies use a variety of media to promote their activities in Chapter 15. In the field of mental health many individual practitioners, as well as entire CAM modalities, tend to advocate that people use their services to 'regain their balance', 'reduce stress', and make other allusions to chronic, but mild, mental health issues. This focus seems to be borne out by various surveys that were done to discover what people use CAM therapies for. For example, Thomas et al. (2001) found that, in a sample of 703 people, 39 per cent of visits to British CAM therapists were for 'stress' and/or 'relaxation'.

Of course, people who experience mental distress may well have their own individual ways of developing an understanding of the meaning of that distress or disruption in their lives. For some it involves exploring spiritual dimensions (Culliford, 2002), while others look for understanding in terms of their upbringing and the development of relationships. Many are also aware of the social conditions that may have led to their distress.

> Many complementary therapies have their origins in lay and folk knowledge so are strongly rooted in a self, and mutual help, non-expert, approach to healing. There is much use of the traditional healing powers of magic, symbolism and ritual in many complementary approaches – the power of which have been neglected and diminished within the rationalism of science but which, used wisely and with care, may have much to offer those who need help in the creative use of irrationality and intuition.
>
> (Mitchell, 2000, p. 335)

Also, using orthodox medical treatment for people with various forms of mental distress could differ fundamentally from the ways in which CAM would be used in such situations. Orthodox psychiatry focuses on symptoms of minor or major distress (see Box 5.2) and may use external chemicals (drugs) to eliminate or diminish the features of underlying mental distress. However, many forms of CAM focus on 'mind–body medicine' (Barrows and Jacobs, 2002), in which the mind and the body are not separated but are seen as part of a single, 'holistic' approach to the individual who has developed a form of distress.

BOX 5.2   IS THERE A FUNDAMENTAL DIFFERENCE BETWEEN 'MINOR' AND 'MAJOR' TYPES OF MENTAL DISTRESS?

Some commentators on mental health issues distinguish between 'major' disruptions that people can face in their mental health status, such as 'schizophrenia' or bipolar disorders, and 'minor' problems, such as mild depression and anxiety. The implication is that 'serious' forms of mental 'illness' should be treated in the domain of professionals, psychiatrists, etc., while complementary and alternative therapies should be used by people with 'minor', 'lifestyle' types of illness. This distinction is used by many psychiatrists and is based on a diagnostic disease model. In the professional domain codes are drawn up to indicate that if a person has a particular set of symptoms then they have a disorder. Many other theorists and commentators argue against this approach and have developed a 'continuum model' (Mechanic, 1999). In this model, types of distress such as depression are on a continuum. People move along the continuum depending on a range of factors, such as life stressors, social support and coping strategies. This approach is more likely to be adopted by CAM practitioners because it implies that complementary and alternative modalities can be used to alleviate the effects of all forms of mental distress.

5.2   Biomedicine and its challengers

During the 20th century the growth and development of 'orthodox' forms of treatment and the classification of mental illness was characterised by the dominance of concepts related to science-based subjects such as biology and neurology. This 'biomedical' approach is based on the fundamental belief that different forms of mental illness are specific diseases of the brain. This approach was described by the prominent biological psychiatrist Nancy Andreasen (1984). She claims to be able to look directly to the brain to understand both normal behaviour and mental illness in terms of how the brain works and how it breaks down. This type of approach is a clear illustration of **reductionism**: in this case, finding the cause and source of mental illness in one site – the brain.

The purely biomedical explanation for the development of mental distress has been challenged and developed by many theorists and practitioners. In particular, George Engels (1980) introduced the concept of the 'biopsychosocial' model, which calls for the consideration of psychological and social influences in addition to those associated solely with changes in brain chemistry. Psychological attention focuses on the individual factors that may produce abnormal thoughts, feelings and behaviours. On the other hand, sociologists look outside the individual person and seek wider explanations within the environmental or social context and may view mental distress as a breakdown in the face of overwhelming environmental stress. In support of a sociological explanation for the development of mental distress, Peggy Thoits states:

> Mental illness is not randomly distributed in the population, but is socially patterned. Patients in treatment are not a random set of individuals, but once again are socially patterned.
>
> (Thoits, 1999, p. 138)

Bracken and Thomas (2002) argue forcefully that people's mental life does not happen only inside their skulls, emphasising the importance of the social and spiritual context:

> We will never be able to understand the various elements of our mental life such as thoughts, beliefs, feelings, and values if we think of them as located inside the brain. Trying to grasp the meaningful reality of sadness, alienation, obsession, fear, and madness by looking at scans or analysing biochemistry is like trying to understand a painting by looking at the canvas without reference to its wider world.
>
> (Bracken and Thomas, 2002, p. 1434)

The biopsychosocial approach is also favoured in the National Service Frameworks for Mental Health (Department of Health, 1999). Box 5.3 is an extract from the frameworks. It demonstrates some of the ways in which current official thinking constructs social explanations for certain types of mental distress.

BOX 5.3　EXTRACT FROM THE MENTAL HEALTH NATIONAL SERVICE FRAMEWORKS

Mental health problems can result from the range of adverse factors associated with social exclusion and can also be a cause of social exclusion. For example:

- unemployed people are twice as likely to have depression as people in work
- children in the poorest households are three times more likely to have mental health problems than children in well off households
- half of all women and a quarter of all men will be affected by depression at some period during their lives
- people who have been abused or been victims of domestic violence have higher rates of mental health problems
- people with drug and alcohol problems have higher rates of mental health problems
- between a quarter and a half of people using night shelters or sleeping rough may have a serious mental disorder, and up to half may be alcohol dependent
- some black and minority ethnic communities are diagnosed as having higher rates of mental health problems than the general population – refugees are especially vulnerable
- there is a high rate of mental health problems in the prison population
- people with physical illnesses have twice the rate of mental health problems compared to the general population.

(Source: DoH, 1999, p. 7)

Sociologists also attempt to focus on the issues concerning the location of **power** when mental health status is being determined:

> It is the medical profession too, by virtue of the power, status, and authority it has achieved, that ensures that psychiatrists are at the top of the hierarchy of the occupational groups involved in the care of the mentally ill; that gives certain exclusive legal powers to psychiatrists *vis-à-vis* their patients – to prescribe drugs, to admit and discharge from hospital against their patients' wishes if necessary, to offer treatment within the NHS and so forth; and it is their identity as doctors that gives psychiatrists a key role in determining the content and character of mental health services ...
>
> (Busfield, 1996, pp. 132–3)

Much sociology in the late 20th century focused on the all-encompassing notion of mental wellbeing. Some writers, such as Wurtzel (2001), criticise the increasing use of psychiatry and the drugs it offers to create wellbeing. These critics argue that doctors prescribe drugs such as Prozac too easily and do not attempt to explore the root cause of the problem. Others, such as Beck (1992), point to the growing depression and anxiety in society as a symptom of a sense of loss of coherence in modern life. Who can people believe or turn to when so many of the institutions that helped structure the pathways through life and a sense of meaning for many people in the past have lost authority? From this viewpoint, mental illness is an everyday response to being in a world devoid of certainty.

In addition, the world view of the medical profession is being challenged by people with personal experience of mental distress, who sometimes describe themselves as 'users and survivors' of the mental health services (Read and Reynolds, 1996; Wallcraft, 1998; Faulkner and Layzell, 2000). Their experiences do not fall into the simplistic diagnostic or treatment categories used by the medical profession. They emphasise that their experience of the phenomenon of mental distress fits into a more pluralistic, multifaceted approach. Indeed, the way in which people who experience a period of significant mental distress become 'labelled' by the biomedically oriented mental health care system is now a source of continued dispute. For example, Scheff (1996) argues that labelling a person with a mental health diagnosis can be more problematic for that person than the underlying mental distress itself. Some people who have had such experiences become campaigners, in order to change the experience for other people who may have to resort to the health care system that 'users and survivors' increasingly consider as damaging (Campbell, 1996).

The World Health Organization also recognises the limitations of the 'medical model':

> Until recently the health professions have largely followed a medical model, which seeks to treat patients by focusing on medicines and surgery, and gives less importance to beliefs and faith (in healing, in the physician and in the doctor–patient relationship). This reductionism or mechanistic view of patients as being only a material body is no longer satisfactory. Patients and physicians have begun to realise the value of elements such as faith, hope and compassion in the healing process.

(WHO, 1998, p. 7)

Political and historical realities

The current profession of psychiatry evolved from its early beginnings in much harsher times, when the prime motivation for treating people with mental disorders was to remove them from the streets and incarcerate them in 'madhouses'. Bedlam Hospital in London was established in 1247 as a 'home for the insane', but the regime within it ensured that the 'inmates' were treated insensitively, even callously. Since those days, of course, attitudes towards people with mental health symptoms have changed enormously.

Ethical developments ensured that much more humane and 'moral' regimes are now the norm in establishments which treat people who have mental distress (Bloch and Pargiter, 2002). Also, the discovery and introduction of many different types of psycho-active medication has given psychiatrists a wide range of treatment options. However, it is hard to escape the fact that there remains a battle for power between the medical profession

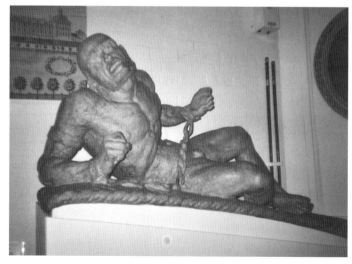

At the door of Bedlam Hospital visitors were confronted by two sculptures commissioned from the Dutch artist Caius Gabriel Cibber (1630-1700): this one of mania or raving madness, the other of melancholy

(especially the psychiatrists) and the proponents of a more 'holistic' or pluralistic approach to the conceptualisation and eventual treatment of mental distress. Thomas (2000) characterises this as 'expertise by experience' versus 'expertise by profession':

> It is quite clear that psychiatry values scientific evidence over and above any other type, especially when it comes to knowing what is effective for people experiencing psychosis or other forms of emotional distress. The problem is that scientific evidence overshadows what is arguably the most valuable source of evidence on effectiveness, the experience of those who use psychiatric services.
>
> (Thomas, 2000, p. 1)

The use (and abuse) of power by the medical profession in the field of mental health work has been well documented throughout history. Despite there being no effective treatment in previous ages for the most florid psychiatric conditions (Porter, 1999), doctors saw the opportunity to become specialists in treating people with 'mental illnesses'. Most 19th-century physicians maintained that insanity was ultimately rooted in the organism, particularly the brain; for that reason therapy had to be incorporated in a medical model, and prescribed by physicians. There followed a dramatic increase in books on insanity, virtually all by doctors; and a growing body of 'mad-doctors' emerged, who were called 'alienists'. What remains largely unchallenged and unchanged since the historical beginnings of the speciality of psychiatry is the clinical and institutional power of psychiatrists, who are largely experienced by users of mental health services as dispensers of medication and potential removers of their liberty.

5.3   Users and survivors of mental health services

The users and survivors of mental health services do not necessarily all want the same outcome. Increasingly, however, people who develop a form of mental distress express the meanings they attach to their condition and the ways in which they believe it should be tackled (Read and Reynolds, 1996; Wallcraft, 1998; Faulkner and Layzell, 2000). Some people who have had a significant time in their lives when their mental equilibrium was challenged or disrupted describe their experience as being part of a 'journey'. Often people can begin to work towards an understanding of the learning and healing that can develop if attention is given to their individual story and their search for meaning in their own lives. Although this 'narrative' approach is common in complementary and alternative forms of therapy, orthodox forms of treatment may not focus on this aspect at all. In particular, many service users are becoming disillusioned with the treatment they are offered by the statutory services:

> The reasons for the shift towards greater use of complementary therapies [by people with mental health problems] are complex and varied. Their appeal seems to extend far beyond any simplistic notions of narrowly defined effectiveness of treatment. The attraction seems to lie in a mixture of their more egalitarian approach to the therapeutic relationship, their recognition of links between lifestyle and illness, the individual nature of the treatments offered and the success of treatments for symptom management, along with a perceived relative lack of noxious side effects. A central and crucial factor is their potential to bring meaning to the experience of suffering by making connections between physical, mental and spiritual circumstances and aspects of people's lives.

> (Mitchell, 2000, p. 334)

How CAM therapies fit into mental health recovery

Although the users and survivors of the mental health system frequently recognise and acknowledge the contribution of CAM therapies, there is often a complex relationship between official services and CAM provision. In the 'Strategies for Living' research (Faulkner and Layzell, 2000), several people who found complementary therapies helpful said they would like easier access to, and greater availability of, them. Two different issues were under consideration here: first, there was the need for the mental health services, and the NHS in general, to recognise the value of complementary therapies and hence make them easily available. The second issue was the simple matter of the cost of private treatments, which are prohibitive to most people living on state benefits.

Some commentators, often speaking from positions of authority within the hierarchies of the medical profession, have questioned whether people who use CAM are more likely to make that choice because they have underlying mental health problems. For example, Holland (1999) questions the stereotype of people who seek help from alternative medicine. He suggests that people using CAM are 'not psychologically strong', and that they may turn to alternative medicine to 'alleviate their distress'. Indeed, he wonders whether CAM could be used as a marker by medical practitioners so that 'the use of such treatments may identify distressed patients'. Sparber and Wootton (2002) examine this point of view in more detail. They raise the following questions:

> Are anxious, depressed people more likely to seek CAM therapies? Or do they seek CAM therapies because they become depressed and anxious about their chronic conditions, and the apparent failure of western medicine to alleviate their symptoms?

> (Sparber and Wootton, 2002, p. 93)

In many ways, the people who position themselves at different points along the spectrum of belief systems about mental health issues can be expected to develop strong views about the people who do not share those views. Thus, for some professional health workers, CAM practitioners and people who use CAM therapies are objects of derision and subject to unwarranted speculation about their views or motives. Some professionals within psychiatry even seem openly hostile to the intrusion of complementary and alternative concepts and practices that threaten their domain:

> Health care professionals, especially, have an obligation to distinguish between remedies that represent the careful consensus of highly trained experts and snake oil.
>
> (Kennedy et al., 2002, p. 6)

It is difficult to tell to what extent such hostility is about care or concern for users rather than an attempt to protect professional power. However, such views appear not to recognise the groundswell of public interest in using CAM for mental health across the spectrum.

5.4   How people with mental distress use CAM

As noted earlier, some people use CAM to maintain their mental equilibrium. CAM approaches appear to be more effective in the prevention and relief of the 'simpler' forms of mental distress than for psychotic or severe and enduring diagnoses. Wallcraft (1998) evaluated the evidence for the claims that a wide range of CAM modalities give effective help for anxiety, depression and insomnia. They include transcendental meditation, acupuncture, nutritional medicine, herbal medicine, homoeopathy, massage and aromatherapy. However, it is not always necessary to experience a problem with mood or thought processes before using some types of CAM intervention. CAM is often used to prevent stress or anxiety; other people turn to CAM when they experience mental distress because of their perception that conventional medical treatments may not be sufficient to help them. Despite certain advances in the treatment of some mental health problems by conventional psychiatry, considerable problems remain:

> Psycho-pharmaceutical developments certainly allow psychiatry itself to function better, but pacifying patients with drugs hardly seems the pinnacle of achievement and any claims as to the maturity of a science of mental disorders seem premature and contestable ...
>
> (Porter, 2002, p. 216)

Dissatisfaction with the medical profession and orthodox medical approaches may have contributed to the growth in demand for CAM. In addition, the increasing knowledge that many drug-based treatments also carry the risk of potentially serious side effects may drive people to try complementary or alternative approaches. If people with mental health needs feel they are not getting help from the statutory services, they will naturally turn to other sources of help (Unutzer et al., 2000). If there is a substantial unmet need for mental health care, people with mental distress might be expected to seek help from alternative providers or therapies outside the formal health care system.

A major survey in the USA looked at the use of alternative medicine by 9585 people who could be considered to have a 'mental disorder' (Unutzer et al., 2000). The use of CAM during the past 12 months was reported by 16.25 per cent of respondents. However, the people using complementary or alternative approaches reported using them in addition to conventional therapies. A further survey of 2055 people in the USA discovered that the use of CAM was centred particularly on people with self-defined anxiety attacks and severe depression (Kessler et al., 2001). Interestingly, only 20 per cent of these people had visited an alternative practitioner, while the majority purchased CAM products over the counter. The survey found that almost nine out of every ten patients with self-defined anxiety attacks who were seen by a psychiatrist also used some form of complementary and alternative therapy to treat anxiety; and more than six out of every ten patients with self-defined severe depression who were seen by a psychiatrist also used a type of complementary and alternative therapy to treat depression. These rates were the same regardless of the wide range of sociodemographic characteristics of patients.

A gender analysis indicates that more women than men use CAM for their mental health needs. Peeke and Frishett (2002) looked specifically at how women use CAM for their mental health needs:

> For years, women have used these medications [anti-depressants to treat mental health problems] without question. They have also suffered from the often-significant side effects they cause. Weight gain, fatigue, nausea, suppressed libido, sleep disturbances, and memory and concentration impairments are examples of the commonly reported adverse reactions to these compounds. It is no wonder that women have responded so enthusiastically to the emergence of new therapeutic alternatives, referred to as alternative or complementary medicine (CAM), that often promise to provide more *natural* treatment with fewer side effects than their pharmaceutical counterparts.
>
> (Peeke and Frishett, 2002, p. 183)

Who uses CAM approaches for their mental health needs?

In the USA, Druss and Rosenheck (2000) studied 1803 people with a 'mental condition' who had seen an alternative practitioner. They reported that the use of CAM was high in this group and 'particularly prevalent among younger, female, and more educated respondents' (p. 712). They found that individuals with 'transient emotional distress' saw CAM practitioners both for reasons associated with the mental condition and for other, entirely separate conditions. They raise the challenging question of whether the 'use of these treatments should be regarded as a marker for emotional distress' (pp. 708–9). In other words, they question whether people who use CAM in other settings are somehow different from other people, and possibly more vulnerable to mental distress.

Russinova et al. (2002), also reporting from the USA, provide evidence of the benefits of CAM perceived by people with 'serious mental illness'. The research was based on the experiences of 157 people with 'schizophrenia', major depression and bipolar disorder (manic depression). Some individuals with severe mental illness seemed to benefit from a variety of alternative practices; and religious or spiritual activities, such as prayer, worship, and religious or spiritual reading, appeared to be practised and experienced as beneficial by people with severe mental illness. Other alternative practices seemed to promote a recovery process beyond the management of emotional and cognitive impairments by also enhancing social or spiritual capacity and promoting the person's own capacity for self-functioning.

The philosophical attraction to approaches used in CAM therapies may also be highly significant. Astin (2000) reviewed evidence from population surveys in the USA and outlined some of the philosophical reasons why people are drawn to CAM therapies. Although he did not survey only people who used CAM for mental health purposes, he found little evidence that people use CAM because they are dissatisfied with conventional medicine, or that they expressed a desire for greater control than users of conventional medicine. Results from his study did, however, support the notion that people use CAM because of a perceived congruence with their own philosophical position and values:

> First, having a holistic belief in the importance of body, mind and spirit in treating health-related matters ... people who have been involved with CAM may have come to modify their health beliefs through contact with these therapeutic systems and the philosophies that underlie them. Second, people who hold a holistic philosophical orientation toward health may be attracted to various CAM practices because they perceive a greater acknowledgement of and appreciation for the role of non-physical factors

(mind/spirit) in creating health and illness. Lastly, belief in the importance of body, mind, and spirit **and** use of CAM may represent a proxy for some higher-order construct such as a general open mindedness to new ideas and concepts.

(Astin, 2000, pp. 106–7)

It is also interesting to consider more overarching reasons for the upsurge in the acceptance and use of CAM at a time when there have been so many apparent advances in medical 'science'. Indeed, why has the dominance of biomedicine in contemporary western society produced its own backlash? Engebretson (2002) notes that complementary therapies are becoming increasingly popular in precisely those cultures dominated by biomedicine. She concludes that the cultural aspects of biomedicine often contrast with those of other healing systems such as traditional Chinese medicine, yoga and shamanic healing. However, some modalities may be extracted from these healing systems to expand the focus of biomedical approaches: for example, away from treating specific episodes of disease towards promoting health. Disease or disruption of health takes different forms in different people, so using the treatment from one culture for a disease that is understood from a different paradigm may be problematic.

| ACTIVITY | PART 1: IS IT ETHICAL TO USE CAM FOR MENTAL HEALTH CONDITIONS? |

Allow 1 hour for all three parts

Read the case study below and make notes about the possible ethical concerns that might arise in this situation.

| VERA: SETTING THE SCENE |

Vera is in her late forties. She recently inherited a very large, detached Victorian house in a rather genteel residential estate to the east of a town on the south coast. She inherited this house and some other capital from her parents who were both killed in a road accident. Vera decided to give up her administrative job in Macclesfield, move into the vacant house and set up a 'bed and breakfast' business. She has no friends or relatives in that part of the country. Indeed, apart from her two cats, she appears to be alone in the world.

Over recent weeks Vera's mood has become increasingly low. As she goes around the house, trying to sort out the rooms, she talks to herself and once neighbours found her wandering towards the sea in the middle of the night in her slippers. Most days she does not leave the house but remains in her nightdress and eats increasingly sporadically. She realises for herself that she is not functioning very well, and certainly has never felt so anxious before. She recognises that she is not thinking as clearly as she usually does and frequently cries herself to sleep at night.

> One day, on the way to the local chemist, she sees a notice in the newsagent's window advertising a crystal healer, James Riddle. She notes down the telephone number and decides to ring him.

What ethical concerns do you have? You will find it useful to refer back to Chapter 4.

Comment

Alarm bells may be ringing on several counts. Vera is in a highly vulnerable state. She apparently does not have any support networks that might help her to make prudent decisions, and she could be open to many different forms of exploitation or even abuse. People in a position where mental distress is a major component can be particularly at risk from unscrupulous practitioners.

How does Vera know what qualifications or training Mr Riddle has? Is he competent? What is the theoretical underpinning of his work and how does he gauge for himself whether it is effective? Does Mr Riddle work to a professional code of conduct and ethical standards? Does he have any competency for the condition that Vera has developed? Would Vera be helped more by other forms of therapy, or by contact with statutory services?

How does the therapist keep up to date? Has he done any recent courses, or does he rely on a weekend course in crystal healing he did many years ago?

ACTIVITY   PART 2: VERA GOES TO THE CRYSTAL HEALER

Read the next part of the case study and make notes on any continuing ethical concerns.

VERA VISITS THE THERAPIST

Vera rings the therapist and makes an appointment to visit him at 7 pm the following Tuesday. He sounds very kind on the phone and this impression is reinforced when they meet in person. Mr Riddle works from home, which is on the estate next to Vera's. His house is reassuringly substantial, but in need of some decoration. He has converted one of the downstairs reception rooms into a therapy room. There are heavy furnishings and a large couch is the central focus of the room. There are various 'New Age' posters on the walls and there is a gentle smell from the incense burner on the mantelpiece. Mr Riddle is about 50 years old. He has a comforting appearance and Vera finds that she can tell him all about herself and her current predicament. The first session lasts well over two hours, during which time Mr Riddle places two translucent crystals on the back of Vera's hands and one on her forehead. Vera is concerned that she has talked 'too much', but Mr Riddle insists that he needed to know exactly how she was feeling, and what she felt about her problems. He refuses to take any payment for the first visit, but suggests that she sees him twice a week for regular therapy sessions.

Comment

Is this practitioner someone who will exploit and/or take advantage of Vera as a vulnerable woman? Or is he a competent practitioner who wants to heal Vera? The contract that he has negotiated might be thought of as rather unorthodox. He has not charged for the initial session. Is this because he wants to make Vera beholden to him in some way, or is it a genuine offer that establishes his good will?

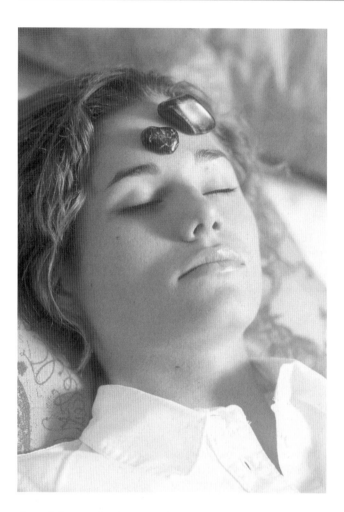

Crystal therapy has been used for centuries and people have tried to harness the energy and purported therapeutic qualities of crystals in many different ways. However, how they are used depends not just on the intrinsic qualities of the stones but also on the ethics and professional standards of the therapist who claims to use them for therapeutic purposes

ACTIVITY   PART 3: THE THERAPY SESSIONS CONTINUE

Now read the final part of the case study and make notes on any ethical concerns.

VERA'S ONGOING VISITS

During the next few months Vera visits the crystal therapist twice each week. On a few occasions he expresses concern for her health and suggests that she has an additional therapy session. Vera has discovered quite a lot about Mr Riddle. Apparently, he has had health problems in the past and she thinks that, therefore, he understands what she is going through. He does not have any paper qualifications, but says he has had lots of success with treating people who feel low. He is also lonely and often feels as though there is nobody who understands him. Indeed, Vera has become a confidante for him in return. Each session costs Vera £30 and, although she can just about afford this money, she is using her savings and has less to spend on preparing her house for the forthcoming holiday season. The therapy sessions have changed in nature recently and Mr Riddle uses more of what he calls 'instinctive touch therapy'.

Comment

This scenario was deliberately chosen to demonstrate the ambiguity of some therapeutic relationships when seen from a neutral standpoint. In these situations, perhaps as a concerned relative, it is important to use some of the ethical guidelines described in Chapter 4. The 'instinctive touch therapy' Mr Riddle claims to use may or may not be a real therapy. Has he trained in it and is he insured to practise it?

What is the nature of Vera's contract with Mr Riddle? Is he being paternalistic in his relationship with her? Does Vera fully understand what is involved and does she have the autonomy to negotiate possible changes to the therapy with the therapist? Is Mr Riddle respecting her confidentiality? Certainly there seem to be some boundary issues because Vera has been the therapist's confidante.

If the situation deteriorates, and professional etiquette is not adhered to, would Vera know how to take action or make a complaint? Who would she complain to?

5.5   Does CAM work for people with mental distress?

> Sometimes it is scientifically impossible to determine which healing art was the primary one in helping an individual regain a sense of health and balance and which were complementary.
>
> (Miller, 2002, p. 640)

The problems and challenges associated with any attempt to discover whether various complementary therapies are effective for particular conditions are considered throughout this book. In the field of mental health and mental distress the search for interventions that 'work' can be particularly problematic (see Box 5.4). The fundamentally 'internal' thoughts and feelings that constitute people's mental health, and whose disruption may cause mental distress, may not be readily amenable to simple notions of evidence-based medicine (Faulkner and Thomas, 2002). Certainly, different people from various professional and lay positions have a wide range of perspectives on the effectiveness of any particular treatment. For orthodox psychiatry, a satisfactory outcome may involve eliminating problematic symptoms and 'improving' particular behaviours. However, users and survivors of mental health services can have very different measures of 'success', including whether the treatment gave them more control and understanding of their situation:

> User-valued outcomes, particularly pertaining to complementary care, may include increased sense of meaning, improved sense of wellbeing, feeling able to cope, having explanations which make sense, being in control of treatment and being respected as a significant individual.

(Mitchell, 2000, p. 343)

BOX 5.4   DOES CAM WORK FOR DEPRESSION?

People have used St John's Wort (SJW) for centuries to treat the symptoms of depression (Nierenberg et al., 2002). A review by Schulz (2002a, b) studied the combined results from over 3000 people taking part in 34 controlled, double-blind trials of the active ingredient of SJW (*Hypericum*). It revealed that the herb is as effective as synthetic anti-depressants in treating depressive symptoms. Although side-effects of taking SJW are remarkably infrequent, and almost invariably mild, there are problems associated with its use alongside certain other types of prescribed medication (Ernst, 2002).

In a more general review of complementary and self-help treatments for the symptoms of depression, Jorm et al. (2002) studied the effectiveness of 37 different treatment modalities. They concluded that the treatments with the best evidence of effectiveness are St John's Wort, exercise and light therapy (for winter depression), and that there is more limited evidence to support the effectiveness of acupuncture, relaxation therapy and yoga breathing exercises.

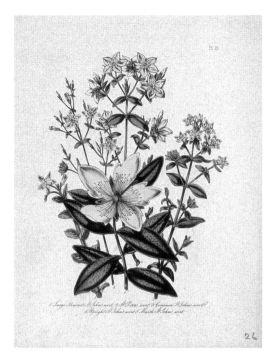

St John's Wort has been considered to have special properties for centuries. Its name *Hypericum* is derived from the Greek meaning 'over an apparition', a reference to the belief that the herb was so obnoxious to evil spirits that a whiff of it would cause them to fly away
(Source: The Wellcome Trust)

> No matter how 'scientific' we aspire to be, clinical decisions always will involve value judgements and it is a serious mistake to pretend otherwise. This makes it essential that psychiatrists reflect critically on the values that underlie the advice they offer and the decisions they make, and that they understand how these values relate to those of patients.
>
> (Faulkner and Thomas, 2002, p. 3)

When deciding what types of evidence of effectiveness may be acceptable or appropriate it is important to recognise the power wielded by certain interest groups, as well as the values attached to particular decisions about mental health issues. Thus certain types of research are prioritised by the medical establishment and by those making policy decisions about the distribution of resources. However, Wallcraft (1998) believes that, in the light of demonstrable consumer demand for a wider choice of less damaging and intrusive therapies for mental health problems, 'lack of proof' should not be a reason for inaction. Much could be done to test, evaluate and monitor the use of complementary therapy in mental health, and the views of mental health service users should be a driving force for innovation.

The current 'gold standard' of research methodology is usually regarded as the **randomised controlled trial** (RCT). In an RCT patients with a particular condition are allocated to two or three groups. One group has the active or new treatment while the second group has no treatment or a standard treatment. The third group may have an apparently similar but inactive (placebo) treatment. The results, or outcomes, from all three groups are compared after a period of time.

A recent review of the 'scientific evidence' using mainly RCTs looked for the therapeutic effects of meditation but failed to find 'proof' of its effectiveness, despite the evidence of centuries of apparently beneficial use of this technique by millions of users throughout the world and in many different cultures (Canter, 2003). The fact remains that many proponents of CAM could not possibly afford to do RCT research of this nature and most CAM modalities could probably not be randomised in this way:

> And besides, many complementary therapists are wary of the constraints of scientific trials. How can you measure something as subtle as Qi, the 'vital force', or 'healing energy'? Is it possible to devise a trial that takes into account treatment that is tailored to individual patients, or rate a result that makes someone feel better, even if they are not cured or even physiologically improved?
>
> (Foster, 2002, p. 15)

If the RCT is usually inappropriate for the study of CAMs, it becomes even more necessary to broaden the types of evidence that can be considered when attempting to assess whether particular forms of mental health intervention may be effective.

Assessing the effectiveness of CAM mental health interventions

If RCTs – the 'gold standard' of scientific proof – cannot always provide the answer to the effectiveness of CAM therapies, Verhoef et al. (2002) argue for the inclusion of qualitative research methods; that is, those not involving numerical data:

> However, [randomised controlled trials] address only one, limited, question, namely whether an intervention has – statistically – an effect. They do not address why the intervention works, how participants are experiencing the intervention, and/or how they give meaning to these experiences. ... Qualitative research can assist in understanding the meaning of an intervention to patients as well as patients' beliefs about the treatment and expectations of the outcome.
>
> (Verhoef et al., 2002, p. 275)

Wallcraft (1998) suggests using a wide range of evidence – including qualitative – to assess the effectiveness of various forms of CAM in mental health work. The six basic types of evidence that she considered are shown in Box 5.5.

BOX 5.5 TYPES OF EVIDENCE IN TESTING THE EFFECTIVENESS OF MENTAL HEALTH INTERVENTIONS

1 Clinical trials, including randomised controlled trials
2 Research reviews including systematic review
3 Outcome studies
4 Evaluated projects
5 Case studies
6 Accounts of personal experience

(Source: adapted from Wallcraft, 1998)

Of course, whether research (quantitative or qualitative) contains numerical data is not the issue. There are many ways of conducting good research into the effectiveness of CAM approaches (Verhoef et al., 2002).

This chapter has tried not to imply that all complementary and alternative approaches used in the mental health field are universally effective or, indeed, without potential problems and pitfalls. It is always important to continue to assess and evaluate the role of CAM approaches in this complex field. This applies both to the need for continued evaluation of the effectiveness of specific therapies and in individual situations. For example, Yager et al. (1999) counsel orthodox health workers to find out more about the CAMs that the people who consult them might be using. They offer the guidelines listed in Box 5.6.

BOX 5.6 GUIDELINES FOR CLINICIANS ON ALTERNATIVE THERAPIES

1 Routinely question patients about alternative therapies
2 Discuss safety and efficacy
3 Discuss merits of alternative treatments
4 Provide information
5 Learn about alternative therapies
6 Determine characteristics of proposed alternative treatments and practitioners

(a) Is the provider credentialed and licensed?
(b) Is the provider's experience in treating the patient based on personal clinical experiences with other patients with similar problems?
(c) What exactly does the therapy consist of?
(d) How many weeks are likely to pass before the patient and provider decide that the therapy is or is not working?

(e) How much will each session cost with or without medications, and what is the anticipated total cost for the specified time period?

(f) What are the potential side effects?

(g) With the patient's permission, is the provider willing to communicate any relevant information to the patient's conventional health care providers?

(h) Are all the interactions being carefully documented?

(Source: adapted from Yager et al., 1999, pp. 1436-7)

5.6 Conclusion

In this chapter the subject of mental health was used to explore in more detail some of the issues explored in Chapters 1 to 4. It has become apparent that complementary and alternative health issues can only be studied in context. That is, CAM therapies and approaches may be considered complementary or alternative only in relation to the dominant 'orthodox medicine', which has achieved primacy in comparatively recent historical times. Many ethical concerns are highlighted by the use of complementary and alternative modalities to help people with some form of mental distress.

This chapter also helped you to start thinking about the effectiveness of complementary and alternative approaches to health.

KEY POINTS

■ Although thought processes happen in the brain, the study of the brain alone is insufficient to explain the nature and scope of mental health problems.

■ Biopsychosocial aspects of mental health add extra dimensions to conceptualising how thoughts and feelings could be ordered or disordered.

■ Complementary and alternative approaches seem to relate more easily to spiritual and cultural considerations of mental health processes than orthodox approaches.

■ The orthodox medical profession may discount or tend to devalue 'unscientific' approaches to the conceptualisation and treatment of mental distress.

■ Users and survivors of mental health services often value the perceived contribution that various complementary and alternative therapies made to their recovery.

■ Even severe forms of mental distress can be helped by complementary and alternative approaches.

■ Research into the 'effectiveness' of various types of therapy is similarly set within the context of competing paradigms and contested outcomes.

■ Complementary and alternative approaches to the treatment of mental distress may not be amenable to the rigours of a 'scientific' research trial, but they may be able to show their effectiveness through other types of research methodology and different end-points.

References

Andreasen, N. (1984) *The Broken Brain: The Biological Revolution in Psychiatry*, New York, Harper & Row.

Astin, J. A. (2000) 'The characteristics of CAM users: a complex picture', in Kelner, M., Wellman, B., Pescosolido, B. and Saks, M. (eds) *Complementary and Alternative Medicine: Challenge and Change*, pp. 101–14, Amsterdam, Harwood Academic Publishers.

Barrows, K. and Jacobs, B. (2002) 'Mind–body medicine: an introduction and review of the literature', *Medical Clinics of North America*, Vol. 86, No. 1, pp. 11–31.

Beck, U. (1992) *Risk Society: Towards a New Modernity*, London, Sage.

Bloch, S. and Pargiter, R. (2002) 'A history of psychiatric ethics', *Psychiatric Clinics of North America*, Vol. 25, pp. 509–24.

Bracken, P. and Thomas, P. (2002) 'Time to move beyond the mind–body split: the "mind" is not inside but "out there" in the social world', *British Medical Journal*, Vol. 325, pp. 1433–4.

Busfield, J. (1996) 'Professionals, the state and the development of mental health policy', in Heller, T. et al. (eds) *Mental Health Matters: A Reader*, London, Macmillan/The Open University (K257 Reader).

Campbell, P. (1996) 'The history of the user movement in the United Kingdom', in Heller, T. et al. (eds) *Mental Health Matters: A Reader*, London, Macmillan/The Open University (K257 Reader).

Canter, P. (2003) 'The therapeutic effects of meditation: the conditions treated are stress related, and the evidence is weak', *British Medical Journal*, Vol. 326, pp. 1049–50.

Caplin, R. (1996) 'Time, faith and encouragement', in Read and Reynolds, pp. 142–5.

Chan, C., Ho, P. S. Y. and Chow, E. (2001) 'A body–mind–spirit model in health: an Eastern approach', *Social Work in Health Care*, Vol. 34, No. 3–4, pp. 261–82.

Culliford, L. (2002) 'Spirituality and clinical care', *British Medical Journal*, Vol. 325, pp. 1434–5.

Department of Health (DoH) (1999) *Mental Health National Service Frameworks*, London, Department of Health.

Druss, B. G. and Rosenheck, R. A. (2000) 'Use of practitioner-based complementary therapies by persons reporting mental conditions in the United States', *Archive of General Psychiatry*, Vol. 57, pp. 708–14.

Engebretson, J. (2002) 'Culture and complementary therapies', *Complementary Therapies in Nursing and Midwifery*, Vol. 8, pp. 177–84.

Engels, G. (1980) 'The clinical application of the biopsychosocial model', *American Journal of Psychiatry*, Vol. 137, pp. 535–44.

Ernst, E. (2002) 'The risk–benefit profile of commonly used herbal therapies', *Annals of Internal Medicine*, Vol. 136, No. 1, pp. 42–53.

Faulkner, A. and Layzell, S. (2000) *Strategies for Living: A Report of User-led Research into People's Strategies for Living with Mental Distress*, London, The Mental Health Foundation.

Faulkner, A. and Thomas, P. (2002) 'User-led research and evidence-based medicine', *British Journal of Psychiatry*, Vol. 180, pp. 1–3.

Foster, Dr (2002) *Good Complementary Therapist Guide*, London, Vermilion.

Holland, J. (1999) 'Use of alternative medicine: a marker for distress?', *New England Journal of Medicine*, Vol. 340, No. 22, pp. 1758–9.

Jorm, A., Christensen, H., Griffiths, K. and Rodgers, B. (2002) 'Effectiveness of complementary and self-help treatments for depression', *Medical Journal of Australia*, Vol. 176, Supplement, pp. S84–96.

Kennedy, S. S., Mercer, J., Mohr, W. and Huffine, C. W. (2002) 'Snake oil, ethics, and the First Amendment: what's a profession to do?', *American Journal of Orthopsychiatry*, Vol. 72, No. 1, pp. 5–15.

Kessler, R., Soukup, J., Davis, R., Foster, D., Wilkey, S., Van Rompay, M. and Eisenberg, D. (2001) 'The use of complementary therapies to treat anxiety and depression in the United States', *American Journal of Psychiatry*, Vol. 158, pp. 289–94.

Mechanic, D. (1999) 'Mental health and mental illness: definitions and perspectives', in Horowitz, A. V. and Scheid, T. L. (eds) *A Handbook for the Study of Mental Health: Social Contexts, Theories and Systems*, pp. 12–28, Cambridge, Cambridge University Press.

Miller, J. J. (2002) Review of *Complementary and Alternative Medicine and Psychiatry*, Muskin, P. R. (ed.), *Psychiatric Services*, Vol. 53, No. 5, p. 6401.

Mitchell, A. (2000) 'Complementary therapies in mental health', in Bailey, D. (ed.) *At the Core of Mental Health: Key Issues for Practitioners, Managers and Mental Health Trainers*, Brighton, Pavilion.

Nierenberg, A., Mischoulon, D. and De Cecco, L. (2002) 'St John's Wort: a critique of antidepressant efficacy and possible mechanisms of action', in Mischoulon, D. and Rosenbaum, J. (eds) *Natural Medications for Psychiatric Disorders: Considering the Alternatives*, Philadelphia, PA, Lippincott, Williams and Wilkins.

Peeke, P. M. and Frishett, S. (2002) 'The role of complementary and alternative therapies in women's mental health', *Primary Care: Clinics in Office Practice*, Vol. 29, No. 1, pp. 183–97.

Porter, R. (1999) *The Greatest Gift to Mankind: A Medical History of Humanity from Antiquity to the Present*, London, Fontana.

Porter, R. (2002) *Madness: A Brief History*, Oxford, Oxford University Press.

Read, J. and Reynolds, J. (eds) (1996) *Speaking Our Minds: An Anthology of Personal Experiences of Mental Distress and Its Consequences*, Basingstoke, Macmillan/The Open University (K257 Set Book).

Rogers, A., Pilgrim, D. and Lacey, R. (1993) *Experiencing Psychiatry: Users' Views of Services*, London, Macmillan/MIND.

Russinova, Z., Wewiorski, N. and Cash, D. (2002) 'Use of alternative health care practice by persons with serious mental illness: perceived benefits', *American Journal of Public Health*, Vol. 92, No. 10, pp. 1600–3.

Scheff, T. (1996) 'Labelling mental illness', in Heller, T. et al. (eds) *Mental Health Matters: A Reader*, London, Macmillan/The Open University (K257 Reader).

Schulz, V. (2002a) 'Clinical trials with hypericum extracts in patients with depression: results, comparisons, conclusions for therapy with antidepressant drugs', *Phytomedicine*, Vol. 9, No. 1, pp. 468–74.

Schulz, V. (2002b) 'Hypericum depression trial study group. Effect of *Hypericum perforatum* in major depressive disorder', *Journal of the American Medical Association*, Vol. 287, pp. 1807–14.

Sparber, A. and Wootton, J. (2002) 'Surveys of complementary and alternative medicine: Part V. Use of alternative and complementary therapies for psychiatric and neurologic diseases', *Journal of Alternative and Complementary Medicine*, Vol. 8, No. 1, pp. 93–6.

Thoits, P. A. (1999) 'Sociological approaches to mental illness', in Horovitz, A. V. and Scheid, T. L. (eds) *A Handbook for the Study of Mental Health*, pp. 121–38, Cambridge, Cambridge University Press.

Thomas, K., Coleman, P. and Nicholl, J. (2003) 'Trends in access to Complementary and Alternative Medicines via Primary Care in England', *Family Practice*, Vol. 20, pp. 575–7.

Thomas, K., Nicholl, J. and Coleman, P. (2001) 'Use and expenditure on complementary medicine in England: a population based survey', *Complementary Therapies in Medicine*, Vol. 9, pp. 2–11.

Thomas, P. (2000) 'Foreword', in Faulkner and Layzell.

Unutzer, J., Klap, R., Sturm, R., Young, A., Marmon, T., Shatkin, J. and Wells, K. (2000) 'Mental disorders and the use of alternative medicine: results from a national survey', *American Journal of Psychiatry*, Vol. 157, pp. 1851–7.

Verhoef, M. J., Casebeer, A. L. and Hilsden, R. J. (2002) 'Assessing efficacy of complementary medicine: adding qualitative research methods to the "Gold Standard",' *The Journal of Alternative and Complementary Medicine*, Vol. 8, No. 3, pp. 275–81.

Wallcraft, J. (1998) *Healing Minds: A Report on Current Research, Policy and Practice Concerning the Use of Complementary and Alternative Therapies for a Wide Range of Mental Health Problems*, London, Mental Health Foundation.

World Health Organization (WHO) (1998) *WHOQOL and Spirituality, Religiousness and Personal Beliefs: Report on WHO Consultation*, Geneva, WHO.

Wurtzel, E. (2001) *Prozac Nation: Young and Depressed in America*, London, Allen and Unwin.

Yager, J., Siegfried, S. L. and DiMatteo, T. L. (1999) 'Use of alternative remedies by psychiatric patients: illustrative vignettes and a discussion of the issues', *American Journal of Psychiatry*, Vol. 156, No. 9, pp. 1432–8.

People and Complementary and Alternative Medicine

Edited by Jeanne Katz

Chapter 6 Understanding health and healing

Julie Stone and Jeanne Katz

Contents

AIMS

- To understand the different meanings of 'health' and 'healing'.
- To debate the relationship between professional and lay concepts in health practice.
- To describe an understanding of relevant models of health, including the biomedical, biopsychosocial, salutogenic and alternative or holistic models.

6.1 Introduction

Since the Second World War, health has come to signify much more than an absence of physical disease for many people in western societies. Interest in health now includes concerns about food, the strength of social networks and the quality of the environment. The stresses of modern living are recognised as a serious health issue. Personal choices are positively or negatively charged, depending on whether they are 'good for you' or 'bad for you'. Most newspapers and magazines publish numerous health-related stories, and television programmes and health journals explain how to lead, or even buy, healthier lifestyles. By giving consumers unprecedented access to health information, the internet has further fuelled people's fascination with health.

This chapter explores people's beliefs about health and illness, focusing on the meanings they ascribe to their health and wellbeing and how these influence their health behaviours. You will consider whether the individual experience of illness contrasts with the disease model underpinning the biomedical approach, and whether this leads some people to seek health advice and treatment from a wider range of sources. The issues of plurality and the multiplicity of ways of both understanding health and responding to it are examined with reference to existing models of health.

You will probe the extent to which the philosophies underpinning various approaches to health provide suitable frameworks for accommodating beliefs about health and healing. As there is relatively little information available about attitudes to using complementary and alternative medicine (CAM), this chapter looks more broadly at health beliefs in general. Chapter 7 explores what people want with regard to their health, and interrogates their decision to use CAM.

6.2   What is health?

What do the words 'health' and 'healthy' mean or imply? Superficially this seems a fairly straightforward question: for example, you may recognise that a house plant does not look too healthy. Does this mean it is diseased or is going to die, or that it requires some attention?

When applied to humans the term 'healthy' is often associated with a variety of other, more elaborate concepts. For example, it may mean that a person looks 'well', as a result of being fit (doing regular exercise), or feeling content with life (being emotionally robust). Older people with mobility difficulties may have different perspectives of 'healthy', compared with an athlete or a young person struggling to make ends meet. Health is a subjective determination – in other words, your own definition of health depends on your cultural background, personal aspirations, physical and mental condition, and situation in life. As life is a course and not static, these aspects fluctuate and the meaning of 'health' is constantly reassessed and re-formed.

ACTIVITY   DEFINING HEALTH

Allow 30 minutes

In 1946 the World Health Organization (WHO) proposed the following definition of health:

> Health is a state of complete physical, mental and social well-being and not merely the absence of disease or infirmity.

(WHO, 1948)

Consider this definition of health and then answer the following questions.

1   Do you think this is a useful definition?

2   Does this definition provide a useful framework for how you think about your own health?

3   In what ways does the WHO definition tally with and/or contrast with your beliefs about your own health?

Comment

You might disagree with the WHO's definition and view health as being the absence of disease; or you may believe health includes emotional and spiritual wellbeing, social functioning, satisfaction, and work/life balance. According to the WHO definition, very few people would describe themselves as completely healthy. It represents an ideal state, and you might not expect to achieve this level of optimum functioning all the time. You probably recognise that most people experience fluctuating levels of health and do not necessarily seek professional help for every episode of illness. You may have considered whether you view health as your responsibility and whether you attempt to self-manage health issues. Certainly, the WHO definition of health seems to envisage an aspirational level of health that goes beyond what the National Health Service (NHS) provides treatment for.

Despite the practical and resource implications of the WHO definition, its vision of health is still valuable, capturing a broader understanding that many people experience about their own health: namely, health is a holistic notion that goes far beyond reductionist explanations of disease. However, this definition has limitations, particularly in relation to measuring health outcomes (Bowling, 1991). To date, health indicators have been primarily mortality and morbidity rates, rates of health service uptake, and subjective indicators, which might include self-reported or collected data about behaviour (such as consulting CAM practitioners, or lifestyle indicators such as smoking). Collecting such data is fraught with difficulties, as health may be seen at one end of the spectrum and death at the other (Bowling, 1991).

It is important to note that there is no universal agreement about the meaning of the terms 'health', 'illness' and 'disease' and that these terms are contested (see Helman, 2001). For the purposes of this chapter, **illness** is the **subjective state** – the behavioural response to which may be noticed by other people – whereas **disease** is the **pathological condition** identified by biomedical strategies (the 'clinical gaze') or technology such as blood tests.

Reviewing the research: how people understand 'health'

Being a contested concept, 'health' is constantly being redefined and re-evaluated. Lay people do not necessarily accept biomedical definitions of health and illness uncritically. Instead they have a complex web of beliefs, constructs and understandings about health and illness. These inform people's health behaviour, including decisions about whether to self-manage, seek help within local or lay networks, or consult a health professional.

Some lay people regard health as the absence of disease. Indeed, in a large study in the UK, Cox et al. (1987) investigated lay views of health and ill health. This health and lifestyle study found that 30 per cent of respondents defined health as 'not ill' or 'disease-free', which could imply different meanings of ill health or disease. One rather crude explanation could be that only certain diseases, which individual lay people cannot manage without professional help, are classified as 'illnesses'. Most people treat their own ill health, whether it is with lay remedies or over-the-counter (OTC) medicines, with or without the advice of a pharmacist, friend or relative.

So how do people build up their knowledge about health and the nature of healing? Stacey (1988) explains that, for much of the 20th century, the main concern when investigating lay concepts was to ascertain how much lay people understood and took heed of 'what biomedicine taught about appropriate health behaviour' (p. 142). Stacey and other medical sociologists have noted that lay concepts are important because they provide information on what:

> people think about and explain to themselves in their own way – ways which they may share with others – the misfortunes which happen to them, the ailments which afflict their bodies and the disorders which enter their lives. Their ideas are taken as logical and valid in their own right, although they may not be consonant with biomedical science or any other organized healing system. Ordinary people, in other words, develop explanatory theories to account for their material, social and bodily circumstances. These they apply to themselves as individuals, but in developing them they draw on all sorts of knowledge and wisdom, some of it derived from their own experience, some of it handed on by word of mouth, other parts of it derived from highly trained practitioners. These lay explanations go beyond common sense in that explanations beyond the immediately obvious are included ...
>
> (Stacey, 1988, p. 142)

People's explanations of health are diverse and can be contradictory, as demonstrated by examples taken from four studies of different populations. Firstly, Herzlich's research (1973) on lay beliefs in middle-class French people identified three distinct ways of conceptualising health:

1 health as **something to be had** – a reserve of strength, a potential to resist illness, which is determined by temperament or constitution

2 health as **a state of doing** – the full realisation of a person's reserve of strength, characterised by equilibrium, wellbeing, happiness, feeling strong, getting on well with other people

3 health as **a state of being** – the absence of illness.

Secondly, Williams' study (1983) of the health histories of older men and women in Aberdeen identified four similar categories of beliefs about health:

1   health as the absence of illness and disease

2   health as stamina – the ability to keep going

3   health as inner strength – a reserve of fitness

4   health as the capacity to cope with illness or endure chronic pain.

Thirdly, Blaxter's survey of health and lifestyles (1983) revealed a multiplicity of meanings of health and distinct differences according to age, gender and class. Her research identified six main definitions of health:

1   health as not being ill

2   health as a functional capacity

3   health as physical fitness

4   health as leading a healthy lifestyle

5   health as a psychological concept

6   health as a reserve.

Lastly, Calnan's research (1987) identified broadly similar categories to the others, but also indicated the need to look systematically at differences between the social classes. He proposed four different concepts of health:

1   health as never being ill

2   health as being able to get through the day – to carry out routines

3   health as being fit – being active, taking exercise

4   health as being able to cope with stresses and crises in life.

In Calnan's study, working-class women were more likely to quote the first two concepts, while the latter two concepts were referred to more frequently by middle-class women. This was true only when the women were asked to talk in general terms about health; the class difference was less apparent when the respondents talked about their own health. To summarise, these four studies show that people work with multiple meanings of health, rather than a single, unitary concept.

Further research shows that people commonly relate ill health to life events such as the death of a close relative, marriage, divorce or job change and do not simply accept or interpret their ill health as being due to objectively verifiable pathogens or disease processes. In a historical study, Herzlich and Pierret (1986) demonstrate that lay people always take a variety of causal factors into account when conceptualising health and ill health, including air, climate and seasons, and poor working conditions. People may switch between professional and lay belief systems to make sense of their personal experience of illness.

6.3 Components and origins of health beliefs

Health beliefs, like other personal beliefs, are learned. Knowledge about health and illness is built up from childhood onwards, from diverse sources including family, social networks, community and religion, and through 'official' government health messages. Individual health beliefs, while rarely 'scientific' in themselves, none the less are grounded in experience, modified over time in the light of that experience, and rational in the light of people's wider belief systems and world views. There can be a dissonance between people's 'lay' beliefs about health, including the appropriate ways of maintaining health, and professional understandings of health and disease. There may be contradictions within the same individual, or health practitioners may 'dispense' advice contrary to their own personal health-related behaviour: for example, encouraging people to stop smoking or drinking alcohol excessively.

Individual accounts of health are sometimes dismissed as naïve and irrational, despite their ability to provide meaning for that person's experience of illness. However, beliefs about health give meaning to personal experiences of illness and how they fit in with unique life stories and world views. These beliefs are so strong that people often cling to them, even when faced with rational scientific explanations to the contrary.

So, people use a variety of constructs, both professional and lay, to make sense of their illnesses. These constructs are socially and culturally determined. In a study of the health beliefs and folk models of diabetes in British Bangladeshi people, Greenhalgh et al. (1998) found that informants wanted to understand and explain the onset and experience of illness. However, this tended to lead not to a systematic search for professional or scientific explanations but, rather, to a reflection on personal experience and the experiences of friends and relatives. Lay sources of information were frequently cited as a major influence on behaviour. While all the Bangladeshi respondents held strong religious (Muslim) views, and often gave explanations in terms of 'God's will', such views were usually held in parallel with accepting individual responsibility and understanding the potential for change. The authors of the study note that the people they interviewed may simultaneously hold both 'traditional' constructs (deeply rooted values and perceptions drawn from their culture of origin) and 'recent' ones (drawn from the host culture and less enduring in the long term).

Thus, people live with, and draw on, multiple realities and paradigms for understanding health. This phenomenon is apparent in all cultures, even seemingly homogeneous ones. Helman (2001) states that modern urbanised societies, whether western or non-western, exhibit 'health care pluralism'. Although different therapeutic modes coexist, they are often based on entirely different premises and may even originate in different cultures, such as western medicine in China or Chinese acupuncture in the modern western world (Helman, 2001).

6.4   Influences on health and illness behaviour

Allow 30 minutes

Drawing on your own experiences of health and illness, answer the following questions.

1   When do you decide you might be ill and need advice?
2   Who do you turn to for health information, advice or treatment?
3   When?
4   Why?

Comment

Different people react in different ways to illness. One person who did this activity said, first, she consults someone close to her - a family member or a friend - wondering whether she should be concerned about the problem. She might also look on the internet - initially she would be concerned about the diagnosis. If this concern persisted, she would consult a doctor; however, if she thought she knew what the problem was, she might do any of the following: treat it herself; go to a pharmacist or doctor; go to another 'conventional' therapist (for example, dentist, chiropodist, optician); or go to an 'alternative' therapist (such as a chiropractor or an osteopath).

Health behaviour is influenced by many factors. Helman (2001) discusses the variety of people in different societies who each offer users their own way of advising on, explaining, diagnosing and treating ill health. As a result, people may decide to rest or take a home remedy; ask advice from a friend, relative or neighbour; consult a local priest, folk healer or wise person; or consult a doctor if one is available. People seek different forms of help and advice depending on the stage and progression of their condition. They may be more likely to seek professional help after other channels of advice and treatment, including self-management, have proved ineffective.

People choose one form of healing rather than another for a variety of reasons, including beliefs, expectations, geographical access, affordability, or congruence with wider cultural beliefs. Research shows that whom people talk to about their health influences what they do and the course of action they take to resolve health problems (Wellman, 2000). The influence of other people varies according to the strength of the tie (whether the advice is given by an intimate friend or merely an acquaintance) and the basis of the relationship (whether it is kinship, friendship or professional). These sources of advice and influence are often described as 'health networks'. Granovetter (1973) argues that weak ties (those between socially dissimilar people, rather than members of the same social circle) transmit a greater range of information, including information about potential alternatives, although strong ties may be more persuasive (Wellman and Wellman, 1992). In making health decisions, people also access and draw on health information from a variety of sources, including self-help groups, health magazines and websites (for example, NHS Direct).

Various models of health and illness behaviour have been devised to answer the question: 'How do individuals come to recognise, understand and cope with health problems?' Four models of health and illness behaviour dominate the literature (Pescosolido, 2000): the Socio-Behavioural Model, the Health Belief Model, the Theory of Reasoned Action, and the Theory of Planned Behaviour. The key features of these models are described in Box 6.1.

BOX 6.1   MODELS OF HEALTH AND ILLNESS BEHAVIOUR

The Socio-Behavioural Model (SBM)

The SBM details three basic categories: need, predisposing characteristics and enabling factors. **Need for care** must be established, which depends on the nature of the illness and its severity (for example, the 'hurt', 'worry', 'bother' or 'pain' that it causes). The SBM considers how people perceive this need and how symptoms are experienced. **Predisposing characteristics** include gender, ethnicity, education and beliefs: that is, the social and cultural factors which shape an individual's tendency to seek care. **Enabling characteristics** recognise that individuals need to act on a desire to receive care, and include the means and knowledge to get treatment (having a source of care, travel time and financial ability, as well as the geographical availability of doctors, clinics, etc.).

The Health Belief Model (HBM)

Whereas the SBM focuses on the influence of the system and issues of access, the HBM examines the meaning of 'predisposing' characteristics and analyses how an individual's specific health beliefs (for example, about the severity of symptoms) and their preferences (for example, the perceived benefits of treatment), as well as their experiences (with health care problems and with providers and their knowledge), affect decisions to seek care and adopt health behaviours.

The Theory of Reasoned Action (TRA)

The TRA concerns **expectancy**: individuals rate how current and alternative actions can reduce their health problems. Like the HBM, this theory focuses on motivations, the individual's assessment of risk, and the desire to avoid negative outcomes. Individuals evaluate whether or not to engage in healthy (for example, taking exercise) or risky (for example, smoking) behaviours and whether to seek preventive as well as curative medical services.

> **The Theory of Planned Behaviour (TPB)**
>
> The TPB evolved from the TRA, but differs by recognising that individuals do not necessarily have control over their behaviour. The amount of behavioural control – or **self-efficacy** – that individuals perceive they have is an important element in this model. Also, 'cues' or 'habits' become an important part of the decisions individuals make to engage in health and illness behaviours.
>
> (Source: adapted from Pescosolido, 2000, pp. 176-7)

Although the four models are practical, Pescosolido (2000) notes some weaknesses: for example, what she calls the 'tyranny of use/no use' created by the strict either/or conceptualisation of choices inherent in these empirical models. She argues that the traditional models do not capture the richness of ethnographic research, which provides deeper understandings of procedures and users. She also notes that focusing on 'illness' overlooks the fact that people may define physical and mental health in terms of moral failure, supernatural punishment, the 'ups and downs' of life, etc., for which seeking medical care is only one of several possible responses. Pescosolido argues that this unnatural separation of illness behaviour from social life is reflected in the reliance of traditional models on rational choice as the underlying mechanism at work. By calling these models 'decision-making' or 'help-seeking' models, the values of rationality and individuality are overemphasised, which are precisely the same values that led to the professional dominance of allopathic medicine.

Having looked at some of the influences on health and illness behaviour, it is clear that users' knowledge of and beliefs about different forms of health care shape their choices about which practitioners to consult in different circumstances. The next section focuses on some models of health care delivery.

6.5   Models of health care delivery

In the quest to understand health and illness behaviour, social and medical researchers have developed various models to explain the different forms of health care delivery. These models emerged because, in the mid-20th century, social researchers began to question not only the position of professions in western countries but also the relationship between professionals and users. Early explorations of the patient's role in health care suggested that it was fairly prescribed (Parsons, 1951), as was that of the physician (Freidson, 1970). However, by the 1980s there was greater awareness of the diversity of ways of receiving healing and health care, particularly in indigenous cultures. Currer and Stacey explain this in their ground-breaking overview of health concepts:

> Any thorough-going critique of health care planning and administration requires the imaginative consideration of modes of healing based upon conceptualisations alternative to the contemporary dominant mode.
>
> (Currer and Stacey, 1986, p. 1)

They also note that even within western cultures there are considerable variations across the population in the ways in which the dominant health care model is conceptualised:

> Members also have access to, and possibly accept concepts derived from, other cosmologies or other modes of healing, and also from earlier formulations of biomedicine itself.
>
> (Currer and Stacey, 1986, p. 1)

The medical anthropologist Arthur Kleinman (1980) notes that all healing systems orient around explanatory models of health and illness. He describes cultural explanatory models as cognitive orientations that determine how disease is named, defined and understood. He identifies the following six universal themes which underpin people's explanatory models.

1 **Aetiology**: the cause of the illness.
2 **Time and mode of onset of symptoms**: the significance of what was happening when the symptoms began.
3 **Pathology**: what the illness is and what is going wrong with the person who is ill.
4 **Course of the illness**: how long the illness might last and how it might develop.
5 **Consequences of the illness**: the possible effects of the illness on the person's life.
6 **Treatment**: what could be done to alleviate or cure the illness.

Four theoretical models are discussed in this section: the biomedical model, the biopsychosocial model, the salutogenic model and alternative or holistic models. Each is a conceptual model which provides a theoretical framework for how health is practised at both an individual practitioner and an institutional level. Eisenberg (1977) explains that models are ways of constructing reality, of imposing meaning on the chaos of the 'phenomenal world'. Each model understands health, illness, the body, and the respective roles of users and healers in different ways. Note that the models described here are **theoretical constructs** (that is, they do not operate in a rigid way), and are not a blueprint for practice. In addition, few practitioners derive their ideas about health and illness solely from the models under discussion.

The biomedical model

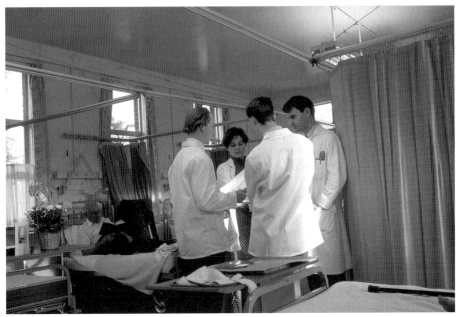

A consultant on a ward round talking to colleagues and leaving the patient isolated

ACTIVITY   THE BIOMEDICAL MODEL

Allow 30 minutes

Read the following description of the biomedical model. Then list what you would consider are (a) the positive and (b) the negative implications of it for lay users.

Biomedicine (which is also known as allopathy, conventional medicine or modern western scientific medicine) is relatively new, unlike some ancient healing systems which have been practised for several thousand years. In the UK biomedicine dominates contemporary and official understandings of health and forms the basis of the NHS and other western health care systems. While the biomedical model is considered the epitome of scientific, objective, reproducible medicine, the actual delivery of health care may be somewhat different in practice. The following statements about biomedicine thus represent an idealised, necessarily artificial version of this model.

- Health is predominantly viewed as the 'absence of disease' and as 'functional fitness'.
- Health services are geared mainly towards treating sick and disabled people.
- A high value is put on the provision of specialist medical services, in mainly institutional settings, typically hospitals or clinics.
- Doctors and other qualified experts diagnose illness and disease and sanction and supervise the withdrawal of service users from productive labour.

The biopsychosocial model

Allow 30 minutes

Read the following description of the biopsychosocial model and make notes on the positive and negative implications for lay users.

While disease dominates biomedical thinking, the biopsychosocial model incorporates social, psychological and emotional factors in diagnosis and treatment. It recognises that illness cannot be studied or treated in isolation from the social and cultural environment. Whereas the biomedical model prioritises professional knowledge, the biopsychosocial model expects health carers and doctors to acknowledge and take into account users' circumstances. This change in focus is reflected in research priorities, in that government departments increasingly respect qualitative research (previously dismissed by the medical research community as 'soft'). (See, for example, ESRC, 2003.)

Medicine practised within a biopsychosocial framework acknowledges the links between socioeconomic deprivation and adverse health. It also considers issues such as improving access to health services and reducing health inequalities as a legitimate and appropriate function of health service provision (Engels, 1980).

Comment

The biopsychosocial model recognises the connection between health and the experience of illness and the physical and social environment. Heart disease and obesity are linked epidemiologically to ethnicity and poverty, and therefore cannot be explained simply in terms of individual self-responsibility and willpower. Rather, definitions of health within a biopsychosocial model consider the way in which people negotiate their way through environmental, social and informational influences (Fulder, 1998). Health is a process concerned with norms of functioning and wellbeing, which are determined by society and professionals, and vary from time to time and group to group. In this sense, health is relative rather than absolute: a process rather than a fixed, defined condition. Fulder describes this process as 'one of dynamic balance where the capacity of the organism to self-repair, self-support, and renewal is not overwhelmed by the interactions with the world within and outside the organism' (1998, p. 152). Within this model, 'the organism' means the community as well as the individual.

The dominance of the biopsychosocial model in western health care is exemplified by the inclusion in medical training of subjects such as medical sociology, medical anthropology and community medicine. None the less, this model is still grounded in scientific method, thus building on the major elements of biomedicine.

The implications of the biopsychosocial model for users and therapeutic relationships include the accommodation of emotional and spiritual aspects of health. Consultations with health professionals who use this model should acknowledge the wider environment, users' social support networks, family support and stress levels. In theory, the biopsychosocial model can generate hypotheses about individual illness which tally with people's broader understandings about why they are ill, in the context of their whole life story. This moves away from professionals deciding what is wrong to a more balanced therapeutic relationship in which users are encouraged to be active partners in health decisions. There may also be scope for more 'caring' therapeutic relationships: some people will value the opportunity to talk about their emotions and broader concerns and may find this therapeutic in itself (a theme explored in Chapter 8).

The salutogenic model

Whereas **pathogenesis** (the way disease processes develop) underpins the biomedical model, the concept of positive health, or **salutogenesis**, focuses on how and why people stay well. Salutogenesis can be seen either as a model in its own right or as an example of the biopsychosocial approach (Antonovsky, 1979, 1987). Antonovsky's salutogenic model was designed to advance understanding of the relationship between stressors, coping and health, with the aim of explaining how some individuals remain healthy despite stressors in their everyday life.

Unlike previous health research on stress, which looked at different kinds of stressors and the conditions most likely to lead to stress, Antonovsky's model highlights the inadequacy of pathogenic explanatory factors and concentrates on the adaptive coping mechanisms underscoring the movement to the healthy end of the 'ease–dis-ease' spectrum. Antonovsky proposed that generalised resistance resources (wealth, ego strength, cultural stability, social support) can promote a **sense of coherence**, which is central to people's ability to cope with stress. Antonovsky defines the sense of coherence as:

> a global orientation that expresses the extent to which one has a pervasive, enduring though dynamic feeling of confidence that (1) the stimuli deriving from one's internal and external environments in the course of living are structured, predictable, and explicable; (2) the resources are available to one to meet the demands posed by these stimuli; and (3) these demands are challenges, worthy of investment and engagement.
>
> (Antonovsky, 1987, p. 19)

Antonovsky describes the substantive structure of the sense of coherence as comprising three components: **comprehensibility**, **manageability** and **meaningfulness**. These develop as people's experiences are influenced by consistency, balancing underload–overload and shaping outcomes respectively. Unlike concepts such as locus of control, self-efficacy and problem-oriented coping, the sense of coherence model is intended to be a influenced by several spiritual schools, in particular Taoism. Ayurveda, a traditional medical system of India, reflects the traditional Hindu world view. Similarly, Tibetan physicians practice Buddhist meditation as an integral part of their medical training.

(Eskinazi, 1998, p. 1621)

CAM therapies originating from a different culture do not have the same potency, value and efficacy when practised in a culture dominated by biomedicine. (This is discussed further in Chapter 11.) Joan Engebretson points out:

As these techniques have been taken out of the cultural context of their historical and geographical or ethnic setting, the techniques are often used without a full understanding of cultural or philosophical underpinnings, beliefs and values.

(Engebretson, 2002, p. 178)

CAM is not homogeneous. Not all practitioners subscribe to every underlying principle. Some therapies claim to be more holistic than others (just as many general practitioners try to practise holistically). Watts (1992) maintains that, while virtually all orthodox medicine is underpinned by the same theoretical foundations, complementary medicine is the product of either many philosophies or none. A bewildering variety of sometimes contradictory ideas coexist, 'their various exponents apparently untroubled by what, to the outsider, seems hopelessly chaotic' (Watts, 1992, p. 106). There is also a dearth of research on the views and beliefs held by CAM practitioners. Individual practitioners may have personal views and philosophies that are at odds with mainstream thought in their particular therapy. The wide variation in practitioners' health beliefs is described in the next section.

6.6 Concepts of healing: philosophies underpinning CAM practice

ACTIVITY   HEALTH BELIEFS IN CAM

Allow 1 hour

Read the following accounts by individual CAM practitioners of four different modalities. These are **personal** perspectives, which may vary from other people's in their disciplines. As you read the accounts note:

1   the positive and negative implications for lay users
2   different approaches to healing among the four CAM modalities.

OSTEOPATHY

Currently osteopathy has no agreed definition. It is a hands-on approach to various health problems which manifest themselves through the neuro-musculo-skeletal system (the moving parts of the body and the associated nerves and blood vessels). This approach embraces a holistic system of diagnosis and treatment involving palpation and manual intervention, complemented by health education. It recognises the primacy of the therapeutic relationship and is based on the philosophy and principles first enunciated by Andrew Taylor Still in 1874:

- Displaced joints may obstruct the free flow of blood – 'the rule of the artery is absolute'.
- All diseases are mere effects, the cause being partial or complete failure of the nerves to conduct the fluids of life properly.
- The body tends to be self-regulating and self-healing.
- All body structures and processes are interdependent.

Therefore, rational treatment is based on the above principles and directs proceedings rather than attempting to effect change directly. Still's therapeutic maxim was to 'find it, fix it and leave it alone' (that is, to diagnose the disorder, treat it, and leave the rest to the spontaneous forces of nature), in recognition of his understanding of the body as an internally organising system.

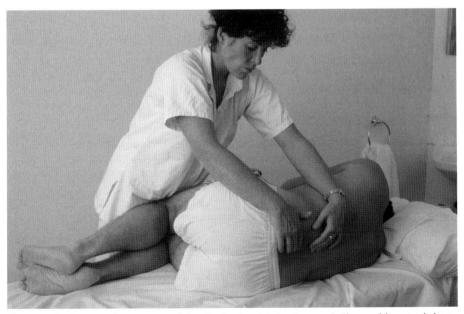

Osteopathy has a unique approach to the body, striving to repair the problem and then leaving the body to heal itself

ACUPUNCTURE

Acupuncture is part of a comprehensive system of health care called 'oriental medicine'. This has a clinical history of at least 2000 years to the present day. Indeed, it is all based on the concept of **qi**, or 'vital energy', a concept that every living organism has energy running through and around it, which enables physical movement, emotional balance and spiritual connection, provided it is in balance and can flow smoothly. This model is based on natural laws and has connections with Maoism. These laws are: the eight principles of yin/yang, deficiency/excess, cold/hot and interior/exterior; the five elements (earth, air, fire, water and wood) and their associations; the causes of disease – internal or external, miscellaneous and secondary; and a different diagnostic language to identify the energetics of each individual patient. Many patients do not want treatment for one complaint, but rather for an apparently disconnected set of complaints or because they do not feel well. Acupuncturists can make connections of the mind, body and spirit for patients and enable them to start making sense of their perceived and experienced 'dis-ease'. Practitioners use a research method of investigation based on looking, asking, feeling and listening (*sizhen*), leading to diagnosis (*bazheng*, or eight rules), then testing the hypothesis in treatment (*ben* and *biao*, or root and branch) and evaluation. In its simplest terms, acupuncture stimulates the body's own healing response and helps restore its natural tendency to balance and harmony by inserting, and manipulating in a variety of ways, fine needles into specific points along the channels of energy (**meridians**). Centuries of observation, analysis and empirical use have resulted in an extensively catalogued location and function of all the points. There are believed to be low-level electrical resistances at these points, but *how* acupuncture works is still not known. Western thought insists on the search for an explanation in scientific terms; eastern thought does not.

HERBALISM

Western medical herbalists are trained in orthodox medical science and use the same technical language as the orthodox medical professions. Although they may use the same labels in terms of pathology, their aim is to support normal physiology and help the ways in which the body heals itself, rather than to treat a named disease. Sometimes users are encouraged to see symptoms such as tiredness or fever as being part of their healing rather than just an aspect of their problem. Herbal medication is seen as having three modes of action:

1 a biochemical pharmacological action
2 a micronutritional effect (plant remedies contain a range of trace nutrients that are often missing from a modern diet)
3 an energetic action.

For any particular required pharmacological action there are several possible herbal remedies. The herbalist has a subjective appreciation of the character of each of them and tries to match the correct remedy to the client's needs.

REIKI

The philosophy of reiki is that everything in the Universe is made of energy, which vibrates at different rates and frequencies on a continuum from the dense, slow vibrations of physical matter to the fast vibrations of spiritual energy, consciousness or light. The human body is made of energy which is dense enough to become physical matter, so it can be seen and touched, but people also have a field of spiritual energy called an **aura**, which surrounds and interpenetrates the physical body. Life-force energy (**qi** or **chi**) flows within the physical body through energy centres called **chakras** and energy pathways called **meridians**, as well as flowing around the body in the aura. Reiki is a spiritual energy vibrating at a very high rate, which helps to break through blockages, flowing through all the affected parts of the aura, charging them with positive energy and raising the vibratory level of the whole energy field. It clears and balances the chakras and straightens the energy pathways, allowing the life force to flow in a healthy and natural way around the whole body. This strengthens and accelerates the body's natural ability to heal itself, and opens the mind, emotions and spirit to an acceptance and understanding of the factors that led to 'dis-ease' in both the physical and the energy bodies.

Comment

For some practitioners, CAM is more than simply about treating disease: an accusation levelled at the biomedical model in its purest form. Individualised user-centred treatment is central to their philosophies. CAM therapists explore and treat underlying causes, not merely control symptoms. CAM therapies sometimes use phenomena that are outside the biomedical understanding of health and disease. For many practitioners, building strong therapeutic relationships is crucial. This includes practitioners' attempts to bridge their own philosophy or cosmology to that of the user, so as to provide an account of illness that resonates for that user. CAM promulgates the view that users promote their own healing, and that the therapist is a conduit for healing energy. While the philosophy of holistic health concerns the user's mind, body and spirit, the treatment is individually targeted.

This chapter introduced four (of many) models of health. Although they were presented as discrete entities, in practice there is considerable blurring of the boundaries between them. Many features of alternative health models are now being incorporated into mainstream medicine and vice versa. For example, a study comparing osteopathic practitioners and doctors in the UK notes that the holistic approach is less confined to osteopathic physicians, especially in speciality hospital care, and is, perhaps, even becoming a trend in the approach to care used in allopathic medicine (Johnson and Kurtz, 2002). As CAM and orthodox medicine continue to integrate, there will probably be further overlap and evolution of health models, reflecting the plurality of ways of knowing about health and dealing with illness.

6.7 Researching health beliefs and CAM users' expectations

People's beliefs about health and illness play an important role in determining whether and when they seek medical care and the extent to which they follow advice and treatment regimes. Beliefs can influence the outcome of treatments (Zola, 1973; Stainton-Rogers, 1991). Therefore, it is important to explore whether users of CAM have different beliefs about and different expectations of health care than non-users.

Adrian Furnham and his colleagues conducted several psychological studies designed to examine the extent to which certain beliefs and attitudes influence the use of CAM, and whether beliefs change as a result of using it. These studies use the Health Belief Model (HBM) as a starting point, which, as you may recall from Box 6.1, suggests that health beliefs can be correlated with behaviour and can differentiate between those who do and those who do not exhibit various health behaviours. Furnham and other researchers have examined whether users of CAM perceive themselves to be more susceptible to disease, whether they have stronger beliefs about self-control, and whether they have different attitudes about the perceived efficacy of biomedical treatment.

The findings vary according to which therapy is studied but they have revealed some statistically significant results. For example, users of homoeopathy were more critical and sceptical of biomedicine (Furnham and Smith, 1988; Furnham and Bragrath, 1992) and were more conscious of their health generally, lending some support for Giddens' description of the more reflexive and sceptical consumer, which was discussed in Chapter 1 (Giddens, 1991). A further study by Furnham and Forey (1994) revealed that users of homoeopathy were also more likely to believe that their health could be improved, had more self and ecologically aware lifestyles, were concerned about ensuring a holistic approach to health care, and were generally more knowledgeable about their bodies than users of conventional health care. Furnham and Smith (1988) and Conroy et al. (2000) also showed that users of CAM did not consider themselves to be more susceptible to disease than non-users and were no more anxious about their health.

A study of people who use acupuncture revealed lower levels of confidence in general practitioners than non-users and a reduced faith in biomedical drugs (Furnham et al., 1995). These levels of dissatisfaction were not present among users of homoeopathy, although a study in the USA found that they were more displeased than people who used chiropractors (Yu et al., 1994). A comparison of users of osteopathy, homoeopathy and acupuncture showed that homoeopathy users valued their involvement in the healing process, while acupuncture users were most concerned about the side effects of biomedical drugs (Vincent and Furnham, 1997). Furthermore, Sirious and Gick (2002) showed differences between long-term and new users of CAM in terms of their values and beliefs, although in both groups health-aware behaviour and dissatisfaction with conventional medicine were the best predictors of use. More importantly, there appear to be as many subtle differences between users of CAM as there are between users and non-users. CAM users should not be considered a homogeneous group with similar beliefs, attitudes and expectations. Nevertheless, this work helps to locate some differences in attitudes and beliefs and suggests reasons for the popularity of CAM. However, and perhaps most interestingly, these studies did not ask the users about their reasons for consulting a CAM practitioner.

Sharma (1992) showed that most CAM users are pragmatic and eclectic. They are interested in whether the therapy might work for them, rather than the theory behind the practice, although Sharma notes that they appreciate explanations which make sense of previously unaccountable experiences or symptoms. She concludes from her research that lay convictions about the causes of health and illness may be relatively unstructured and that patients will try any treatment that seems to work or has worked for people they know. This might account for users expressing satisfaction with a variety of CAM therapies based on mutually exclusive models. Sharma also suggests that a therapy could be said to 'work' in that the practitioner's discourse provides meanings and interpretations that are more satisfactory to the user than orthodox explanations. One attraction for users is that CAM practitioners can give an explanation of health and illness that is more congruent with their own account:

> Complementary practitioners may have explanations that make sense to patients – such as describing illness as a result of environmental factors or as a physical expression of emotional patterns. Conventional medicine may have problems with such explanations if they have no scientific justification, but sociological research shows that patients consider them beneficial when they reinforce their own beliefs and expectations.
>
> (Zollman and Vickers, 1999, pp. 1487–8)

Watts asked what users wanted and found that:

> Many people get more out of being told that their inner being is out of balance than they do out of knowing that their haemoglobin level is low. The latter may mean little to them; but even sceptics will recognize the former as a kind of metaphorical description of the feelings that may have driven them to seek help in the first place.
>
> (Watts, 1992, p. 105)

How far will users go along with the therapist if the treatment is strange and unusual and not what they were expecting? Sharma's study suggests that CAM users do not necessarily seek out practitioners who share similar beliefs about health and healing to their own. Users can often be persuaded to try out new ideas:

> I suspect that sick people who find the treatments offered altogether too bizarre or counter to their own notions of what will make them better drop out before the treatment has gone too far. Others can be cajoled into accepting unfamiliar, time-consuming or even painful regimes because the therapist is prepared to explain the treatment and provide moral support, for which the orthodox doctor has little time and sometimes no inclination.
>
> (Sharma, 1992, p. 168)

Sharma suggests that, even if some users start out using CAM believing they are no different from non-users, their exposure to therapists' ideas may affect their health beliefs over time. Sharma speculates that this is more so when the use of one non-orthodox type of medicine leads users to experiment with other forms of CAM, thus increasing their exposure to alternative beliefs:

> There is no reason to suppose that therapist and patient always share beliefs about health and illness, but equally there is no reason to suppose that the one may not influence the other as they interact.
>
> (Sharma, 1992, p. 88)

Sharma's study of CAM practitioners researched the extent to which they explicitly and consciously offer alternative explanations of health and illness, and whether the encounter between practitioner and user is used as an opportunity to socialise users into new ways of interpreting what happens to their bodies – an issue that is returned to in Chapter 9. Sharma asks whether practitioners treat their special knowledge as a source of dominance: a resource they are not prepared to share. She wonders whether there is an element of control in practitioners trying to bring round users to their way of thinking (Sharma, 1992, p. 168). One homoeopath said it was not so much about getting users to comply with the advice of medical authority (the doctor or practitioner), but rather it was more about getting users to a stage where they take responsibility for their own health (Sharma, 1992).

The practitioners in Sharma's study rejected the notion of professional mystique: that is, that they would give away too much power if they explained too much about the therapy and how it works. None the less, practitioners were not always keen to give detailed explanations of what they did and why. Sharma (1992) also found that practitioners had ways of accounting for therapeutic failures that made sense within their own theories of healing: 'the patient was clinging to his/her illness, s/he was not the kind of patient who could easily accept homoeopathy, the patient did not give the treatment long enough to work.'

Clearly, researching people's beliefs and expectations about CAM, and their motivation for using it, reveals a variety of findings. While some people are attracted to a specific philosophy or set of beliefs, others seem content to pursue a therapy if they believe it will work for them. Researchers acknowledge the methodological difficulties of trying to analyse individuals' health choices and behaviours retrospectively.

6.8   Conclusion

The biomedical model that dominated health professional–user interactions for the past 100 years or so marginalised and appeared to devalue certain aspects of the individual and personal experience of illness. However, health care provision is now more user-centred in the prevailing biopsychosocial model. Despite the diversity of health beliefs, the edifice of modern medicine is built on a dominant scientific perspective, which promotes a certain world view at the expense of other cosmologies. CAM offers a diverse array of other philosophical approaches to health and healing. This chapter showed that the enterprise of health and healing is far broader than the world view encompassed by biomedicine. Cultures and societies produce profoundly different beliefs about health. Where the mainstream health care provision is insensitive towards lay understandings of health and illness, people seek out healing practices that are more congruent with their experiences, belief systems and culture. Whereas in the past this always involved folk and traditional healing, increasingly it includes the use of CAM. The question of who uses CAM, in what situations, and for what conditions is explored in the next chapter.

KEY POINTS

- The ways in which people understand health and illness vary considerably, lay understanding often conflicting with professional understanding of disease.

- People may hold multiple and conflicting beliefs about health.

- Individuals' health beliefs are not constant and fixed, but reflect their life experiences and acquisition of knowledge from a variety of sources.

- People's health beliefs influence their health behaviours, including the decision about when and whom to consult for health advice.

- Models of health provide understanding on the basis of different cosmologies. These models are not fixed but overlap and continuously evolve.

- The biomedical model has gradually given way to a broader biopsychosocial understanding of health. This is reflected in both medical training and clinical practice.

- CAM can provide ways of understanding the body that accord with and give meaning to people's lay understanding.

- Despite a greater professed interest in the balance between people and their environment, CAM treatments may promote an individualistic analysis of health.

- There is no single CAM philosophy. CAM therapists work in a variety of ways, some being more holistic than others, some working with philosophies that can be accommodated within a biomedical understanding of the body (e.g. osteopathy) and others that cannot (e.g. acupuncture).

- Users of CAM are not necessarily drawn to therapists because of their particular philosophy.

References

Antonovsky, A. (1979) *Health, Stress and Coping: New Perspectives on Mental and Physical Well-Being*, San Francisco, CA, Jossey-Bass.

Antonovsky, A. (1987) *Unraveling the Mystery of Health: How People Manage Stress and Stay Well*, San Francisco, CA, Jossey-Bass.

Blaxter, M. (1983) 'The causes of disease: women talking', *Social Science and Medicine*, Vol. 17, No. 2, pp. 59–69.

Bowling, A. (1991) *Measuring Health*, Buckingham, Open University Press.

Bury, M. (1997) *Health and Illness in a Changing Society*, London, Routledge.

Calnan, M. (1987) *Health and Illness: The Lay Perspective*, London, Tavistock.

Conroy, R. M., Siriwardena, R., Smyth, O. and Fernandes, P. (2000) 'The relation of health anxiety and attitudes to doctors and medicine to use of alternative and complementary treatments in general practice patients', *Psychology, Health and Medicine*, Vol. 5, No. 2, pp. 203–12.

Cox, B. D., Blaxter, M., Buckel, A. L. J., Fenner, N. P., Golding, J. F., Gore, M., Huppert, F. A., Nickson, J., Roth, M., Stark, J., Wadsworth, M. E. J. and Whichelow, M. (1987) *The Health and Lifestyle Survey*, London, The Health Promotion Trust.

Currer, C. and Stacey, M. (eds) (1986) *Concepts of Health, Illness and Disease*, Leamington Spa, Berg.

Eisenberg, L. (1977) 'Disease and illness. Distinctions between professional and popular ideas of sickness', *Culture, Medicine and Psychiatry*, Vol. 1, No. 1, pp. 9–23.

Engebretson, J. (2002) 'Culture and complementary therapies', *Complementary Therapies in Nursing and Midwifery*, Vol. 8, pp. 177–84.

Engels, G. (1980) 'The clinical application of the biopsychosocial model', *American Journal of Psychiatry*, Vol. 137, pp. 535–44.

Eskinazi, D. (1998) 'Factors that shape alternative medicine', *Journal of the American Medical Association*, Vol. 280, No. 18, pp. 1621–3.

ESRC (Economic and Social Research Council) (2003) 'Therapeutic practitioners lifecourses', *Lifestyle and Health* [online], www.esrc.ac.uk/esrccontent/publicationsList/Thematic/Themefirst.html [accessed 1 June 2004].

Freidson, E. (1970) *Profession of Medicine: A Study of the Sociology of Applied Knowledge*, New York, Harper and Row.

Fulder, S. (1998) 'The basic concepts of alternative medicine and their impact on our views of health', *The Journal of Alternative and Complementary Medicine*, Vol. 4, No. 2, pp. 147–58.

Fulder, S. (2002) 'Extinction and diversity in alternative medicine', *The Journal of Alternative and Complementary Medicine*, Vol. 8, No. 4, pp. 395–7.

Furnham, A. and Bragrath, R. (1992) 'A comparison of health beliefs and behaviours of clients of orthodox and complementary medicine', *British Journal of Clinical Psychology*, Vol. 32, pp. 237–46.

Furnham, A. and Forey, J. (1994) 'The attitudes, behaviours and beliefs of patients in conventional versus complementary medicine', *Journal of Clinical Psychology*, Vol. 50, pp. 458–69.

Furnham, A. and Smith, C. (1988) 'Choosing alternative medicine: a comparison of the patients visiting a GP and a homoeopath', *Social Science and Medicine*, Vol. 26, pp. 685–7.

Furnham, A. and Vincent, C. (2000) 'Reasons for using CAM', in Kelner, M., Wellman, B., Pescosolido, B. and Saks, M. (eds) *Complementary and Alternative Medicine: Challenges and Change*, Amsterdam, Harwood Academic Publishers.

Furnham, A., Vincent, C. and Wood, R. (1995) 'The health beliefs and behaviours of three groups of complementary medicine and a general practice group of patients', *Journal of Alternative and Complementary Medicine*, Vol. 1, pp. 347–59.

Giddens, A. (1991) *The Consequences of Modernity*, London, Polity.

Granovetter, M. (1973) 'The strength of weak ties', *American Journal of Sociology*, Vol. 78, pp. 1360–80.

Greenhalgh, T. and Hurwitz, B. (1999) 'Why study narrative?', *British Medical Journal*, Vol. 318, pp. 48–50.

Greenhalgh, T., Helman, C. and Chowdhury, A. M. (1998) 'Health beliefs and folk models of diabetes in British Bangladeshis: a qualitative study', *British Medical Journal*, Vol. 316, pp. 978–83.

Helman, C. (2001) *Culture, Health and Illness* (4th edition), London, Arnold.

Herzlich, C. (1973) *Health and Illness*, London, Academic Press.

Herzlich, C. and Pierret, J. (1986) 'Illness: from causes to meaning', in Currer, C. and Stacey, M. (eds) *Concepts of Health, Illness and Disease*, Leamington Spa, Berg.

Johnson, S. and Kurtz, M. (2002) 'Perceptions of philosophic and practice differences between US osteopathic physicians and their allopathic counterparts', *Social Science and Medicine*, Vol. 55, pp. 2141–8.

Jones, L. J. (1994) *The Social Context of Health and Health Care*, Basingstoke, Macmillan.

Kaptchuk, T. J. and Eisenberg, D. M. (2001) 'Varieties of healing. 1: Medical pluralism in the United States', *Annals of Internal Medicine*, Vol. 135, No. 3, pp. 189–95.

Kleinman, A. (1980) *Patients and Healers in the Context of Culture*, Berkeley, CA, University of California.

Parsons, T. (1951) *The Social System*, New York, Free Press.

Pescosolido, B. (2000) 'Rethinking models of health and illness behaviour', in Kelner, M., Wellman, B., Pescosolido, B. and Saks, M. (eds) *Complementary and Alternative Medicine: Challenge and Change*, Amsterdam, Harwood Academic Publishers.

Sharma, U. (1992) *Complementary Medicine Today: Practitioners and Patients*, London, Routledge.

Sirious, F. S. and Gick, M. L. (2002) 'An investigation of the health beliefs and motivations of complementary medicine clients', *Social Science and Medicine*, Vol. 55, pp. 1025–37.

Stacey, M. (1988) *The Sociology of Health and Healing*, London, Unwin Hyman.

Stainton-Rogers, W. (1991) *Explaining Health and Illness. An Exploration of Diversity*, London, Harvester Wheatsheaf.

Vincent, C. A. and Furnham A. (1997) *Complementary Medicine. A Research Perspective*, Chichester, Wiley.

Watts, G. (1992) *Pleasing the Patient*, London, Faber and Faber.

Wellman, B. (2000) 'Partners in illness: who helps when you are sick?', in Kelner, M., Wellman, B., Pescosolido, B. and Saks, M. (eds) *Complementary and Alternative Medicine: Challenges and Change*, Amsterdam, Harwood Academic Publishers.

Wellman, B. and Wellman, B. (1992) 'Domestic affairs and network relations', *Journal of Social and Personal Relationships*, Vol. 9, pp. 385–409.

Williams, R. G. A. (1983) 'Concepts of health: an analysis of lay logic', *Sociology*, Vol. 17, No. 2, pp. 185–204.

World Health Organization (WHO) (1948) Preamble to the Constitution of the World Health Organization, as adopted by the International Conference, New York, 19–22 June 1946. Available online at www.who.int/about/definition/en [accessed 1 June 2004].

Yu, M. M., Vandiver, V. L. and Farmer, J. (1994) 'Alternative medicine and patient satisfaction: a consumer survey of acupuncture, chiropractic, and homoeopathic health care services', *International Journal of Alternative and Complementary Medicine*, Vol. 12, No. 9, pp. 25–8.

Zola, I. K. (1973) 'Pathways to the doctor: from person to patient', *Social Science and Medicine*, Vol. 7, pp. 677–89.

Zollman, C. and Vickers, A. (1999) 'ABC of complementary medicine: complementary medicine and the patient', *British Medical Journal*, Vol. 319, pp. 1486–9.

Chapter 7 Understanding why people use complementary and alternative medicine

Sarah Cant

Contents

AIMS

- To assess the reasons why people choose CAM practitioners as opposed to consulting conventional health workers.
- To recognise and understand the possible hidden patterns of CAM use and why they are difficult to access for auditing and research.

7.1   Introduction

The decision to consult a complementary and alternative medicine (CAM) practitioner or buy a CAM remedy is not a new phenomenon. For instance, it has been possible to see a homoeopathic practitioner and buy homoeopathic remedies in London since 1850, when the first homoeopathic hospital was opened in Golden Square in Soho (Campbell, 1984). Nevertheless, the burgeoning successes of orthodox medicine meant the majority of the population chose to visit biomedical practitioners, particularly once the National Health Service (NHS) was established in the UK in the 1940s, providing free biomedical treatment. However, from the late 1970s through to the present day, medical practitioners, non-medical practitioners (who gradually set up their own training schools and professional associations) and, of course, consumers have been increasingly interested in CAM. The range of complementary and alternative medicines available to the paying public proliferated during this period, including not simply the revival of therapies that had existed since the NHS was created but also therapies imported from abroad (Cant and Sharma, 1999). In 1993 the BMA estimated that there were at least 160 **distinctly different** therapies available to users (BMA, 1993); since then many more have developed.

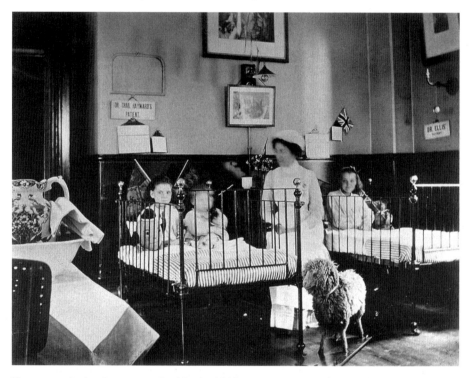

Homoeopathy has been practised in the UK for many years and not only in London, as shown by this photograph from 1910 of the Hahnemann Hospital and Homoeopathic Dispensaries in Liverpool (Source: Wellcome Historical Images no. L0029312)

Understanding consumers' renewed and sustained interest in CAM and the motivations, wants and preferences of this ever-increasing body of users is the basis for this chapter. The decision to consult a CAM practitioner is significant, as the person must pay (with some exceptions), potentially contradict the advice of their medical practitioner, and submit themselves to practices and medication that have not necessarily been rigorously scientifically tested. Using CAM therapies constitutes a significant 'leap in faith' (Giddens, 1991, p. 23) with a financial cost to the consumer.

What people want from CAM has generated significant interest, leading to inquiries by the government (House of Lords, 2000), the medical profession (BMA, 1993) (as noted in earlier chapters) and social scientists (for example Furnham and Bagrath, 1992; Cant and Sharma, 1999). Yet it is notoriously difficult to explore the question of what people want from CAM, not least because they can choose from a vast array of therapies. This begs a further question: why are some particular therapies chosen more frequently than others? In this chapter several sources of data are used to try to answer these questions, including profiles of the people who choose CAM; an examination of the ways in which they access the services and what happens to their use of orthodox medicine; and an exploration of the attitudes, beliefs and expectations of users as opposed to non-users and their qualitative descriptions of their experience of consultations with CAM practitioners.

ACTIVITY   EXPERIENCES OF USING CAM

Allow 15 minutes

If you have ever consulted a CAM practitioner or bought CAM remedies from a chemist or health food shop, reflect on your experiences and note down your answers to the following questions. If you are a regular CAM user, you might reflect on the first time you consulted a practitioner. Conversely, if you have never used CAM, ask a few friends or colleagues about their experiences.

1   What advice, if any, did you gather from friends, family or the medical profession?

2   What were the reasons for your decision to consult a practitioner or buy remedies?

3   What were your expectations before visiting the CAM practitioner and did they match your experiences?

When you have completed this activity, keep your observations or notes to hand to compare with the findings later in this chapter.

Comment

People who have done this activity recounted diverse expectations and experiences. For example, a medical practitioner discussed her sore knee with a friend who practised massage. Despite having no expectations that her friend could 'cure' the problem, she agreed to let her friend 'treat' it and was amazed by the rapidity of its recovery. Another person was advised to see an acupuncturist for chronic back problems, was expecting an instant cure, and was disappointed there was no difference after the treatment.

This chapter will show that it is very difficult to generalise about users' expectations and experiences of CAM. Users of CAM constitute a cross-section of the population who have a vast and complex array of ideas, beliefs and expectations, which in turn can change as contact with a therapy and/or a practitioner increases and the understanding of their illness alters. Exploring these expectations and experiences gives clues to some of the attractions of CAM but also warns that preferences are neither uniform nor fixed.

ACTIVITY   REASONS FOR CHOOSING CAM

Allow 25 minutes

The five descriptions below are about CAM users. Read each one and make notes on why each person sought CAM treatment and why they chose to continue that treatment.

1   Susan has back pain after the birth of her third child, which limits her physical mobility. Although painkillers offer temporary relief, she is concerned about the effects of long-term use. As a result of six, 20-minute consultations with a chiropractor her pain has lessened.

2   John has had chronic eczema for 15 years. He is reluctant to continue applying steroid creams and noted that his condition worsens when he is under stress at work. After visiting a homoeopath he understands that his eczema is affected by his emotional wellbeing and can be related to several events he experienced during his childhood. He now visits the homoeopath for a range of other conditions.

3   Angela has downloaded two sets of material from the internet, the first about the importance of immunising her child with the MMR vaccine and the second outlining the possible links between the MMR vaccine and autism. In an hour-long consultation, the homoeopath listens to Angela's concerns and offers a remedy for her child to take alongside the vaccine to protect the child from any ill effects.

4   Aidan is in good health and has not visited a biomedical practitioner for 15 years. However, he uses a range of CAM therapies such as reflexology, herbalism and spiritual healing to maintain his good health.

5   Helen was concerned about how much her new baby was crying post-delivery and visited a cranial osteopath to assess the extent of post-birth trauma. She now also attends baby massage classes and has started seeing a chiropractor and acupuncturist for her own asthma.

Comment

People choose to see a CAM practitioner for several reasons, including the 'quick fix' of a recurrent health problem, to explore new understandings of body and self within a holistic framework, to discuss health concerns in depth, and to explore the interconnections of their history with the onset of illness. There is also evidence of a distrust of orthodox medicine, in particular, concerns about the side effects of biomedical medication. This chapter will establish the importance of each of these factors.

The factors influencing a decision to use CAM are complex and vary from one setting to another. While most of this chapter concentrates primarily on consultations with a practitioner in the private sector, it is also the case that many people choose to self-prescribe CAM. Herbal and homoeopathic remedies are widely available in supermarkets and chemists. Again, this use varies, ranging from the one-off use of a 'rescue' remedy during labour, to the routine use of remedies in times of illness or injury – for example, the application of arnica (a homoeopathic remedy) to bruises – to the daily supplementation of a diet with vitamins.

In studying biomedical treatment, social scientists have revealed that the experience, explanation and judgement of states of health, illness and sickness are historically, culturally and socially located (Zola, 1973; Davey and Seale, 1996). The decision to seek some form of medical intervention is influenced by gender, class and ethnicity and (as discussed in Chapter 6) by expectations of what it means to be healthy or, conversely, unwell. Thus, deciding to seek help for a medical condition is complicated. It is not based on a simple assessment of the severity of medical signs and symptoms; it is affected by the person's life situation and personal circumstances (Blaxter, 1983, 1990), by beliefs about health and illness (see Chapter 6; also Herzlich, 1973; Pill and Stott, 1982; Blaxter, 1983) and the opinions of friends and family (Freidson, 1970). In the UK since 1948, the NHS has provided access to biomedical practitioners free at the point of delivery, but choice about which practitioner to consult can still be exercised according to a range of criteria, such as sociodemographic characteristics (for example gender and class), the personality of the practitioner, and perhaps their approach to medical practice. Choice may be constrained by the accessibility and availability of particular practitioners and some users choose to bear the costs of a biomedical consultation by seeking care in the private sector (Calnan et al., 1993).

How, if at all, is the situation different when the decision to consult or self-prescribe is taken within CAM? People's choices in CAM are far more diverse and complicated. There is a huge range of therapies available, with differing philosophies, claims and treatments. At the same time, most CAM is in the private sector and requires some financial investment, prohibiting many people from using it. An examination of how many people use CAM and their sociodemographic profile highlights some of the inequities associated with CAM use, but it also offers some insights into the reasons for stepping outside the biomedical realm.

7.2 The demography of CAM use

The number of people choosing to consult a CAM practitioner is consistently increasing (Harris and Rees, 2000). It is estimated to have trebled between 1981 and 1997 (Zollman and Vickers, 1999). In 1993, a national study in the UK estimated that 33 per cent of the population had used some form of complementary therapy and 10 per cent had consulted a complementary practitioner (Thomas et al., 1991). In 1998 the study was repeated and the number of consultations with practitioners of eight therapies and the extent of self-care, as indicated by the purchase of over-the-counter (OTC)

Several important factors are missing from Table 7.1. For example, it does not reveal long-term or sporadic use of CAM: what about people who have used CAM since birth and are possibly the second generation in their family to do so? Nor does it reveal which therapies women are likely to seek. Also, it says little about the use of CAM for children in the UK, although there is some evidence from studies in other countries that parents are increasingly purchasing remedies and requesting consultations. Gross-Tsur et al. (2003) in Jerusalem and Loman (2003) in the USA both estimate that 33 per cent of children in their studies had experienced CAM. In some countries legal restrictions limit the use of CAM for minors: for instance, in Sweden it is illegal for young people under 16 to be given CAM. The information about older age groups is also problematic, not least because the age bands are relatively wide. An ethnographic study of older users suggests that the finding that older people are less likely to use CAM may be too simplistic (Andrews, 2003). Instead, the use of CAM in this group may increase, as members of the baby boom generation become the older users of the future.

There is also evidence that CAM users are more likely to be middle class (RSGB, 1984; MORI, 1989), covered by private health insurance (Lloyd et al., 1993) and more highly educated (Lloyd et al., 1993; Astin, 1998). There is a dearth of information about the ethnicity of users as none of the national studies included relevant questions such as the use of OTC Chinese, Asian, ayurvedic or West Indian herbal remedies, nor has there been sufficient research into therapies and practices that are linked to religious and cultural beliefs but do not yet attract users from all ethnic groupings.

Overall, the available data about CAM use is not too surprising, as it corresponds to the usage patterns of biomedical services. Women are more likely to experience chronic illnesses, generally have higher levels of morbidity, and are more likely than men to consult biomedical services. Although 90 per cent of users pay privately for CAM (Thomas et al., 2002), the fact that they have higher incomes is not especially revealing, except to warn of the financial barriers to use for some sections of the population.

All the British studies showed there are regional differences in use. Northern England and Scotland generally have much lower rates of consultation (MORI, 1989), but this may reflect the greater number of training schools and practitioners in Southern England (Fulder and Munro, 1981; Thomas et al., 1991). Cant and Sharma (1994) note in their study of chiropractors, reflexologists and homoeopaths that the training schools are clustered in the south and that practitioners, once qualified, tend to choose to practise in the same area. For instance, the highest concentration of chiropractors was in Bournemouth, the location of the largest chiropractic training college in Europe. However, there has subsequently been a burgeoning development of complementary health studies in further and higher education colleges all over the UK. It is relevant to note here that studies have shown general practitioners from affluent areas are becoming more interested in providing complementary medicine (Wharton and Lewith, 1986; White et al., 1997).

This issue of accessibility is important, suggesting not simply geographical inequalities but also that demand may be limited by supply and that usage would increase if there was more even coverage of practitioners across the country.

7.3   The conditions CAM is used for

An examination of which therapies are the most popular, and which conditions users most often present with, also gives an insight into what people want from CAM. Studies in the UK and elsewhere show that a relatively small group of therapies attracts the most popular support: namely, acupuncture, homoeopathy, herbalism, osteopathy and chiropractic (Thomas et al., 1991; Sharma, 1992; Fulder, 1996; Zollman and Vickers, 1999; House of Lords, 2000). Reflexology and aromatherapy are also increasingly supported (NAHAT, 1993; Fulder and Munro, 1981; Fisher and Ward, 1994). The most popular therapies have also attracted the greatest research interest and, consequently, knowledge of what people want from other, less widely used, therapies is comparatively sketchy.

Most patients present with chronic rather than acute conditions: in other words, with health problems where the effectiveness of orthodox medicine is currently limited (Sharma, 1992; Cant and Calnan, 1991). Sharma (1992) identified pain (especially back pain) and allergies as the most frequently presented problems. Osteopaths and chiropractors are used extensively throughout the world for lower back pain (Thomas et al., 1991), the area they have identified as their speciality. Acupuncture is used for chronic pain and migraines, whereas homoeopaths tend to see more non-specific conditions, allergies and stress-related illnesses and diseases resulting from inadequate immunity. In Mintel's survey in 2003, most respondents considered back pain (28 per cent) and sleep problems and stress (25 per cent) to be suitable for treatment by CAM. There is also extensive evidence of the increased use of CAM after the diagnosis of specific diseases such as AIDS and cancer (Greenblatt et al., 1991; McGinnis, 1991; Lerner and Kennedy, 1992).

The association between chronic illness and CAM is interesting, not least because many studies have established that people with chronic illnesses are generally very knowledgeable about their condition, and want to be included in any decision making (West, 1976). For instance, Cox et al. (2003) studied women with endometriosis and found that complementary therapies were instrumental in enabling them to be more assertive, take control and decide how to manage their disease.

informed themselves about various therapies and possible cures for their problems, but that the choice of practitioner was made on the basis of advice from 'significant others'. Similarly, in Australia, Lloyd et al. (1993) found that, after personal recommendation (64 per cent), personal assessment of practitioners after shopping around was the next most frequent means of identifying a therapist, and 78 per cent of users had accurate and detailed knowledge of their practitioners' qualifications. This seems to suggest a degree of active consumerism and that users are knowledgeable and informed, but this may be more likely for people who do not act on personal recommendation.

Overall, is illness behaviour any different among users of alternative medicine? In terms of lay referrals and gathering advice from local networks, it arguably merely replicates seeking help in the biomedical sector. There seems to be evidence that users do gather advice about their condition and shop around, but this could be a feature of having a chronic health problem.

This section revealed some interesting findings in the demography and patterns of CAM use. A wide range of people use CAM services, most notably for chronic and intractable conditions, and there is some evidence of active consumerism. Questions should also be asked about levels of equity and how much communication there is between GPs and their patients about CAM. However, the more fundamental question is why has there been a resurgence in the popularity of CAM in recent years? While the increasing prevalence of chronic illnesses might be one explanation, the exploration of this question also requires some engagement with theories of contemporary social change, which should give some insight into why people want CAM.

7.6 Theorising the CAM renaissance

The next activity shows how the decision to use CAM derives from changing ideas about health and illness, and changing expectations about what doctors can and should deliver. Specifically, it is important to consider what social and cultural processes underpin these shifts in preference and expectation (political processes were examined in Chapter 3).

ACTIVITY   WHY THE RESURGENCE OF INTEREST IN CAM?

Allow 15 minutes

Read the following extracts and then list all the factors you can think of that may have facilitated the renewed interest in CAM.

> [R]ecent transformations in the economy have been paralleled by changes in cultural practices. This is manifest in the increased general awareness of 'green' issues and the rejection of 'modernism' in all its forms including the industrialised therapies of biomedicine which are seen to

exacerbate rather than resolve public health problems. … popular
dissatisfaction with biomedicine has increased and … the cultural gap
between biomedical practitioners and their patients has become much
more visible in recent times.

(Bakx, 1991, p. 20)

[A]t any one time, there is substantial, sometimes radical, disagreement
within the medical professions about risk factors as well as about the
aetiology of major health hazards … In the face of such complexity, it is
not surprising that some people withdraw trust from virtually all medical
practitioners.

(Giddens, 1991, p. 121)

A decision to go along with conventional or high-tech medicine, for
example, is likely to be only partly a matter of informed choice:
ordinarily it also 'says something' about a person's lifestyle. …
To opt for a form of alternative medicine … might signal something
about, and actually contribute to, certain lifestyle decisions which a
person then enacts.

(Giddens, 1991, p. 141)

Comment

These extracts suggest that lay members of the public are taking a more active
and critical role as consumers of health care and are increasingly sceptical about
the value of science (Giddens, 1990) and orthodox medicine in particular (Gabe
et al., 1994). This is especially true since consumers have become better informed
through information on the internet. However, as Giddens (1991) suggests, the
changes are not simply related to scepticism about biomedical knowledge: they
also relate to lifestyle choices and the search for alternative experiences that CAM
might offer (see Chapter 1). In other words, the consumption of goods and
services, of which health care is no exception, is imbued with cultural meaning.
It is important to examine the extent to which CAM users hold different beliefs,
values and expectations about what sort of experience should be derived from a
medical consultation.

Understanding why ideas have changed requires an examination of the
contemporary social world. Both Giddens (1991) and Beck (1992) identified
the importance of **manufactured risk**: those risks that are a consequence of
human intervention, often as a result of deploying knowledge that was
intended to bring about positive change and progress. The risks or side effects
of drugs and medical interventions constitute a type of manufactured risk, as
they were not designed to have ill or iatrogenic effects. However, the
evidence of such unintended consequences is the source of much anxiety and
concern. As people become more aware of these types of risk, their faith in
scientific knowledge and those who manage this knowledge (in this case the
doctor) can be reduced. Thus, an inevitable consequence of risk being

an American study found homoeopathic users were more displeased than those seeking treatment from chiropractors (Yu et al., 1994). The comparison of users of osteopathy, homoeopathy and acupuncture (Vincent and Furnham, 1996) showed homoeopathic users valued their involvement in the healing process more and users of acupuncture were most concerned about the side effects of biomedical drugs. Furthermore, Sirious and Gick (2002) showed differences between long-term and new users of CAM in terms of the values and beliefs they hold, although in both groups health-aware behaviour and dissatisfaction with conventional medicine were the best predictors of use. Importantly, there appear to be as many subtle differences among CAM users as there are between users and non-users, and users should not be treated as a homogeneous group with similar beliefs, attitudes and expectations. Nevertheless, this work helps locate some differences in attitudes and beliefs and provides clues about the popularity of CAM. However, and perhaps most interestingly, these studies did not directly ask users why they consulted a CAM practitioner.

7.7   Users' explanations for using CAM

This chapter has started building up a set of explanations for why people decide to use CAM. Furnham's studies (quoted above) demonstrate that users have a complex and differing range of beliefs. But exactly which beliefs are most predictive? Orthodox medicine may have failed to offer solutions for chronic health problems, but how satisfied are users with the treatment they get from CAM? Specifically, how many users continue to use CAM? Are they simply the 'worried well' or does CAM offer a valuable and different approach to legitimate health worries? What are users' explanations for the attractions of CAM and their dissatisfaction with orthodox medicine? The research suggests that, in practice, individuals do not simply weigh up the costs and benefits of use in a calculated way. Rather, the decision-making processes are complex and ever changing, incorporating altered perceptions of health and illness and a desire for inclusion and power in the healing process. People want a reflection of their personal experiences but are also tied to changing social and cultural conditions.

In 1999, the BBC conducted a telephone survey of 1204 randomly selected British adults (Ernst and White, 2000). Although the survey did not specify which therapies should be classed as CAM, respondents were asked what was their main reason for accessing CAM.

Allow 20 minutes

Study Table 7.2, which is from the BBC survey, and then:

1   List the reasons that refer to positive aspects of CAM.

2   List the reasons that refer to negative aspects of orthodox medicine.

TABLE 7.2   REASONS FOR USING CAM

Reason	Percentage using CAM
Helps or relieves injury/condition	25
Just like it	21
Find it relaxing	19
Good health/wellbeing generally	14
Preventative measure	12
Do not believe conventional medicine works	11
Doctor's recommendations/referral	11
To find out about other ways of life/new things	11
Way of life/part of lifestyle	8
Cannot get treatment on NHS/under conventional medicine	7

(Source: Ernst and White, 2000, p. 35)

Comment

Care is needed when analysing these results, which are based on a small and not necessarily representative sample of the British population. Also, note that using CAM because of a friend or relative's recommendation, which is often a main reason for using it, was not an option in this study. Nevertheless, a range of diverse explanations for using CAM are given that are challenging and broaden understanding about what consumers demand of health provision, extending far beyond a medical cure. For example, the BBC survey identified several positive attributes of CAM: that respondents 'like it', 'find it relaxing' and that it helps their sense of 'good health/wellbeing'. In the vignettes earlier, in the second activity in Section 7.1, Susan represents the type of user who turns to CAM for a cure, as a second resort for a condition where orthodox medicine has failed her. However, consideration of the less used therapies reveals different reasons for seeking such care. For instance, in the UK reflexologists do not make any public claims to offer cures (Cant and Sharma, 1996); instead, the emphasis is on relaxation and enhancing the patient's feeling of wellbeing. Similarly, many beauty treatments are included in the category 'alternative medicine' because they are concerned with care rather than cure. Also users will visit practitioners for preventive medicine and to maintain good health, especially as they extend their understanding of the potential of CAM. In another of the vignettes, Aidan is a good example of this type of longer-term user. In addition, users may find that CAM offers them treatments and solutions for conditions and anxieties that would not be recognised by a biomedical practitioner. A cranial osteopath sees many newborn babies and gently 'works' the skull to alleviate any trauma associated with delivery yet, biomedically, these babies would not be regarded as in poor health. In the last vignette, Helen's expectations and needs are at odds with medical definitions and CAM offers her another option.

The analysis of the BBC survey suggests a balance sheet can be drawn up of positive and negative experiences of CAM and biomedical practice. This is not a novel approach for interpreting why people use CAM. Sharma's study (1992) offers ample evidence of the costs and benefits of using alternative and orthodox medical services. First, the use of alternative medicine can be linked to wider concerns about modern science. Specifically, many consumers seem genuinely concerned about the side effects of drugs. They are anxious about taking medication that seems to contain artificial substances and chemicals. In the vignettes, Susan and John were concerned about the biomedical treatments they had taken for a period of time. However, users are also increasingly knowledgeable about potential side effects. Consider the example of Angela in the vignettes: she could not decide whether to immunise her child because her information was contradictory and complex (partly because of the debate within orthodox medicine). Increased access to the internet could exacerbate this problem. In contrast to the possible side effects of some biomedical treatments, the apparent harmlessness of alternative medicine and its concentration on natural products is clearly an attraction. This may help explain the increased purchase of OTC remedies.

Much of the labelling on health products exudes naturalness and health. It often shows pictures of plants or 'healthy looking' people, but does not necessarily portray them as any more potent than photographs of apples on labels for conventional supermarket apple sauce. Many products carry health warnings about the possible dangers to pregnant women or children of using these remedies.

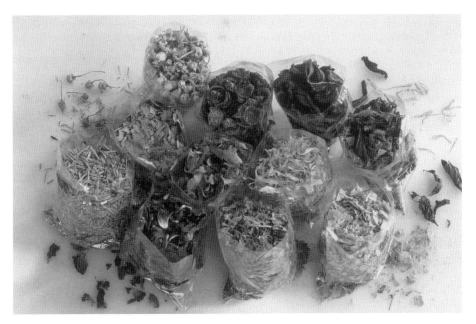

Health products are often packaged to look attractive and convey the message that their consumption will promote health. These herbs convey a more 'natural' or 'organic' message

ACTIVITY   IS CAM SAFE OR RISKY?

Allow 15 minutes

Ursula Sharma held in-depth interviews with 30 users of CAM (Sharma, 1992). Consider the following extract from her research and relate Jason's mother's concerns to ideas of CAM safety as opposed to allopathic medicine.

> Jason had a very bad skin rash which would not clear up, and I thought it might be eczema. The doctor prescribed cortisone creams and steroids, which I thought was rather drastic. We went to a homoeopath who dealt with the problem more or less. It was a relief not to have put cortisone cream and stuff like that all over his hands ... I was always worried about having medicine in the house and I was relieved that homoeopathic medicines are non-poisonous. If you take a whole bottle full you are not going to die even though it may be labelled 'belladonna' or something like that.
>
> (Sharma, 1992)

Comment

It is interesting that CAM is automatically associated with safety and naturalness: a further display of users' 'leap in faith'. Although they subsequently revised their views about CAM as an endeavour, the BMA identified the potential harm that might arise from consulting alternative practitioners (BMA, 1986). This harm included alternative practitioners failing to identify serious medical conditions and the side effects associated with alternative medical products. Some products have been associated with harmful toxicity and face being banned from use. For instance, the herb comfrey is poisonous if ingested in very large quantities; St John's Wort is often marketed as a 'natural Prozac' but questions have been raised about its safety when used with other prescribed medicines (DoH, 2000); and the herbal ingredient kava has been linked to liver toxicity (DoH, 2002). As CAM products become more popular they will inevitably be increasingly subject to research studies to evaluate their safety and, in turn, will get a more sceptical reaction from consumers.

Surveys of users found widespread satisfaction with CAM (House of Lords, 2000), but what is the basis for this satisfaction? In a *Guardian* survey (1996), all but four of 386 CAM users claim to have experienced some improvement in their condition, suggesting that the clinical efficacy of the treatment is important. However, satisfaction levels are probably also based on more complex measures than outcome alone, including the time and attention given by CAM practitioners.

All studies reveal that consumers are drawn to consultations where they have more opportunity to discuss their problem in depth. Usually the time given by CAM practitioners exceeds that of the biomedical clinic:

> [Complementary practitioners] give you more time. Obviously most of them charge you so they would do. But most of them treat the individual symptoms as the individual's problem not just some Latinised name.
>
> (Sharma, 1992)

The first consultation with an alternative practitioner tends to last well over an hour (Cant and Calnan, 1991; Sharma, 1992), although some therapies do not require as long with the patient, as in chiropractic where consultations usually last between 15 and 20 minutes (Cant and Sharma, 1999).

The amount of time spent with a practitioner is an attraction for users, but is time alone important or is it also how that time is spent? To answer this question it is necessary to enter the consulting room and hear what users say about their experiences. In an Australian study, Lupton (1995) found that users of orthodox medicine judged their experience with doctors on the basis of interpersonal features. This was rated over and above their medical knowledge and expertise, particularly 'their ability to listen and communicate' and their willingness to 'spend time with you' and 'talk things over'. In the longer CAM consultations, people have the opportunity to give more information about their complaint and absorb information provided by the practitioner. Qualitative studies reveal that people respond to being treated as an equal and want a more participative relationship with their practitioner (Hewer, 1983). This possibility derives from the fact that most alternative medicine proposes a form of holism, which rejects the treatment of symptoms in isolation and instead seeks to understand them in the context of a person's total health profile. Such an approach requires both an individualistic approach to treatment and the need to extract detailed information from the patient about the circumstances of their illness and their feelings about it. Consequently, the user is given the position of 'expert', having valuable knowledge about their self. This notion of the therapeutic relationship being central to CAM encounters is discussed in Chapters 8 and 9.

Most studies suggest that users feel they participate more equally in a CAM encounter. According to Taylor (1984), this shift links more to changes in the political rather than the medical culture and to demands for the democratisation of decision making. This view resembles Giddens' discussion of the growing disillusionment with the expert, the processes of re-skilling by the public, and the opportunity to reflect on their own health and experiences. The in-depth and confessional nature of many holistic consultations allows for self-reflection and individualism.

The holistic emphasis of many CAM consultations also gives some further clues to the attractions of CAM. In the vignettes earlier, John began to see his eczema in a broader framework, recognising the links between stress and onset. As noted in Chapter 6, contemporary medical practitioners recognise and understand the impact of emotional and spiritual influences on physical symptoms, but there is often little time to discuss them in detail and most treatments aim to relieve symptoms rather than the underlying causes. In homoeopathy, for instance, the choice of remedy is based on a range of physical symptoms and emotional factors, and users are questioned about their family, lifestyle and environment. This holistic emphasis in much CAM prescribing is visible in the descriptions of remedies that are given on the internet for self-prescription.

ACTIVITY   CHOOSING AN APPROPRIATE TREATMENT

Allow 20 minutes

Read through the descriptions in Box 7.1 of four (out of a possible eleven) homoeopathic remedies for eczema. Make notes on the relationship between the remedy, the physical symptoms and the personality and emotional disposition of the person. How is this approach different from one that a biomedically trained specialist might use?

BOX 7.1   HOMOEOPATHIC REMEDIES FOR ECZEMA

Antimonium crudum

People likely to respond to this remedy have eczema with thick, cracked skin and are also prone to indigestion. They are usually sensitive and sentimental, love to eat (craving pickles, vinegar, and other sour things), and may be overweight. Children can be shy and irritable, insisting that they not be touched or looked at. Itching is worse from warmth and sun exposure. *Antimonium crudum* is often indicated for impetigo, plantar warts, and calluses, as well as eczema.

Arsenicum album

People who need this remedy usually are anxious, restless, and compulsively neat and orderly. The skin is dry, itches, and burns intensely. Scratching can make the itching worse, and applying heat will bring relief. Indigestion with burning pain and a general feeling of chilliness are often seen when *Arsenicum* is indicated.

Graphites

People likely to respond to this remedy have tough or leathery skin with cracks and soreness, and often have a long-term history of skin disorders (impetigo, herpes, etc.). The areas behind the ears, around the mouth, or on the hands are often cracked, with a golden oozing discharge that hardens into crusts. Itching is worse from getting warm in bed, and the person will often scratch the irritated places till they bleed. Difficulty concentrating, especially in the morning, is often seen in a person who needs *Graphites*.

Mezereum

A person who needs this remedy often has strong anxiety, felt physically in the stomach. Intensely itching eruptions start as blisters, then ooze and form thick crusts, and scratching can lead to thickened skin. Cold applications often help the itch (although the person is chilly in general). A craving for fat and a tendency to feel better in open air are other indications for *Mezereum*.

(Source: Numark Pharmacists, 2004)

Comment

This example provides an insight into the way a homoeopathic practitioner makes diagnostic decisions and how dependent the practitioner is on the client to give her or him vital information for that diagnosis. So the user plays a vital role in the consultation (see Johannessen, 1996) and, moreover, a very different role from that played out in most biomedical consultations. In addition, this form of individualised prescribing (linking the prescription to the specific profile of the user) means many of these practices are difficult to evaluate by a randomised controlled trial.

Holistic questioning and prescribing potentially allows users to ascribe more meaning to their condition, linking their illness to wider cultural, personal and social frameworks. The lay public use a wide range of frameworks to make sense of episodes of illness – such as a previous experience or the health of other family members – which the biomedical doctor does not generally draw on. As noted in Chapter 6, Helman emphasises the sense-making potential of CAM, especially in relation to suffering:

> Many patients have an unfulfilled sense of wanting to be connected, once again to some wider context, to locate their suffering in a wider framework – even to somehow contain themselves within the many cycles of nature ... Complementary practitioners often help people make sense of their situation in a more meaningful way than does medicine, often utilising, more traditional modes of dealing with misfortune ... many of them utilise traditional cultural beliefs in order to explain to the patient why they have been affected by that particular illness at that particular time.
>
> (Helman, 1992, p. 12)

There seems to be some evidence that patients believe alternative medicine helps them make sense of their situation, even if it is by simply linking their health problems to their family's. As one respondent in Sharma's study outlined:

> I had to do a massive questionnaire about my family background. No-one had ever asked me to do this before. I had to ring my mother and go back to bronchial asthma in my family before the turn if the century ... all this seems to come together and it was **my** body and **my** temperament.
>
> (Sharma, 1992)

Thus, CAM may offer new ways of looking at health and illness that move beyond reductionist accounts and allow for more varied and holistic interpretations. In Busby's study of users of Chinese chi kung (1996), she argues that individuals have the opportunity to know themselves and become experts of their own bodies and health. This practice gives them an alternative framework for knowing their own bodies, and the opportunity to construct multiple possibilities for comprehending the relationship between their body, their self and the social context. Similarly, Lloyd et al. (1993) found that users were concerned about having a healthy lifestyle (also, see Table 7.2) and Crawford (1980) notes a connection between healthism and CAM, described as the desire to retain and maintain perfect health.

7.8 Conclusion

Understanding what people want from CAM is highly complex. The positive attractions of CAM can be compared with the dissatisfactions with orthodox medicine. The time, the relationship with the CAM practitioner and the holistic emphasis can be contrasted with possible side effects, rushed consultations and reductionist diagnosis and treatment. However, balancing positive and negative aspects is too simplistic to explain the complexities of the wants, preferences and decision-making processes of CAM users. Moreover, it creates a false dichotomy between orthodox medicine and CAM, which does not hold true in practice. The fact that most CAM users continue to see orthodox practitioners signals the dangers of drawing conclusions based on this type of balance sheet and suggests that, even if scepticism and mistrust of orthodox medicine are increasingly prevalent, this is not universal. The use of CAM has become part of 'normal' health and illness behaviour: something that a significant proportion of the population contemplate. Yet users are not homogeneous and choosing and using CAM has different meanings for different people.

Nevertheless, some generalisations are possible. The social context in which decisions to use CAM are made reveals some influences and reasons for use. The financial cost of buying CAM products and services and the geographical barriers to access suggest that more people might want CAM than the surveys suggest. As noted in Chapter 6, cultural and religious background and experience may influence the use of CAM but this remains an under-researched area. The relatively recent revival of interest in CAM points to the importance of broad social changes and the changing health profile of the population, especially the prevalence of chronic illness. Certainly, the widespread availability of information about healthcare options and the knowledge of risks associated with many medical interventions may have led to a more reflexive and questioning consumer and seems to resonate with the themes highlighted by Giddens (1991).

There is some mileage in examining whether what people want has changed, and whether consumers now have different expectations. This may relate to the amount of involvement they want and expect in the consultation and subsequent healing process, and to the desire for such concerns to be taken seriously. Of course, such explanations do not describe the experiences of all users. While some may consult because they have particular health ideologies, very clear understandings of health, illness and their body, and require a spiritual engagement with their practitioner, others may simply want symptomatic relief. Some users may believe they are truly consumers of health in CAM, being taken seriously, and exercising choice and power. More research needs to focus on the extent to which the relationship between a practitioner and a user is or can be equal. Paying for a consultation clearly offers more choice but, again, the extent of 'consumerism' differs according to which therapy is accessed. More investigation is needed of whether or not a new value system has emerged (Bakx, 1991; Coward, 1989), in which people hold very different ideas about science, individual responsibility and consumerism.

What people want is ever changing. Orthodox medicine is learning from CAM, and may adapt its own practices. Yet CAM offers certain aspects of a healing relationship that may not be incorporated in orthodox medicine, particularly in a state-funded setting. Time is not the only issue here: the inclusion of a much broader understanding of what constitutes health and illness necessarily challenges some of the assumptions of pathology and physiology. CAM offers treatments, relief and different possibilities for consumers, if they choose to access them.

KEY POINTS

■ It is difficult to make generalisations about what people want from CAM. There are many ways of using CAM and different therapies mean different things to different people.

■ Information about what people want from CAM is based on studies of people who use it. Given that most use requires some financial investment, the sample is necessarily skewed. There are also inequities regionally. If access were more even, use would probably increase.

■ Survey data are problematic: for example, questions about ethnicity have not been asked and it is difficult to compare studies because their methodologies and samples vary. There is little information about why people choose not to use CAM or discontinue using CAM.

■ It is far too simplistic to list the advantages of CAM versus a list of disadvantages of orthodox medicine. People's reasons for using CAM are complex, ever changing and not simply set against orthodox medicine. Nevertheless, there appears to be a more critical stance towards medical expertise and a desire to be included more fully in the healing process, even if this fracturing of trust does not involve rejecting orthodox medicine per se.

■ There is some evidence that, as CAM becomes more widespread, users can increasingly make judgements about which types of therapy to use for particular conditions. This gives users a sense of knowledgeability and expertise, and they are more informed and reflexive. This knowledgeability does not extend to orthodox medical practitioners, who currently have no way of knowing which CAMs are being used, unless their patients tell them.

■ There is much evidence that users hold a different set of values and beliefs from non-users, although this information is complex and in some cases contradictory. Clearly, more research is necessary on the impact of wider cultural values and the influence of lifestyle, especially to ascertain whether any users are drawn to the philosophies and values of CAM. Current research findings do not answer these questions.

References

Andrews, G. J. (2003) 'Placing the consumption of private complementary medicine: everyday geographies of older people's use', *Health and Place*, Vol. 9, No. 4, pp. 337–49.

Astin, J. A. (1998) 'Why patients use alternative medicine. Results of a national study', *Journal of the American Medical Association*, Vol. 279, pp. 1548–53.

Bakx, K. (1991) 'The "eclipse" of folk medicine in western society', *Sociology of Health and Illness*, Vol. 13, No. 1, pp. 20–38.

Beck, U. (1992) *Risk Society: Towards a New Modernity*, London, Sage.

Blaxter, M. (1983) 'The causes of disease: women talking', *Social Science and Medicine*, Vol. 17, pp. 59–69.

Blaxter, M. (1990) *Health and Lifestyles*, London, Tavistock.

BMA (1986) *Alternative Therapy Report of the Board of Science and Education*, London, British Medical Association.

BMA (1993) *Complementary Medicine. New Approaches to Good Practice*, London, British Medical Association/HMSO.

Busby, H. (1996) 'Alternative medicines/alternative knowledges: putting flesh on the bones using traditional Chinese approaches to healing', in Cant, S. and Sharma, U. (eds) *Complementary and Alternative Medicines: Knowledge in Practice*, London, Free Association Books.

Calnan, M., Cant, S. and Gabe, J. (1993) *Going Private. Why People Pay for Their Health Care*, Buckingham, Open University Press.

Campbell, A. (1984) *The Two Faces of Homeopathy*, London, Jill Norman.

Cant, S. and Calnan, M. (1991) 'On the margins of the medical marketplace? An exploratory study of alternative practitioners' perceptions', *Sociology of Health and Illness*, Vol. 13, pp. 34–51.

Cant, S. and Sharma, U. (1994) *The Professionalisation of Complementary Medicine*, Project report to the Economic and Social Research Council, Swindon.

Cant, S. and Sharma, U. (1996) *Complementary and Alternative Medicines: Knowledge in Practice*, London, Free Association Books.

Cant, S. and Sharma, U. (1999) *A New Medical Pluralism? Alternative Medicine. Doctors, Patients and the State*, London, Routledge.

Coward, R. (1989) *The Whole Truth: The Myth of Alternative Health*, London, Faber and Faber.

Cox, H., Henderson, L., Wood, R. and Cagliarini, G. (2003) 'Learning to take charge: women's experiences of living with endometriosis', *Complementary Therapies in Nursing and Midwifery*, Vol. 9, No. 1, pp. 62–8.

Crawford, R. (1980) 'Healthism and the medicalisation of everyday life', *International Journal of Health Services*, Vol. 10, No. 3, pp. 365–88.

Davey, B. and Seale, S. (1996) *Experiencing and Explaining Disease*, Buckingham, Open University Press.

DoH (2000) CMO urgent communication, CEM/CMO 2000/4.

DoH (2002) CMO urgent communication, CEM/CMO 2002/10.

Eisenberg, D. M., Kessler, R., Foster, C., Norlock, F., Calkins, D. and Delbanco, T. (1993) 'Unconventional medicine in the United States', *New England Journal of Medicine*, Vol. 328, No. 4, pp. 246–53.

Ernst, E. and White, A. (2000) 'The BBC survey of complementary medicine use in the UK', *Complementary Therapies in Medicine*, Vol. 8, pp. 32–6.

Fisher, P. and Ward, A. (1994) 'Complementary medicine in Europe', *British Medical Journal*, Vol. 309, 9 July, pp. 107–11.

Freidson, E. (1970) *Professions of Medicine*, New York, Harper and Row.

Fulder, S. (1996) *The Handbook of Alternative and Complementary Medicine*, Oxford, Oxford University Press.

Fulder, S. and Munro, R. (1981) *The Status of Complementary Medicine in the United Kingdom*, London, Threshold Foundation.

Furnham, A. and Bagrath, R. (1992) 'A comparison of health beliefs and behaviours of clients of orthodox and complementary medicine', *British Journal of Clinical Psychology*, Vol. 32, pp. 237–46.

Furnham, A., Vincent, C. and Wood, R. (1995) 'The health beliefs and behaviours of three groups of complementary medicine and a general practice group of patients', *The Journal of Alternative and Complementary Medicine*, Vol. 1, pp. 347–59.

Gabe, J., Kelleher, D. and Williams, G. (eds) (1994) *Challenging Medicine*, London, Routledge.

Giddens, A. (1990) *The Consequences of Modernity*, Cambridge, Polity Press.

Giddens, A. (1991) *Modernity and Self-Identity. Self and Society in the Late Modern Age*, Cambridge, Polity Press.

Greenblatt, R. M., Hollander, H., McMaster, J. R. and Henke, C. J. (1991) 'Polypharmacy among patients attending an AIDS clinic: utilisation of prescribed unorthodox and investigational treatments', *Journal of Acquired Immune Deficiency Syndrome*, Vol. 4, No. 2, pp. 136–43.

Gross-Tsur, V., Lahad, A. and Shalev, R. S. (2003) 'Use of complementary medicine in children with attention deficit hyperactivity disorder and epilepsy', *Paediatric Neurology*, Vol. 29, No. 1, pp. 53–5.

The Guardian (1996) 'Back to our roots', *The Guardian*, 9 January.

Harris, P. and Rees, R. (2000) 'The prevalence of complementary and alternative medicine use among the general population: a systematic review of the literature', *Complementary Therapies in Medicine*, Vol. 8, Issue 2, pp. 88–96.

Helman, C. (1992) 'Complementary medicine in context', *Medical World*, Vol. 9, pp. 11–12.

Herzlich, C. (1973) *Health and Illness: A Social Psychological Analysis*, London, Academic Press.

Hewer, W. (1983) 'The relationship between the alternative practitioner and his patient: a review', *Psychotherapy and Psychosomatics*, Vol. 40, pp. 172–80.

House of Lords (2000) *Science and Technology. Sixth Report*, Science and Technology Committee, 21 November, London, The Stationery Office.

Johannessen, H. (1996) 'Individualised knowledge: reflexologists, biopaths and kinesiologists in Denmark', in Cant, S. and Sharma, U. (eds) *Complementary and Alternative Medicines. Knowledge in Practice*, London, Free Association Books.

Lerner, I. and Kennedy, B. J. (1992) 'The prevalence of questionable methods of cancer treatment in the United States', *Cancer*, Vol. 42, pp. 181–5.

Lloyd, P., Lupton, D., Wiesner, D. and Hasleton, S. (1993) 'Choosing alternative therapy: an exploratory study of socio-demographic characteristics and motives of patients resident in Sydney', *Australian Journal of Public Health*, Vol. 17, No. 2, pp. 135–41.

Loman, D. (2003) 'The use of complementary and alternative health care practices among children', *Journal of Pediatric Health Care*, Vol. 17, No. 2, pp. 58–63.

Lupton, D. (1995) *The Imperative of Health: Public Health and the Regulated Body*, London, Sage.

MacLennan, A., Wilson, D. and Taylor, A. (1996) 'Prevalence and cost of alternative medicine in Australia', *The Lancet*, Vol. 347, pp. 560–73.

McGinnis, L. (1991) 'Alternative therapies 1990', *Cancer*, Vol. 67, pp. 1788–92.

Mintel (2003) 'Consumers put their faith in complementary medicines' [online], www.mrweb.com/drno/frmemail.htm [accessed 22 May 2003].

MORI (Market and Opinion Research International) (1989) *Research on Alternative Medicine* (conducted for *The Times* newspaper), London, MORI.

National Association of Health Authorities and Trusts (NAHAT) (1993) *Complementary Therapies in the NHS*, Birmingham, NAHAT.

Numark Pharmacists (2004) 'Homeopathic remedies for eczema' [online], www.numarkpharmacists.com/hn/Homeo/Eczema [accessed 14 July 2004].

Ooijendijk, W., Makenbach, H. and Limberger, A. (1981) *What is Better?*, Netherlands Institute of Preventative Medicine and The Technical Industrial Organisation London, translated and published by the Threshold Foundation, London.

Pill, R. and Stott, N. C. H. (1982) 'Concepts of illness causation and responsibility: some preliminary data from a sample of working class mothers', *Social Science and Medicine*, Vol. 16, pp. 43–52.

Research Surveys of Great Britain (RSGB) (1984) *Omnibus Survey on Alternative Medicine*, London, RSGB.

Sawyer, C. and Ramlow, J. (1984) 'Attitudes of chiropractic patients: a preliminary survey of patients receiving care in a chiropractic teaching clinic', *Journal of Manipulative and Physiological Therapeutics*, Vol. 7, No. 13, pp. 157–63.

Sharma, U. (1992) *Complementary Medicine Today: Practitioners and Patients*, London, Routledge.

Sirious, F. S. and Gick, M. L. (2002) 'An investigation of the health beliefs and motivations of complementary medicine clients', *Social Science and Medicine*, Vol. 55, pp. 1025–37.

Stevenson, F. A., Brittan, N., Barry, C., Bradley, C. and Barber, N. (2002) 'Self-treatment and its discussion in medical consultations: how is medical pluralism managed in practice?', *Social Science and Medicine*, Vol. 57, No. 3, pp. 513–27.

Taylor, C. R. (1984) 'Alternative medicine and the medical encounter in Britain and the United States', in Salmon, W. J. (ed.) *Alternative Medicines. Popular and Policy Perspectives*, London, Tavistock.

Thomas, K., Carr, J., Westlake, L. and Williams, B. (1991) 'Use of non orthodox and conventional health care in Great Britain', *British Medical Journal*, Vol. 302, 26 January, pp. 207–10.

Thomas, K. J., Nicholl, J. P. and Coleman, P. (2002) 'Use and expenditure on complementary medicine in England: a population based survey', *Complementary Therapies in Medicine*, Vol. 9, No. 1, pp. 2–11.

Vincent, C. and Furnham, A. (1996) 'Why do people turn to complementary medicine? An empirical study', *British Journal of Clinical Psychology*, Vol. 35, pp. 37–48.

West, P. (1976) 'The physician and the management of childhood epilepsy', in Wadsworth, M. and Robinson, D. (eds) *Studies in Everyday Medical Life*, Oxford, Martin Robertson.

Wharton, R. and Lewith, G. (1986) 'Complementary medical and general practice', *British Medical Journal*, Vol. 292, pp. 1498–1500.

White, E., Resch, K. and Ernst, E. (1997) 'Complementary medicine. Use and attitudes amongst general practitioners', *Family Practice*, Vol. 14, pp. 302–6.

Yu, M., Vandiver, P. and Farmer, J. (1994) 'Alternative medicine and patient satisfaction. A consumer survey of acupuncture, chiropractic and homoeopathic health care services', *International Journal of Alternative and Complementary Medicine*, Vol. 12, No. 9, pp. 25–8.

Zola, I. K. (1973) 'Pathways to the doctor: from person to patient', *Social Science and Medicine*, Vol. 7, pp. 677–89.

Zollman, C. and Vickers, A. (1999) 'ABC of complementary medicine: users and practitioners of complementary medicine', *British Medical Journal*, Vol. 319, pp. 836–8.

Chapter 8 The therapeutic relationship and complementary and alternative medicine

Julie Stone and Jeanne Katz

Contents

AIMS

- To explore the meanings of the term 'therapeutic relationship'.
- To demonstrate how different ideas of holism underpin the therapeutic relationship in CAM.
- To identify the key components of effective therapeutic relationships.

8.1 Introduction

This chapter explores what is meant by the term 'therapeutic relationship'. You will be asked to draw on your own experiences to identify characteristics of both good and bad therapeutic relationships. Many people think the nature of therapeutic relationships in complementary and alternative medicine (CAM) largely accounts for its popularity. Some even attribute any successful therapeutic outcomes not to any specific treatment given by CAM practitioners, but to the therapeutic relationship itself. This chapter considers the work of Kelner (2000) and of Mitchell and Cormack (1998). In the light of their work, some of the principles and components of effective therapeutic relationships will be outlined, drawing on comments given by individual CAM practitioners from diverse modalities on their understanding of the therapeutic relationship. This chapter focuses predominantly on therapeutic relationships in CAM as it is commonly practised in contemporary British society. Remember, however, that therapeutic relationships take many forms within cultures and between cultures. This gives rise to a multiplicity of understandings and expectations of what the therapeutic relationship is and what therapeutic relationships can deliver.

8.2   What is a therapeutic relationship?

The term 'therapeutic relationship' has several meanings. Probably the most common one is descriptive, namely that the therapeutic relationship is the relationship between a health care practitioner and a person seeking treatment: that is, a relationship in which therapy is delivered. A second meaning is a more idealised version: the particular rapport established between a care giver and a care seeker (which exists alongside any technical skills being delivered). A third use of the term, commonly found in CAM, takes this idea further and sees the therapeutic relationship as being intrinsically beneficial and a possible catalyst for self-healing.

ACTIVITY   WHAT IS A THERAPEUTIC RELATIONSHIP?

Allow 10 minutes

How would you describe a typical therapeutic relationship between a CAM practitioner and a person who attends for a therapy session? Make brief notes and then compare them with the comment below.

Comment

A therapeutic relationship can be described as a relationship between a care giver and a care receiver that is intended to bring about a healing effect. In this descriptive sense, a therapeutic relationship is established whenever a person seeks treatment and a care giver agrees to treat them. In CAM, establishing a relationship between the practitioner and user is often considered paramount and central to the therapeutic encounter (Mitchell and Cormack, 1998). When such an encounter generates trust and confidence, it can form the basis for a positive therapeutic process and outcome (Thorlby and Panton, 2002). The main focus of interest in this chapter is the therapeutic relationship between CAM practitioners and CAM users, but it is important to recognise that therapeutic relationships arise in a wide variety of contexts and settings, including both formal (the doctor's surgery or the CAM practice) and informal ('tea and sympathy' from a friend, or a massage or home remedy administered by a loved one).

Another way of conceptualising the therapeutic relationship is as something that goes beyond practitioners' technical skills and the interaction between practitioners and their clients. In this sense, the therapeutic relationship involves the whole therapeutic encounter with a user where, ideally, the entire therapeutic process exerts a beneficial and empowering effect.

The term 'relationship' usually implies a connection that evolves over time. This presupposes that a user will have more than one encounter with a practitioner. In most cases, users see CAM practitioners for several sessions over an extended period of time. Of course, not all therapeutic encounters are successful. Someone who has a bad therapeutic experience may not attend a follow-up appointment. Chapter 9 explores what might be termed 'failed therapeutic relationships'.

Therapeutic relationships in health care are usually between two people, although sometimes a parent or carer is also involved: for example, in the case of young children or adults with severe learning disabilities. In the earliest stages of a therapeutic relationship, both practitioners and (adult) clients need to consider whether they are sufficiently well suited to pursue such a relationship. This requires good communication at the outset of therapy. Critically, a therapeutic relationship is not the same as a friendship. While there should be mutual respect between practitioners and clients, a successful therapeutic outcome may not depend on the parties liking each other (although active dislike is probably not a good basis for a therapeutic relationship!).

To enable clients to know what they are getting into, practitioners must be explicit about how they work, the scope and style of their practice, and the principles informing their therapeutic basis. Both partners in the relationship should be clear about what the therapy can and cannot deliver. Of course, this implies that service users have some level of choice about whom they consult, which may not always be the case. Therapeutic relationships occur in a social context. As future chapters will show, characteristics and expectations of the healing relationship may vary according to geographical location, demographics and different illness populations. Cultural expectations may have particular significance. As Mitchell and Cormack (1998) point out, CAM practices may have some positive healing effect because the therapies they use are meaningful to the people they treat. Furthermore, many cultures socially value and even venerate people who are healers. People who choose to use them may have strong expectations of relief from symptoms, which can affect outcome.

One precondition for establishing a therapeutic relationship may be that practitioner and client share a fairly similar idea about the relationship between them and what it can deliver. Where user-centred treatment and responsibility are featured, both practitioner and user should be prepared to participate actively in the therapeutic relationship. In creating the conditions for such a relationship, the practitioner sets the stage for a therapeutic partnership to develop. This involves responsibilities not only on the part of the practitioner but also, simultaneously, on the part of the user, who, by entering into the relationship, implicitly agrees to participate actively in the healing process.

Therapeutic relationships must operate within both common law and established ethical principles. As Chapter 4 showed, this presupposes that a practitioner has a duty of care to benefit and not to harm the client, as well as a duty to respect and promote their autonomy. Ideally, the health care relationship is at the heart of the therapeutic encounter. It is founded on the principles of benevolence and trust. As with all relationships, not all encounters between health practitioners and health users are positive. At best, the therapeutic relationship itself can exert a powerful healing force. At worst, it can be disempowering and destructive, with the potential to seriously harm the user. Learning how to forge effective therapeutic relationships is an essential part of professional training. It should also form an ongoing part of a practitioner's reflective practice, continuing professional development and supervision.

'Healing' as a broader concept than 'curing'

Chapter 6 showed that different people seek different results from the health care interaction. Broadly speaking, people have therapy because they want to feel better. For some people this means the alleviation of symptoms; for others it is being able to cope better with their situation. Not all people who consult CAM practitioners are 'ill'. People also seek CAM treatment to maintain their health and general wellbeing.

To find a meaningful definition of the therapeutic relationship, it is necessary to consider what is meant by a **healing effect**. Ideally, a therapeutic relationship seeks to improve a person's wellbeing by bringing about not merely a transitory but a sustained sense of relief. Healing implies effecting a change in the person's situation. This may be achieved in the following (possibly overlapping) ways:

- curing or alleviating the user's symptoms
- helping the user to live satisfactorily with chronic symptoms: for example, by modifying their behaviour or changing their expectations
- improving the user's mental outlook, making their experience of illness more manageable
- providing support and encouragement to a person who is feeling ill
- bolstering the user's resources to prevent or minimise the likelihood of symptoms recurring
- establishing a healthy balance within and between individuals
- helping the person to believe they can look after themselves.

Critically, the therapeutic relationship is **not just about removing a person's symptoms**. People can be healed without necessarily being cured. Similarly, curing disease does not in itself render a person healthy (Mitchell and Cormack, 1998). A successful therapeutic relationship restores a sense of integrity and wholeness. Cassell (1978) defines healing as a process of restoring a person's sense of connectedness, indestructibility and control (similar to Antonovsky's 'sense of coherence' – see Chapter 6). This may require considerably more than the use of technical skills. Since healing is about change, the therapeutic relationship also involves seeking a person's participation in healing and, ideally, working with them in a therapeutic alliance:

> Central to the osteopathic relationship with patients is the primacy of the patient as an individual with an emphasis on interpersonal skills in which the patient's voice is paramount. In this way, patients' needs, concerns and expectations are validated and addressed as a key part of the healing process. Osteopaths adopt a holistic approach, treating the individual patient rather than just their disorder. This approach recognises that psychosocial factors as well as physical factors may influence patients' health.
>
> (BL, an osteopath, personal communication)

It is possible to imagine that the more holistic the practitioner's orientation, the more likely the therapeutic relationship is to pay attention to all aspects of the user's suffering (physical, emotional and spiritual):

> The classical tradition emphasizes deep inner stillness, calm and reflection, being at the still centre of the wheel, in order to better attune in a somatic sense to our patients, to ourselves and the healing process. Our medicine is based on the interdependence, interrelatedness and transformation of all things.
>
> (DE, an acupuncturist, personal communication)

CAM practitioners claim that they treat the whole person and that orthodox doctors are more interested in treating symptoms. However, as noted in Chapter 6, the move within orthodox medicine away from a mechanistic model of the user towards a biopsychosocial model recognises that disease does not exist in a vacuum. All health carers are increasingly being taught to focus on the person's illness, as they experienced it, and not just on the disease. Similarly, health carers increasingly seek to involve users in health care decisions and encourage people to take responsibility for their health, to the extent that they can. This is enshrined in government policy as well as at the level of individual encounters (see, for example, DoH, 1998.)

The therapeutic relationship can be seen as being derived specifically from **therapeutic intent**. At the centre of all healing encounters, across all cultures, there is the desire to bring about relief from suffering. While informal relationships may do this unintentionally, therapeutic intent separates casual, if beneficial, interventions from therapeutic interventions. The relationship between healer and user is deliberate. It does not 'just happen' when a practitioner treats a person. Nor is the therapeutic relationship an optional 'add-on extra' to the delivery of a technical

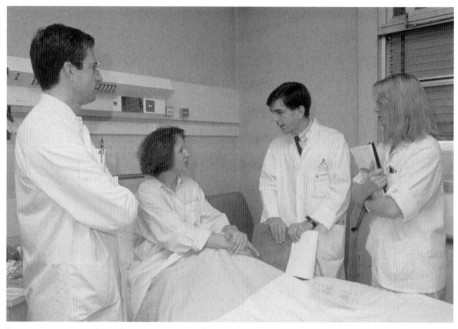

In contrast to patients' experience in the past, where they felt that their views about their illnesses were not taken seriously by their doctors, practitioners now try to involve patients in decision making

intervention. Creating the conditions for therapeutic relationships to develop is part of a practitioner's duty of care. This requires specific skills, which must be learned and refined. Creating good therapeutic relationships is about more than having good 'people skills'.

ACTIVITY   CHARACTERISTICS OF HEALING RELATIONSHIPS

Allow 30 minutes

Reflect on the therapeutic relationships you have experienced as either a user or a provider of therapy. On the basis of your experience, make notes on the following questions.

- What aspects or characteristics made this experience a useful therapeutic experience?

- What factors are important to a successful therapeutic relationship?

- If you have had a bad experience of therapy, what made the encounter harmful or uncomfortable?

Comment

Certain principles seem to be integral to a successful therapeutic relationship. Some of them are listed in Box 8.1.

> ## BOX 8.1   THE PRINCIPLES OF GOOD PRACTICE
>
> ■ The generation of a supportive therapeutic environment of openness and partnership conducive to self-awareness, growth and healing.
>
> ■ A contract, which should be negotiated between the therapist and the client and which details the therapeutic process and potential outcomes, thus empowering the client to remain autonomous.
>
> ■ Sound, relevant advice based on all available research evidence to facilitate the client's decision-making process, including consent to treatment or the opportunity to decline if they so wish.
>
> ■ An individualized holistic approach to treatment with personal time for the client is made explicit as the philosophical and caring basis of the [therapeutic] interaction.
>
> ■ The therapist should work within the Professional Code(s) of Practice as the framework for safe effective practice, recognizing the boundaries as well as the potential of [the therapy].
>
> ■ Adequate preparatory and continuing education, as well as mentor support and clinical supervision of ongoing practice.
>
> (Source: Thorlby and Panton, 2002, pp. 92-3)

This activity may have elicited uncomfortable feelings about experiences of bad therapeutic relationships. The failure of a relationship that is intended to bring about healing can leave people feeling particularly vulnerable and abandoned. The ability to create a safe space and to maintain appropriate boundaries is central to a good therapeutic relationship. The more practitioners encourage their users to divulge deeply personal information about their emotional and spiritual states, the greater the need for appropriate skills to contain and support them. Whether the setting for the therapeutic encounter is formal (in a consulting room in a natural health centre) or informal (in a room in the practitioner's home), the practitioner is responsible for acting sensitively and ethically at each stage of the therapeutic relationship.

Therapeutic relationships may be inhibited by the following factors.

■ The treatment is painful and the user has not been warned about this.
■ The practitioner fails to answer the user's direct questions.
■ The user thinks the treatment was a waste of time (for example, because they were led to expect immediate relief but do not feel any better).
■ The practitioner imposes an explanatory belief which the user disagrees with.
■ The practitioner is dismissive of the user's views of their illness.
■ The practitioner is a poor communicator or is judgemental or non-empathetic.

- The practitioner is overly empathetic to the point of burdening the user with stories of his or her own pain or suffering.
- The practitioner appears to blame the user for becoming or staying ill.
- The practitioner oversteps boundaries: for example, by making sexual innuendoes or touching a user inappropriately.
- The practitioner fails to give the user his or her full attention: for example, by taking telephone calls during the consultation.

(Source: adapted from Stone, 2002)

If you have experienced a bad therapeutic encounter, you will appreciate that the effects can range from disappointment to considerable emotional distress and/or feelings of self-blame and self-doubt. The extent to which the therapeutic relationship can cause harm is explored in greater detail in Chapter 9.

Interestingly, most factors that have been identified relate to factors that the practitioner rather than the user controls. This may be because of the paradigmatic therapeutic relationship that most people see as the 'doctor–patient' relationship. Historically, this is stereotypically a one-sided affair, in which the professional has the power and the patient is the passive recipient of treatment from a beneficent practitioner. Such ideas are now outmoded, because the delivery of health care has changed dramatically since the 1970s and health carers, in general, adopt a more user-centred approach. Along with this increased focus on users' rights, there are expectations about users' responsibilities. These changes have altered the nature and, possibly, the expectations of the therapeutic relationship.

Expectations of the therapeutic relationship

One difference between most orthodox medical and many CAM therapeutic encounters is that people using CAM for the first time do not necessarily know what to expect, especially what techniques the therapist will use. Unless they have contacted a reputable professional organisation before the consultation, users will probably have got their information by word of mouth or from the media. They are unlikely to know whether what the practitioner does is usual practice. Consider the following, somewhat contradictory, quotations from a homoeopath and a reiki practitioner.

> It is important to retain some clarity and agreement with the patient as to why they are seeking treatment and what expectations as to outcomes might be. It need not be a fixed agreement, but some boundaries regarding prognosis and outcome may be required.

(TD, a homoeopath, personal communication)

> Most people who come for a reiki treatment want help with a specific
> physical problem, from frequent headaches or a frozen shoulder to more
> serious complaints, although some simply want to be able to relax and cope
> better with the stresses of modern life – you don't have to be ill to benefit
> from the deep relaxation which is the normal result of receiving reiki!
> However, most conditions can be treated, but I encourage clients to rid
> themselves of specific expectations of what it will do, and how fast it will
> perform.
>
> (PQ, a reiki practitioner, personal communication)

As noted in Chapter 6, some users approach CAM practitioners because they
are dissatisfied with their relationships with orthodox practitioners. Evidence
suggests that people want more personal, less distant relationships with
practitioners: more sharing of information; more time for considering their
individual needs, including psychosocial issues; and more opportunities to
participate in decision making. Dissatisfaction in these areas increases the
likelihood of users shopping around for relationships which better meet these
needs (Kelner, 2000).

> Eliciting a great deal of personal information does have implications for the
> therapeutic relationship. Many of my patients who have attended for
> chronic illnesses have told me 'I have never told anyone about that before'
> when revealing historical or emotional aspects of their lives. It is common
> for patients to cry or experience strong emotions during a consultation, or to
> remember events that had been forgotten. It appears that the nature of the
> homoeopathic consultation differs greatly from what a patient generally
> experiences with his or her GP. This has implications for the interaction
> between the practitioner and patient.
>
> (TD, a homoeopath, personal communication)

People may seek a variety of therapeutic relationships at different times for
different purposes. A person with a chronic condition may look for a
practitioner who understands how this condition affects their life and
involves them in decisions about how to live with the condition and
minimise its disruptive effect. This requires a practitioner with skills such as
the ability to listen, the willingness to engage with the person, and the ability
to offer practical tips to help them to help themselves.

> While a patient may often approach a herbalist wanting a 'medicine' as a
> quick fix for an illness, their encounter with a herbalist may actually
> encourage them to place their symptoms and their recovery in a wider
> context ... Herbalists are trained in orthodox medical science and use the
> same technical language as the orthodox medical professions. Although
> they may use the same labels in terms of pathology, their aim is to support
> normal physiology and aid the ways in which the body heals itself rather

than to treat a named disease ... The patient will be encouraged to observe patterns in their illness, to observe both current habits and diet and also their own history. A relatively minor condition will be seen as a chance of averting more serious illness in the future by attention to diet, exercise and emotional needs in the present.

(B, a herbalist, personal communication)

Kelner (2000, pp. 80–2) describes three models of therapeutic relationship between health care workers and users, whom she terms 'patients' in the original description:

1 **Paternalistic model**
   - Doctor is the technical expert; user is the passive recipient of treatment.
   - User's knowledge is largely irrelevant (although seen to have some expertise in relationship to their own chronic illness).
   - User adopts the 'sick role', which exempts them from certain responsibilities, providing the user agrees to comply with the doctor's advice.
   - Doctor periodically overrides user's choices if they think it is for the user's own good.
   - Considerable power imbalance: the user is not told about their condition and the doctor evades direct questions about the choice of treatment.

2 **Shared decision-making model**
   - Mutual participation in decision making.
   - Practitioner has technical knowledge, but user is the acknowledged expert on their own condition.
   - Practitioner helps user choose the most appropriate approach to managing their condition.
   - User accepts responsibility for making necessary lifestyle changes.
   - Ongoing dialogue between practitioner and user.
   - Collaborative enterprise between practitioner and user based on consultation and sharing information.

3 **Consumerist model**
   - Decision making is firmly in the hands of the user.
   - Practitioner is the service provider, rather than the expert.
   - Assumes users can exercise choice when given facts.

- Assumes equal power between practitioners and users.

- Emphasises user self-determination but may overlook the extent to which pain, distress and fear compromise a person's ability to make effective choices about treatment.

These models provide a useful framework for analysing the interactions between the practitioners and users of CAM. You may have identified aspects of all three models in your own experiences of CAM. Kelner explains that these models reflect a variety of therapeutic relationships and assume different degrees of importance, depending on what is happening in society as a whole:

> As values shift, information explodes, chronic illnesses increase and health care costs keep rising, models that were useful for understanding therapeutic relationships in the past, become less applicable. Now they need to be modified and expanded in order to more accurately reveal the dynamics of these relationships in the current environment.
>
> (Kelner, 2000, p. 80)

Although Kelner's three models could be said to represent a continuum from professional-led practice to user-led practice, aspects of each of them may be therapeutic at different points during a person's illness. Paternalism is not necessarily 'wrong' for all users all of the time, any more than shared decision making is necessarily 'right' for all users all of the time. People's expectations of their practitioners differ, as do their own roles in the healing process. For example, some older users may not want to be actively involved in their treatment process and may deliberately seek a practitioner with a paternalistic approach (Blaxter and Patterson, 1982). Some practitioners (and indeed users) believe that a degree of benevolent paternalism is warranted and required at the outset of the therapeutic relationship, when the user needs to depend on the practitioner, but this should give way to shared decision making once the user can exercise their autonomy (Stone, 2002).

At first sight, the paternalistic model seems anathema to describing CAM relationships, where users are supposedly encouraged to take responsibility for their own health. However, not all CAM practitioners explain to the user what they are doing or why, and may not give users answers to their questions. Similarly, not all users want to take an active part in their own healing. Some users expect to be the passive recipients of health care, even within CAM. Consider the following quotation from a reiki practitioner:

> Many clients go to a complementary or alternative health practitioner with the same intention as they do to a conventional medical practitioner – to get 'fixed' – however unrealistic this assumption may be.
>
> (PQ, a reiki practitioner, personal communication)

Chapter 7 showed that CAM users want their views to be respected, particularly if they have a long experience of living with a chronic condition which may not have a 'cure', but they could be given advice on how to manage it. CAM users want to be listened to, given time to explore their feelings about their illness, be given answers to their questions and be treated as individuals. All these notions are consistent with the shared decision-making model. As CAM users normally pay for their treatment, they also expect value for money and will not be satisfied with only time and attention if the treatment does not work. In this case, users might shop around until they find what they are looking for. This seems to tie in with the consumerist model.

The three models of therapeutic relationship are not static. As Kelner indicates, they reflect broader social trends and are in a continual state of flux. Thus, the move away from paternalism reflects the growing emphasis on individual rights, the civil rights and feminist movements, and the general rise of consumerism. The erosion of medical authority must be seen in the broader context of attempts to move towards a more egalitarian society and the challenge to professionalism in many spheres of life, not just in health care (Mitchell and Cormack, 1998). The consumerist model, which in some ways is posited as the opposite of the paternalistic model, is not realistic if socioeconomic and structural forces prohibit individuals from exercising real power and control over their situation (Lupton, 1996). Many users have limited financial resources to shop around indefinitely. Others are less able to negotiate the terms of their health relationships in the way the consumerist model implies, perhaps through illness or lack of social and educational opportunity.

Kelner's study (2000) compared a sample of CAM users with GP patients. Her project was designed to investigate the health beliefs and practices of 300 respondents during 1994–95 in Toronto, Canada. These people were consulting either family physicians (GPs) or one of four types of alternative practitioner: chiropractors, acupuncturists or traditional Chinese doctors, naturopaths and reiki healers. People consulted their GPs about more acute health problems and CAM practitioners about more chronic problems (which is consistent with research findings in other countries). Kelner's research produced some interesting findings about whether people seeking CAM want substantially different outcomes from people seeking conventional treatment. In the extracts from Kelner's study in Box 8.2, note the similarities and differences between the therapeutic relationships between (a) physician and patient and (b) CAM practitioner and patient.

> **BOX 8.2   FINDINGS FROM A STUDY OF THERAPEUTIC RELATIONSHIPS**
>
> *The physician-patient relationship*
>
> This group of patients reported good working relationships with their family physicians. Almost all of them (90%) said that their physician had fully met their expectations. The vast majority (88%) reported that their family physicians were always willing to answer their questions and over three-quarters of them (78%) said they were given clear and complete explanations about treatments. Most (83%) felt that their physician understood their perspective on their health problem.
>
> When it came to explaining the potential side effects of recommended therapies, satisfaction was not as high; only 58% said that their family physician always did this. Under half (48%) of the patients felt that their physicians were willing to involve them in decision-making about their health care. Nevertheless, an overwhelming majority (92%) said they would recommend their doctor to others with similar problems.
>
> (Source: Kelner, 2000, p. 86)
>
> *The CAM practitioner-patient relationship*
>
> Like the family physician patients, the CAM patients expressed high levels of satisfaction with their current practitioners; 86% of the total group felt that their practitioner was fully meeting their expectations. There were, however, some variations between the CAM groups; more of the patients of chiropractors (90%) and Reiki practitioners (98%) reported that they were fully satisfied than did the other CAM patients.
>
> Most CAM patients (85%) said that their practitioner always was willing to answer their questions; close to three-quarters of them (71%) reported that their practitioners always gave them clear explanations about their health problems; just under half of them (47%) found that their practitioner always explained the side effects of their treatments; most (82%) felt that their practitioner understood their perspective very well and 60% reported that their practitioner always involved them in the decisions about their treatment. Almost all (94%) agreed that they would recommend their practitioner to others with similar problems.
>
> (Source: Kelner, 2000, p. 88)

In this small sample, GPs exhibited many of the traits people are believed to associate with CAM practitioners. Thus, Kelner's findings challenge the supposition that it is primarily the more intimate and sympathetic style of interaction used by CAM practitioners that explains their popularity. If anything, family doctors enjoyed just as good relationships with their patients as CAM practitioners, and patients cited the rapport they had with their GP as contributing to the healing effect. A higher proportion of GP patients cited faith in their doctor's technical skills, even though only a small percentage of them were getting positive results from their current treatment. The patients in Kelner's study did not seem to find their doctors impersonal or lacking in interest, even though this is widely assumed to be a reason why people look outside conventional medicine to CAM.

On the other hand, the CAM users placed most emphasis on positive results such as less pain and discomfort. Their relationships with their practitioners were largely pragmatic: if the practitioners could help them, they would continue to see them; if not, they would move on to try another practitioner or another kind of therapy. The attraction of CAM was not solely the quality of the therapeutic relationship. Moreover, the findings showed that CAM practitioners were less willing than the GPs in providing information about side effects. Only 60 per cent involved users in decisions, implying that 40 per cent of the CAM practitioners did not routinely involve users in decision making, challenging the notion that CAM practitioners are never paternalistic. Kelner's research disputes some fairly basic assumptions about the different nature of the therapeutic relationship in CAM and suggests that a good therapeutic relationship is important in all health care contexts.

To assess the relevance of these models, or analyse what goes on in a CAM therapeutic encounter, some of the distinct features and shared characteristics of CAM relationships must be considered, since they may have a fundamental impact on the content of the therapeutic relationship, the respective roles of practitioners and users, and the user's expectations.

8.3 Characteristics underpinning CAM therapeutic relationships

Several researchers have investigated the distinguishing features of the relationships between users and CAM practitioners. Mitchell and Cormack (1998, p. 10) summarise the main ones as follows.

- CAM is holistic: that is, the mental, physical and spiritual aspects of a person are seen as interdependent.
- Symptoms may be assessed only in relation to a particular person.
- A broad definition of health is used.
- There is an emphasis on treating chronic disorders.
- There is a relatively low risk of side effects.
- Patients are expected to do what they can to help themselves.
- There is an emphasis on the patient's perspective.

It is not easy to reduce a phenomenon as complex as CAM therapeutic relationships to a list of generalised headings. Not all CAM practitioners subscribe equally to all of the above descriptors, nor do all therapies subscribe with equal enthusiasm to each of the above principles. None the less, the list gives a broad outline of some of the main factors of CAM, which have important implications for the therapeutic relationship.

Interpretations of holism and the CAM therapeutic relationship

Many CAM practitioners describe themselves or the way in which they work as 'holistic'. Although holism has more than one meaning, most practitioners believe that the holistic way of viewing the user and the world is a key aspect of their therapeutic relationship.

Many complementary disciplines aim not only to relieve symptoms and restore wellness, but also to help individuals in a process of self-healing within a holistic view of health. According to this view, individuals are more than just mind, body and spirit in a social, family or work environment: as well as promoting wellness, some complementary medicine has a philosophy that everything is interconnected and, consequently, intrinsically bound in a therapeutic relationship between the individual and the practitioner (Wright and Sayre-Adams, 2001).

CAM therapeutic relationships are often referred to as 'holistic' (Mitchell and Cormack, 1998), a term used in a variety of ways in the literature. Generally, holism means an understanding of reality in terms of integrated wholes, whose properties cannot be reduced to smaller units (Capra, 1982). Holism describes an approach that considers the whole picture rather than the function of small fragmented aspects in isolation from one another. The term 'synergy', which holism is sometimes confused with, means an action or effect in which the whole is more effective than the sum of the individual fragmented parts.

The commonly understood meaning of **holistic healing** is the notion that problems of ill health or 'dis-ease' involve a person's mind, body and spirit. The term **holistic medicine** is thus used to describe a therapeutic approach that aims to treat the whole person:

> Holistic medicine is indeed about whole-person medicine but its strength and vitality lie in the fact that its definition of what constitutes a 'whole' person is drawn from a number of different disciplines and not solely the biological sciences.
>
> (Pietroni, 1990, p. 25)

In health care, Mitchell and Cormack (1998) suggest that holism can have three implications:

> First, holism acknowledges that the person's spirit, mind and body interact together to produce an individuality which goes beyond any one single aspect of the self. Thus holism requires a transcendence of the mind–body split which is implicit in reductionist scientific medicine.

Second, holism recognizes that the individual person exists in a context. The physical, social and cultural worlds in which the person lives determine, and in turn are determined by, the nature of the individual's life and experiences.

[Third,] holism suggests that treatment, or the healing act, is also more than the sum of its component parts. The various aspects of treatment are considered to work together, synergistically creating a complex dynamic system in which each component builds on, and interacts with, the contribution of other components.

(Mitchell and Cormack, 1998, pp. 5–6)

While some practitioners may adhere to a therapeutic approach that seeks **to treat all levels** of a user's problem, this is not usual. The more common understanding is that a therapeutic intervention on one level will have a beneficial effect on other levels. The term 'holistic' is often used to denote a perceived contrast between CAM relationships, which are said to be interested in treating the whole person, and relationships in orthodox health care, which are often characterised as being more interested in the symptoms than the person. Adjectives such as 'reductionist' and 'mechanistic' may be used pejoratively to reinforce this distinction. Yet, these polarised terms mask the complexity of the CAM therapeutic relationship. Some CAM therapies are more holistic than others; and some CAM practitioners are more holistic than others. Simply calling a relationship 'holistic' does not necessarily make it holistic. Nor are the principles of holism restricted to CAM practitioners. Many orthodox practitioners view the people who come to see them, and their work, holistically.

CAM and self-healing

A central theme of CAM is promoting the body's capacity to self-heal (Fulder, 1996). CAM views the healing process as the facilitation of the forces for getting better that already exist in the person seeking treatment and in their social world (Mitchell and Cormack, 1998). The extent to which the user, rather than the healer, brings about healing has a fundamental effect on how the therapeutic relationship is construed, and the extent to which self-responsibility is likely to be required and promoted within a therapeutic partnership.

The nature of the relationship between complementary therapists and their clients is based on different premises to the conventional doctor/patient relationship. Unlike the conventional model, which sees patients largely as the passive recipients of beneficent practice, complementary medicine views the healing process as something substantially different. The therapist acts as a conduit through which the patient's own self-healing mechanism may kick-in. Within this relationship, greater reliance may be placed on self-responsibility, change coming from within patients themselves. Thus, the patient's consent and co-operation is not something which the therapist needs in order to be allowed to do something to the patient, rather, it is central to the process of healing, in which the patient is an active participant.

(Stone and Matthews, 1996)

On this basis, the model of interaction most likely to characterise CAM would be the shared decision-making model. If CAM is about self-healing after all, surely there is less emphasis on the technical skills of the practitioner and more on the input of the user. The following quotation gives an interesting insight into respective responsibility according to the personal view of this practitioner:

Channelling reiki into a client simply starts a healing process, and this process is entirely dependent upon the individual client, because essentially all healing is self-healing, and the client is encouraged to take responsibility for their own health and wellbeing. The practitioner is not a healer (although some people would refer to him or her as such), but merely a channel for healing energy, helping the client to help themselves ... Ultimately if they want the healing to be permanent they have to take responsibility for healing the cause. This may mean changing how they think or the way they relate to other people, or even altering their whole lifestyle, from their diet and home environment to their close relationships, job or career.

(PQ, a reiki practitioner, personal communication)

In what ways can users be seen as helping themselves in the CAM relationship? Some writers argue that users exercise self-responsibility by seeking health care outside orthodox medicine. Others suggest that paying for treatment is therapeutic in itself, since it denotes a commitment to improving your own health. Stone (2002) identifies some of the responsibilities that users incur by entering into a therapeutic contract with a CAM practitioner. These include agreeing to:

- attend appointments
- consider reasonable advice from the therapist – for example, about exercise or changes in lifestyle – and to introduce such changes as are possible
- pay for missed sessions, if this was agreed at the outset of therapy
- respect the therapist's personal and professional boundaries and rights as an individual.

However, does self-healing, in the sense that CAM practitioners use it, depend on a greater level of user self-responsibility? There needs to be a distinction between **self-healing** and **self-responsibility**. Much of CAM is based on pre-Cartesian thinking, which is mentioned in Chapter 9. The philosopher René Descartes (1596–1650) proposed that the mind and the body are distinct phenomena. In CAM, the mind and the body are not seen as separate and divided. It would be wrong to assume, therefore, that the sort of self-healing referred to by some CAM therapists implies that the user's rational will or volition, or indeed the user's deliberate actions, bring about healing.

Rather, the idea of self-healing underpinning many CAM therapies is that the body, under healthy conditions, heals itself. The conscious, health-seeking activities of the user should not be assumed to bring about the healing. This is not to say that taking self-responsibility does not have a beneficial effect: for example, increasing the user's sense of empowerment and control. However, it can potentially be destructive to the user's wellbeing to assume that self-healing will only happen if the user 'does their bit'. By confusing the body's capacity for self-healing with self-responsibility, opportunities for victim blaming arise, where an incompetent healer can blame a lack of improvement on the user not making enough effort to get well. This is discussed in greater detail in Chapter 9.

Even though the distinct ideas about self-healing versus self-responsibility are sometimes conflated, the ability to take an active part in the healing process seems to be one reason why users are attracted to CAM. A shift in the locus of control from external (reliance on the skills of a technically proficient practitioner) to internal (bolstering the user's **belief** that they can bring about changes in their health status) is believed to be part of what might bring about healing (Kelner, 2000).

8.4 Effecting change within the CAM therapeutic relationship

ACTIVITY   COMPONENTS OF THERAPEUTIC RELATIONSHIPS

Allow 5 minutes

Do you think that it is possible, helpful or necessary to identify which components of the therapeutic relationship bring about healing?

Comment

Scientists argue that it is vitally important to identify which part or parts of the encounter are beneficial so that they can be refined and improved. They also argue that, unless a therapy is compared with a control group, there is no way of knowing whether the apparent benefits would not have occurred anyway. Many sceptical doctors and scientists dismiss any benefits that the CAM relationship might have as being a placebo effect. Thus, controlled trials tend to concentrate on searching for the specific effects of treatment. However, as discussed above, holistic practitioners believe that the sum of all the components of a therapeutic relationship are more powerful than the isolated components (including any possible placebo effect) and thus are wary of researching specific effects, rather than looking at the total intervention.

Mitchell and Cormack (1998) maintain that, to understand how the therapeutic relationship brings about healing, the whole range of actions and interactions involved in the healing encounter must be considered. They do this by breaking down the treatment act into four separate dimensions.

1   Technical aspects of treatment: dealing with disease.
2   Theoretical aspects of treatment: the formulation of a story – dealing with illness.
3   Practical aspects of treatment: self-help and social actions – dealing with sickness.
4   Relationship aspects of treatment – dealing with the ill person.

There is little research correlating how much each particular aspect is responsible for effecting therapeutic outcomes. Mitchell and Cormack (1998) recognise that these four categories may not be neatly reflected in clinical practice, where all four dimensions are most likely to work synergistically, but their intention is to use them to build a framework, in which the significance of each can be accommodated within the treatment as a whole. These aspects of the therapeutic relationship are considered in more detail in the rest of this section.

Technical aspects of treatment: dealing with disease

The technical aspects of treatment are the focal or specific methods by which the practitioner addresses the user's symptoms. The techniques include prescribing medicine or remedies, manipulating the spine, channelling energy or making psychological interpretations. The modes of action of the treatment techniques fall into the following broad categories.

- **Ingestive:** where the patient takes in a substance or substances such as foods, drugs, remedies or aromatherapy oils.

- **Invasive:** where the patient's body is entered with the use of tools as in surgery, acupuncture needling, vaccination, ... forceps deliveries.

- **External:** where the patient's body is touched on the outside using particular manipulations such as osteopathic or chiropractic thrusts, massage.

- **Remote:** where the patient and practitioner do not necessarily have any kind of direct contact as in some forms of spiritual healing.

- **Mental:** where the patient and the practitioner communicate to alter the patient's beliefs and ideas, as in the various types of psychotherapy and in some forms of shamanism.

(Adapted from Buckman and Sabbagh, 1993, by Mitchell and Cormack, 1998, p. 31)

The appropriate use of techniques can bring about specific healing effects, especially where there are clear causal determinants for symptoms. The choice of technique reflects the practitioner's theoretical orientation. For example, following the principle that like cures like, a homoeopath may prescribe a remedy based on an allergen to a person who has allergic reactions:

> In many other CAMs the therapeutic relationship might be perceived as being based on something which the therapist **does** to the client, such as a massage, or **gives** to the client, such as a homoeopathic remedy, and these elements are expected to produce certain responses, albeit within a given range of results.
>
> (PQ, a reiki practitioner, personal communication)

Professional techniques are taught within complex theoretical knowledge systems. Their use is jealously guarded by practitioners who are skilled and trained in the particular theory. Techniques become approved within a broader process of legitimisation. Techniques also symbolise the therapist's power to effect change.

Theoretical aspects of treatment: the formulation of a story – dealing with illness

This part of the therapeutic relationship seeks to impose some meaning on the illness experience. (Why me? Why now? Why this particular illness?) Kleinman (1988) identifies six universal themes underpinning people's explanatory models:

- **Aetiology:** ideas about the cause of illness.

- **Time and mode of onset of symptoms:** ideas about the significance of what was happening when the symptoms began.

- **Pathology:** ideas about what the illness is and what is going wrong with the person who is ill.

- **Course of illness:** ideas about how long the illness might last and how it might develop.

- **Consequences of illness:** ideas about the possible effects of the illness on the person's life.

- **Treatment:** ideas about what could be done to alleviate or cure the illness.

(Adapted from Kleinman, 1988, by Mitchell and Cormack, 1998, p. 33)

In this aspect of the therapeutic relationship, the practitioner ascertains what the user's explanatory model is and offers some alternative ideas, which perhaps can be used to reframe the user's ideas in a way that makes sense to the user and allows them to develop new strategies for coping (possibly including being subjected to technical interventions).

> In my own practice I felt that my training did not equip me well enough to deal with the emotional needs of my patients, nor with skills to help people overcome habits that were perpetuating their illness. To address this I have undertaken training in various forms of counselling and therapy and my approach to patients is now very influenced by my interests in neuro-linguistic programming and process-oriented psychology. One way in which this affects my communication with patients is that I am very interested in their metaphors for their illness, and the way in which they describe their symptoms. I aim to respond to patients in ways that make sense within their own world view and their own understanding of their illness.
>
> (B, a herbalist, personal communication)

An ideal therapeutic relationship proposes an explanatory model that is both useful and relevant to the user. A model of treatment which focuses on disease (for example, the biomedical model) is unlikely to generate a story that promotes healing if it fails to take account of personal and social meanings of health. Users want to make sense of their problems. The accuracy of that model (that is, its correctness in accordance with some criterion of truth) may be less important than orthodox doctors think:

> What conceptual frames of reference clients learn, how they integrate new information with their own pre-existing world view, and how basic values and philosophies are communicated in clinical interaction is largely unknown at present. What views of problems are most productive for therapy is a largely unanswered question. But it may not matter greatly what world view is adopted. It may be that any coherent system that provides clients with clear rubrics for understanding their own behaviour, and that of other persons, will introduce into their lives a greater sense of predictability and stability, with a consequent increase in their sense of well-being.
>
> (Wills, 1982, p. 396, quoted in Mitchell and Cormack, 1998, p. 35)

This might account for users' expressions of satisfaction with a variety of CAM therapies based on mutually exclusive models. Indeed, as Sharma comments, a therapy may be said to 'work' to the extent that the practitioner's discourse provides meanings and interpretations which are more satisfactory to the user than orthodox explanations (Sharma, 1992).

Practical aspects of treatment: self-help and social actions - dealing with sickness

This element of the therapeutic relationship concerns giving practical advice about the day-to-day management of sickness, so as to promote self-healing, facilitate convalescence and prevent further recurrence. Giving practical advice and information helps users to regain a sense of mastery and control over their illness. Self-help allows users to manage the consequences of their illness in their social world. It involves discussion of whether and how long they should avoid work or moderate their activities, considering relevant resources such as self-help groups, voluntary agencies, and potential support which may be drawn from family and social networks. These practical strategies are an essential element of making the treatment coherent, relevant and of maximum benefit to the particular user.

> I pay careful attention to the patients' experiences, illness explanations, and expectations so that I not only address their physical disorder, frequently back pain, but also their psycho-social needs. This interaction recognises that each patient is not only biologically unique but also experiences their problem in their own individual way and has their own method of coping. Therefore, in the therapeutic relationship, I attempt to identify and treat their biological disorder and also attempt to address their psycho-social problems. This approach is intended to deal with the problem as presented and allow each patient to understand and deal more effectively with the current problem and any future similar events.
>
> (BL, an osteopath, personal communication)

Relationship aspects of treatment: dealing with the ill person

Here, the relevant aspects are the use of the relationship to persuade the user to accept the practitioner's method of help and as a therapeutic device, whereby the experience of being cared for contributes to the healing. This requires convincing users that they are cared for by the practitioner, which contributes to users 'feeling better in themselves'.

> For the herbalist to formulate an effective remedy she or he will have to both correctly diagnose the patient's condition and make enough of a connection with the patient to ascertain which will be the most effective combination of herbs for that person. My measure of having made a

connection with the person will be gauged by having a sense of being in the present with them, of there being no pretence between us. My hope for the patient's measure of this is that they will leave the room feeling better than when they entered.

(B, a herbalist, personal communication)

The relationship aspect involves listening to users, imagining their world view, acknowledging feelings about their illness, and being sensitive to their needs as these change throughout the course of treatment. This may, for example, require a practitioner to switch between a paternalistic model of care at the outset of treatment, when a user might be overwhelmed by the illness experience and want to depend on the practitioner's wisdom to make choices on their behalf, and a shared decision-making power model, when the user has the resources to engage positively in their own healing process. For this dimension of the therapeutic relationship, practitioners rely heavily on their own sense of self and powers of persuasion, conveying hope and enhancing morale about the possibilities for improvement.

Mitchell and Cormack (1998) posit that healing occurs within a therapeutic relationship when all of these dimensions are present and interact. In this way, the therapeutic relationship balances the technical and the personal, the art and the craft, and the expert and the lay approaches. A genuinely holistic practitioner would understandably be less interested in or impressed by isolating the effective parts of a therapy. Nevertheless, if professional practice is to develop and practitioners are to be trained to a high standard, it may be necessary to research both the specific effects of CAM therapy as well as the effectiveness of interventions as a whole with a view to eliciting how practitioners effect healing. This is the only way scientists will be convinced that any benefit is not merely due to a placebo effect, and practitioners will have the opportunity to demonstrate the enhanced benefits of studying a clinical intervention as it is used in practice.

ACTIVITY   COMPETENCIES WITHIN THE THERAPEUTIC RELATIONSHIP

Allow 20 minutes

Make a list of the particular competencies you think a CAM practitioner should bring to the therapeutic relationship.

Comment

You might have listed some of the following competencies.

- ■ Technical skills
- ■ Ability to demonstrate warmth, empathy, openness, genuineness and a non-judgemental nature

- Demonstrable respect for the person as an individual, including listening to what the person is saying and respecting their view of the world and, specifically, views about their illness
- The ability to convey confidence, both in oneself as a practitioner and in the efficacy of the therapy being offered
- Good communication skills
- Motivational skills to encourage the person to pursue health-seeking behaviour

Some CAM practitioners argue that reducing their skills to a list of competencies risks making their practice mechanistic and reductionist. Also, it can be extremely difficult to determine competencies in CAM because of the range of underlying philosophies within and between CAM therapies and the considerable diversity in training standards. None the less, several well-established therapies have now defined specific competencies. These enable education and training institutions to identify which proficiencies are required for safe practice. Competencies are also useful for revalidation purposes, so that registering bodies can ensure periodically that practitioners' skills remain up to date. In addition, competencies may enable regulators to determine whether practitioners have fallen short of the professional duties expected of them.

8.5 Conclusion

This chapter explored some of the meanings of therapeutic relationships, as they are understood by users and practitioners. Although users and practitioners may have different understandings of the term 'therapeutic relationship', certain characteristics seem to promote and inhibit effective therapeutic outcomes. While many CAM practitioners pride themselves on the quality of the therapeutic relationships they establish with their clients, research shows that different models of relationships (such as paternalism and consumerism) also exist within CAM relationships, and that there is a considerable degree of consistency surrounding what people want out of health care relationships, whether they are with a CAM practitioner or orthodox practitioners. 'Real world' therapeutic relationships are subject to many constraints. For example, GPs may espouse a holistic approach to their users' problems but, because of time constraints and institutional bureaucracy, they have to treat users symptomatically. None the less, the biopsychosocial approach underpinning orthodox health care education is consistent with the adoption of a holistic approach. Although many CAM practitioners reject a competence-based approach as being unduly mechanistic, there is a trend towards identifying competencies for good practice, including the skills required for forging effective therapeutic relationships. Further research is necessary to demonstrate how far the therapeutic relationship has intrinsic value over and above the specific effects of therapy.

KEY POINTS

■ The term 'therapeutic relationship' has several meanings, ranging from descriptive (the relationship between a health carer and a user) to an idealised relationship that can effect specific therapeutic benefits.

■ Expectations of the therapeutic relationship vary within and between cultures, locations, user groups and demographics.

■ Models of therapeutic relationships include: paternalistic, shared decision-making and consumerist. Aspects of all three models can be identified in both CAM and orthodox health care.

■ Certain features characterising CAM relationships have distinct implications for the therapeutic relationship, notably the holistic nature of CAM, the emphasis on self-healing and the requirement that users help themselves (not only by complying with practitioners' advice but also by taking active steps to control and manage their condition, to the extent that this is possible).

■ Effective outcomes are thought to result from a complex interaction of technical and non-technical skills, although the intrinsic value of the therapeutic relationship has been inadequately researched.

References

Blaxter, M. and Patterson, E. (1982) *Mothers and Daughters: A Three Generational Study of Health Attitudes and Behaviour*, London, Heinemann Educational Books.

Buckman, R. and Sabbagh, K. (1993) *Magic or Medicine? An Investigation into Healing*, London, Macmillan.

Capra, F. (1982) *The Turning Point*, London, Flamingo.

Cassell, E. J. (1978) *The Healer's Art*, Harmondsworth, Penguin.

DoH (1998) *Modernising Health and Social Care: National Priorities Guidelines 1999/00–2001/2*, Health Service Circular HSC (98)189, London, Department of Health.

Fulder, S. (1996) *The Handbook of Alternative and Complementary Medicine* (3rd edition), Oxford, Oxford University Press.

Kelner, M. (2000) 'The therapeutic relationship under fire', in Kelner, M., Wellman, B., Pescosolido, B. and Saks, M. (eds) *Complementary and Alternative Medicine: Challenge and Change*, Amsterdam, Harwood Academic Publishers.

Kleinman, A. (1988) *The Illness Narratives*, New York, Basic Books.

Lupton, D. (1996) *Your Life in Their Hands: Trust in the Medical Encounter*, Cambridge, Blackwell Publishers.

Mitchell, A. and Cormack, M. (1998) *The Therapeutic Relationship in Complementary Health Care*, Edinburgh, Churchill Livingstone.

Pietroni, P. (1990) *The Greening of Medicine*, London, Victor Gollancz.

Sharma, U. (1992) *Complementary Medicine Today: Practitioners and Patients*, London, Routledge.

Stone, J. (2002) *An Ethical Framework for Complementary and Alternative Therapists*, London, Routledge.

Stone, J. and Matthews, J. (1996) *Complementary Medicine and the Law*, Oxford, Oxford University Press.

Thorlby, M. and Panton, C. (2002) 'Exploring the therapeutic relationship', in Mackereth, P. A. and Tiran, D. (eds) *Clinical Reflexology: A Guide for Health Professionals*, Edinburgh, Churchill Livingstone.

Wills, T. A. (1982) 'Non-specific factors in helping relationships', in Will, T. A. (ed.) *Basic Processes in Helping Relationships*, New York, Academic Press.

Wright, S. and Sayre-Adams, J. (2001) 'Sacred space: the right relationship in health and healing: not just what we do but who we are', in Rankin-Box, D. (ed.) *The Nurses' Handbook of Complementary Therapies* (2nd edition), London, Baillière Tindall.

Chapter 9 Critical issues in the therapeutic relationship

Geraldine Lee-Treweek and Julie Stone

Contents

> **AIMS**
>
> - To explain how therapeutic relationships have changed in recent decades.
> - To discuss and debate reasons for the diversity of patients' experiences within the CAM therapeutic relationship.
> - To identify how the philosophy and principles of CAM therapeutic relationships have been critiqued by social scientists.

9.1 Introduction

This chapter examines the main areas of criticism of the therapeutic relationship in complementary and alternative medicine (CAM). Both social scientists and media commentators have extensively critiqued what some people call a 'therapy culture'. Many critics have questioned the dependency that some users develop in their use of CAM and voice concerns about the ways in which the therapeutic relationship can be abused. In challenging some of the assertions made on behalf of CAM practitioners, you will be able to reflect once more on your own experiences and expectations of therapeutic relationships, and consider the strength of these arguments.

The chapter begins by introducing a range of users' experiences of the therapeutic encounter in CAM. It illustrates how these experiences can be very diverse, with both positive and negative effects for users.

Then there is a more critical analysis of CAM therapeutic relationships by looking at how therapeutic relationships have changed, and re-evaluating possible therapeutic responsibilities held by users and practitioners of CAM. The work of Rosalind Coward (1990) is used to illustrate the views of a growing group of social commentators who believe social factors that contribute to ill health are often rejected by CAM in favour of emphasising the individual's responsibility for their own health and illness.

The next section explores how CAM practitioners, as well as doctors, may try to impose on the user an understanding of illness that robs them of their own views, making them feel disempowered. Even though CAM can occasionally give the user helpful ways of reconceptualising their body and their illness, both 'reductionism' and 'holism' can reduce them to a mere pawn in the practitioner's paradigm, minimising rather than facilitating the user's sense of control.

Next the controversial debate is raised about whether the success of the CAM therapeutic relationship is a powerful form of placebo. Critics using biomedical approaches to health often argue that the placebo effect is both the reason for CAM working and its weak point. They say that healing in CAM is often a result of the powerful effects of the therapeutic encounter and users' and practitioners' belief that the therapy will work.

The next section discusses what happens when the therapeutic encounter fails. It looks at four ways in which therapeutic relationships can be said to fail: clinically, interactionally, through a mismatch of expectations or as a breach of boundaries. This section also considers how far users can challenge practitioners when they believe the therapeutic relationship has been unsuccessful.

Finally, this chapter briefly examines some factors that may alter the nature of therapeutic relationships in CAM in the future, including a greater integration of CAM into orthodox care, a growing litigation culture, and future advances in science.

9.2 Users' experiences of the therapeutic relationship

As noted in Chapters 7 and 8, CAM users may seek a very different type of therapeutic relationship from those they experience with orthodox practitioners. Some people may want to spend more time with a CAM practitioner than they do with their GP, to have more say in determining the frequency of access to practitioners, to have more control over what happens in the consultation room, and to have more choice about the treatments they are given.

In any therapeutic encounter, people want to be treated with respect, to be listened to, and to have a sense of importance in relation to knowing about their own health. This seems to apply whatever the therapy, setting or level of formality.

Many people can have good and bad therapeutic relationships within the same CAM modality; that is, they may have had a range of experiences within, say, osteopathy or shiatsu. This suggests that some practitioners are better than others at developing healing therapeutic relationships. It could also suggest that some therapeutic styles suit some users more than others and that these users are attracted to particular styles. For example, some users may want the practitioner to take control of the interaction, asking direct questions and seeking answers. Other users might prefer to talk at length about their health problems as they understand them while the practitioner listens.

Patterns of interaction change within the therapeutic encounter according to the stage of illness being treated, which means that relationships between user and practitioner can be fluid. Some users choose a therapy almost at random, without having a clear idea, or realistic expectations, of what it can offer them. Lack of communication about what the therapy is and does leads to dissatisfaction and the person is unlikely to return for further treatment. The same applies when a person feels they have been cheated, either because the practitioner did not seem sufficiently skilled, or because the treatment had no obvious effect.

A practitioner and a client may simply not get on with one another. People who pay for therapy are likely to shop around until they find a practitioner with whom they can have a rapport. A decision not to pursue therapy with a practitioner does not necessarily indicate that the therapeutic relationship has failed, nor does it necessarily cast aspersions on the practitioner.

9.3   Changing notions of the therapeutic relationship and responsibility

The shift in practitioner–patient relationships in the last 30 years was described earlier in this book. In addition, Budd and Sharma note that in industrialised societies the nature of the majority of illnesses presented to doctors has changed from acute to chronic and, along with this, the nature of the healing relationship has also changed (1994, p. 11). For many long-term conditions, orthodox treatment can provide only short-term gains. Instead, the key issue is the management of symptoms. In many cases, a person takes on the role of being an expert in that they direct and know the best ways of dealing with episodes of ill health. This type of person is what the government terms 'the expert patient' (DoH, 1999, 2001). At the same time, everyone is presented in health policy ideology as a new consumer of health care services under the NHS, whether they are chronically ill or not. People have rights about their own health and obligations to look after it, while state-provided health services claim to be more patient-centred.

Changes in the therapeutic relationship can be seen in the way in which the training of doctors, nurses and the professions allied to medicine now pays more attention to social and psychological aspects of care. The shift from paternalism to shared decision making, as noted in Chapter 7, is perhaps most apparent in primary care services and is witnessed by the growing interest in narrative-based medicine, which puts the patient's story centre stage (see, for example, Greenhalgh and Hurwitz, 1998). Despite the rhetoric of patient-centredness, change is slow because of entrenched attitudes about the appropriate roles of practitioners and patients. For patients to gain greater power and control, professionals have to relinquish **their** power and control. Real change requires a complete restructuring of health services and health roles. However, in theory, if not fully in practice, there is a definite shift towards sharing therapeutic responsibility (for a discussion of this, see Coulter, 1999). This includes giving people the information they need to make decisions and be an active partner in the therapeutic alliance. To what extent this idea of partnerships of responsibility is a reality depends on both the individuals (users and practitioners) and the settings, situations and health matters involved.

Patients and therapeutic responsibility

ACTIVITY   THERAPEUTIC RESPONSIBILITY

Allow 15 minutes

Based on your own experience, and using the evidence you have read about and heard, answer the following questions.

- Do you believe there has been a significant shift towards shared decision making during therapeutic encounters with CAM practitioners?

- What impact do you think more equal relationships might have on shared therapeutic responsibility?

Comment

Whereas, in the past, responsibility for successful outcomes was exclusively the practitioner's, people are now encouraged to accept a far greater level of self-responsibility in the therapeutic relationship. How far this extends to taking some responsibility for therapeutic outcomes should also be considered.

In CAM, outcomes and expectations may not be just about a narrow definition of health. Patients may seek happiness or wellbeing, a new understanding of their health or their lives, education about a particular topic, a feeling of pleasure and relaxation, or even the fulfilment of a sense of curiosity (Budd and Sharma, 1994, p. 2). The aims of CAM therapy are not, therefore, limited to a cure or the management of symptoms. Given this diversity, the question is whether the models of therapeutic responsibility used in other settings, such as orthodox health care, are useful or appropriate for discussing CAM. Stone and Matthews (1996) argue that, even though CAM relationships stress the centrality of patient self-responsibility, courts and professional bodies still place the entirety of the burden of therapeutic responsibility on the practitioner:

> [T]he law is not prepared to impose duties of self-responsibility on patients. Patients are not held personally responsible in a legal system which is shaped more by the Hippocratic medical tradition than one which sees the legitimacy of health professionals as deriving solely from the patient's rights and the patient's consent to be treated. ... there is little room for contributory negligence in a medical negligence action. Is there anything wrong with the status quo? The answer in relation to cases concerning allopathic medical practitioners is probably not. The technical expertise base of most of modern medicine is such that it probably is justifiable to regard the practitioner as the expert, and the patient as the grateful, and often passive, recipient of health care who expects not to be harmed by unreasonable errors, and expects to find legal redress should such errors occur.
>
> (Stone and Matthews, 1996, p. 213)

In orthodox medicine, where doctors assume a high degree of professional expertise and successful therapeutic outcomes are attributed to a range of interventions, doctors should arguably be held accountable when things go wrong, because the person on the receiving end of that professional expertise cannot contribute much to professional wisdom, and so depends entirely on responsible professional judgement being used. The more power that a single party holds, the fairer it seems to place all the liability on that one party because, in essence, the disempowered party cannot significantly influence the outcome of the therapeutic exchange. Stone and Matthews (1996) argue that, as health care becomes more patient-centred, this way of thinking about therapeutic responsibility will become increasingly outmoded. This model is not appropriate for a therapeutic relationship which depends for its success on the client's active participation. They cite psychotherapy as an example of how existing legal and professional models of accountability may be ill-suited to analyse patient-centred encounters. In psychotherapy, they argue, the therapist gives the client space to realise their potential. If the client fails to do so, no one would expect this to be expressed through the law: for example, 'I'm suing you because you promised to make me happy.' Where the efficacy of a therapy depends on both the patient **and** the practitioner exercising self-responsibility, the practitioner should not be held accountable if the patient fails to fulfil their part of the deal.

Stone and Matthews go on to argue that, unless and until the law shifts towards a contractual model founded on mutual responsibility, the notion of patient self-responsibility will amount to little more than lip service. Patient-centred rhetoric is one matter, but backing up patient-centredness with the force of law denotes a significant shift in how practitioner–patient relationships are conceptualised:

> Suggesting this model has profound political implications. If we are to expect patients in this context to make responsible choices and to take steps to promote their own health, then this relies on the patient having access to a far greater amount of information than the law currently requires.
>
> (Stone and Matthews, 1996, pp. 292–3)

Responsibility for the causes of ill health

Doyal and Pennell (1979) write from the perspective of political economy and argue that there is a continual state of conflict hidden within health experiences and health care relationships. Society produces ill health through an unrelenting drive towards profit and a failure to put the health and wellbeing of individuals first. Work and everyday social life are bound up with taking risks. Many workers experience stress and some occupations involve the risk of physical injury. Social class groupings, affluence or poverty, gender, age and ethnicity can all impact on the likelihood or not of an individual becoming ill. Some occupations are associated with diseases, such as miners and industrial workers (white finger), hairdressers (eczema) and typists (carpal tunnel syndrome). From the perspective of political economy, the development of more 'caring', and allegedly equal, therapeutic relationships in orthodox health care settings is little more than an attempt to gloss over the inequalities that lead to ill health in the first place. For all the talk about patients' rights, and the shared responsibility between doctor and patient, it is the patient who carries the risk and burden of industrial and work-related stress, illness and disease. Orthodox medicine has arguably done little to address these underlying causes of illness. While a small proportion of doctors will take on an advocacy role for their patients, the politics of ill health remain outside the surgery door.

Should CAM therapists be expected to be more overtly political? Poverty, social deprivation and overwork are key stressors for people in modern society. Much CAM business involves helping individuals whose health has been adversely affected by these types of problem. Critics of CAM, such as journalist and social commentator Rosalind Coward (1990), argue that CAM practitioners do not really deal with the social causes and aspects of ill health. Thus, while a hypnotherapist is happy to help a client learn to deal with stress at work (and charge the going rate for this service), hypnotherapists are not marching to Parliament en masse to complain about poor workplaces, heavy workload, bullying and interpersonal aggression, which can lead to people seeking help for stress-related problems. In other words, CAM does not attribute much importance to the political context of illness. Instead it compounds the view that the individual is responsible for dealing with their damaged health.

It can be argued that CAM practitioners perpetuate an unhealthy obsession with perfect health. Because practitioners offer to treat people's minds, bodies and spirits, the quest for perfect health may, for some, become a relentless preoccupation. When treatment is extended beyond illness to wellbeing, people may feel they could always do more to enhance their health. This might reflect a more general concern with control over their life which people in western industrialised societies are encouraged to feel they should have.

CAM and the 'tyranny of health'

Some commentators criticise the very idea of the 'therapy culture'. The issue for them is not how to get people more involved with their health and the therapeutic relationship, but the unhealthy attitude many people have towards seeking perfect health in the first place. How healthy is it for people to constantly turn to professionals or therapists for advice on health care and lifestyle? Should people believe that being in the best of health is the main concern in their lives? The cultural acceptance of purveyors of the various kinds of health knowledge can be interpreted as suggesting a growing dependency on 'experts' to deal with everyday, normal problems of living. Health may become an unending quest for feeling good, balance and a sense of being understood. As everyone's life involves some degree of conflict, problems, sad and upsetting events, and adaptation to difficult circumstances, when will the quest ever end? Rather than health being a fluid experience of the body and mind, Michael Fitzpatrick (2000) argues that it is now sought and valued above all else. He coined the term 'tyranny of health' to describe the moral imperative that everyone faces to take good health seriously and seek it at all costs.

There are consequences of living in a world focused on 'good health'. Lee-Treweek (2003) uses the term 'tyranny of healing' in developing Fitzpatrick's original concept to indicate how many people who have chronic health problems are pressurised never to give up seeking their former health. Friends, family and colleagues who want to support a person with a chronic illness often encourage them to keep trying new CAM, herbal and vitamin products, etc. Also some CAM modalities and practitioners are more than happy to advertise being able to help with a multitude of symptoms and ills. In the marketplace of claims about health products and CAM, it can be hard to accept that healing may not occur; and other people may even interpret such acceptance as the chronically ill person 'giving up'. However, in some circumstances, chasing the dream of total healing is psychologically and emotionally distressing, economically unviable and 'unhealthy' in itself.

9.4   Ownership, control and ideas about the body

This section focuses on the extent to which a person becomes invisible when a practitioner rigidly adheres to a specific view of health and disease, and fails to accept that others (specifically the person they are treating) may have different ideas about illness or, indeed, about their body. The imposition of a fixed view of illness and disease can be extremely disempowering for people seeking help.

ACTIVITY   CONFLICT OVER TREATMENTS

Allow 25 minutes

Think about times when you visited orthodox health care practitioners and CAM therapists or were a hospital inpatient. Make notes on situations when you thought the treatment you received was not what you wanted, or you were 'out of control', or your personal views and wishes were ignored.

Comment

At some time in their lives most people experience unease at receiving medical treatment or advice they are not very happy with. It can feel as though you have disappeared behind your symptoms, especially if what you say is not taken seriously or you are left out of discussions about your own body. Also, it can be hard to insist on what you want when the 'professionals' seem to have a fixed view about what is the appropriate form of treatment. Examples of this include being prescribed drugs you are not happy with; being forced to submit to examinations or procedures that you do not want; and being treated in a way that makes you feel your body and your symptoms, rather than you as a person, are of much more interest to the practitioner.

Reductionism and 'ownership' of the body

Social scientists interested in changing relationships between workers and users of health care often draw attention to what is termed the **loss of ownership** or **loss of governance** of the body. These terms mean that a person's body is treated in some health situations as more important than the person themselves. It is almost as if they are purely a case, an example of a type of disease, or a set of symptoms. Traditionally, such criticisms were levelled against biomedical approaches to the body, and medical historians sought to demonstrate that power over the body is central to the development of medical authority. The work of the sociologist and historian David Armstrong is important to debates in this area (Armstrong, 1987, 1993). He argues that modern medicine developed its power in society through its knowledge of the body and through mapping physiology, anatomy and the biology of disease processes. As the inside of the body was investigated, medicine could claim knowledge about how it worked, giving medicine a monopoly over these new understandings. The science of the body and of disease became the preserve of the medical establishment. The study and treatment of the ill and diseased body moved into medically dominated settings such as hospitals and clinics (Foucault, 1973).

One effect of this focus on the diseased body and the medical 'case' was that the individual person could easily become hidden behind a disease label or a set of medical notes. The focus on parts of the body, rather than the whole person, is called **reductionism** (as you may remember from earlier chapters). A reductionist attitude towards healing and treatment means the patient becomes little more than an object of medical treatment and a battleground on which to fight disease. How patients feel about their treatment and the role of the patient's mind and emotions while in health care settings become side issues to the imperative of treating the body.

As noted in Chapter 8, reductionist medicine is a direct product of Cartesian ideas about the body, specifically, the long-held view that the mind is separate from the body. The philosopher René Descartes (1596–1650) argued that minds and bodies are made of totally different substances: minds are spiritual matter and bodies are material matter. Within conventional scientific thinking, there was no way to link the activities of the mind with the functions of the body. As Mitchell and Cormack explain:

> As translated into biomedical practice, there has been a focus on the physical aspects of illness, with diseases being understood as biological phenomena in which signs and symptoms are manifestations of underlying pathology. Social and psychological aspects of illness may have been recognized and viewed as significant in themselves, but there has been no philosophical or theoretical framework for links between the psychosocial and the physical.
>
> (Mitchell and Cormack, 1998, pp. 63–4)

In theoretical terms, concerns about the limitations of the reductionist biomedical model gave rise to the emergence of the biopsychosocial model of health and illness, proposed by Engels (1980) and discussed in Chapter 5 and Chapter 6. This model, which now underpins conventional training and practice, recognises that behaviours, thoughts and feelings influence a person's physical state. Engels argues that psychological and social factors influence biological functioning and also play a role in health and illness. However, even the biopsychosocial model fails to provide a scientific basis for exploring treatments or approaches to considering the patient as a whole. The discovery in the 1980s of a rich supply of nerves linking the brain with the immune system led to a new branch of science: **psychoneuroimmunology** or PNI (Evans, 2003). Finally, a theoretical basis was established to support a relationship between the brain and the immune system, which some CAM practitioners cite in support of their philosophy that the mind can influence events in the body. The science of PNI is in its infancy, but developments in this area will be highly influential in the shift away from biomedical approaches in which personal meaning and bodily processes are viewed as distinct and separate.

Holism and ideas about the body

Reductionist medical approaches have been criticised for providing a fixed, mechanistic view of the body, which fails to capture the patient's experience. The power associated with biomedical diagnoses and expertise means that patients' explanations for their illnesses are often overlooked or dismissed. Does holism, which seeks to treat the mind, body and spirit, fare any better in giving patients a sense of control or ownership of what their illness means? This question is often reframed in terms of patient-centredness:

> All healthcare practitioners, conventional or complementary, aim to tailor their interventions to the needs of individual patients. However, conventional practitioners generally direct treatment at the underlying disease processes, whereas many complementary practitioners base treatment more on the way patients experience and manifest their disease, including their psychology and response to illness. Treatment is 'individualised' in both cases, but patients' personalities and emotions may be more influential in the latter approach.
>
> (Zollman and Vickers, 1999, pp. 1486–7)

However, claiming that a treatment is holistic and user-centred may not make the user feel more in control, as the following hypothetical example shows.

CONTROL AND CAM TREATMENT

A 30-year-old man visits a chiropractor, having had numerous experiences of care in the NHS, some of them upsetting and, he feels, humiliating. The first visit to the chiropractor includes an hour-long, extensive initial interview and he leaves feeling very satisfied and that, at last, someone is listening. However, on subsequent visits the appointment is much shorter (15 minutes), he undresses, receives a back treatment and leaves. This happens

> on several occasions and, although there is improvement, he believes the chiropractor is now more interested in treating his back and not in treating him as a person. He leaves and goes to another chiropractor who seems to spend time each session assessing how he is doing overall health-wise.

None the less, CAM does offer various ideas or explanatory models about what the body is and how it becomes ill, some of them opposing traditional biomedical notions of anatomy and physiology:

> Teresa ... had sought acupuncture treatment ... to help with back pain which was thought to be associated with secondary cancer in her liver ... she expected to have needles inserted in her back ... where she had experienced pain, [but] she also had needles inserted on her calves and feet, areas considered unrelated to back pain in Western anatomy and physiology ... her acupuncturist ... explained that these were points on a liver meridian.
>
> (Busby, 1996, p. 141)

Teresa's practitioner offered a view of the body according to traditional Chinese acupuncture (TCA) that she had not encountered before. In particular, the idea of energies moving around the body through meridian lines provided a different form of treatment and, doubtless, a different way of thinking about her illness. Busby (1996) goes on to discuss the way in which the notion of the body as 'energy' fits with some of Teresa's ideas about her own body. That is, some of the concepts of TCA were congruent with how Teresa experienced her body and thought about illness. Other therapies that explain health states by relating to energies in transit around the body include shiatsu, reiki healing, vortex healing and all healing systems that use the notion of **chakras** (energy centres positioned at various points on the body). With energy-based therapies, some people gain much from seeing themselves through the framework provided by the practitioner – that is, as having an energy imbalance which led to illness – rather than through the frameworks provided by GPs or orthodox medical specialists.

Other CAM therapies also provide different frameworks for understanding and thinking about bodies and disease or illness, which include the following.

- **Mechanical view of pain and dysfunction in the body** – for instance, some osteopathic and chiropractic approaches.
- **Illness or disease as the product of imbalance in their systems** – homoeopathy and many traditional healing systems, such as ayurvedic medicine.

- **Illness or disease as the product of stress, negative thinking or no longer useful subconscious processes** – hypnotherapy and guided imagery therapies.
- **Emotions and shocks are held in the body and require healing** – some osteopathic approaches, homoeopathy, massage and probably all the energy-healing modalities.

This list of different ways of conceptualising the body and illness or disease is not exhaustive, but it demonstrates the way in which CAM appears to offer a variety of ways for individuals to think about health, the body, the mind and the causes of disease. Patients can be **empowered** through having a sense of congruence and control in CAM therapy that they perhaps do not have in orthodox forms of medical care.

ACTIVITY   WHO BENEFITS FROM DIFFERENT VIEWS OF THE BODY?

Allow 15 minutes

Note down some reasons why health care users might gain from a different view of their bodies. Are there any ways in which a different view of their body may be damaging or distressing for a user?

Comment

Some users' health problems may not 'fit' orthodox care services, or their conditions may not be treated easily by orthodox means. Complementary therapy may be a chance to develop a therapeutic relationship with someone who does not even use the illness categories of orthodox care and is prepared to help with difficult symptoms when orthodoxy has perhaps 'given up'. For instance, people diagnosed with the rheumatic illness fibromyalgia, which can lead to debilitating muscle pain in various parts of the body, often find that orthodox services have little to offer them and that some orthodox practitioners even doubt the authenticity of their symptoms. CAM may therefore give a sense of practitioner acceptance and support after what is a journey through orthodox care that is sometimes confusing, harmful or less than supportive.

So far in this chapter the discussion has been about how CAM approaches to the body offer alternatives to the traditional biomedical approaches that have been criticised for making people feel out of control. From a positive perspective, new ways of seeing the body can enable users to choose those most congruent to their own personal ideas. A holistic view of the body and more equal relationships between practitioner and user could lead to a more empowering experience for the user.

However, is this experience of empowerment and congruence a feature of all CAM therapeutic relationships? Arguably, users can feel as out of control in a CAM encounter as in a conventional encounter. Numerous critics of CAM point to the way in which some CAM modalities leave little room for users' own views and can create their own sense of 'loss of ownership' of the body. Individuals have varying experiences of the CAM therapeutic relationship and what some people experience as empowering can for others be overbearing, bizarre or at odds with their own views of the world.

The issue of congruence and blame is very important. Some therapies are founded on the idea that different parts of the body relate to how the person feels inside. For example, the New Age 'guru' Louise Hay sees the body and its ailments as reflecting more general problems in a person's life and thinking (Hay, 1984). She believes the nature of illness yields clues about the person's problems. For instance, illness involving the eyes may indicate that the patient does not like what they see in their own life. Likewise, skin problems may indicate difficulties with anxiety, fear or being threatened. These views of illness or bodily malfunctions are open to a wide range of interpretations by individuals who are exposed to them. Some people use these pronouncements metaphorically, to help them see their condition in a new light and take active steps to 'heal their life'. However, for others such an approach is at odds with how they feel and Hay's theory may seem intimidating or threatening. Some may also consider this approach to be 'victim blaming' in that it somehow suggests that people exhibit illness precisely because of their approach to themselves and their lives. The individualisation of illness that is helpful to some people may also demonstrate a gap between CAM practitioners' views on health or illness and how the person receiving 'therapy' or advice feels.

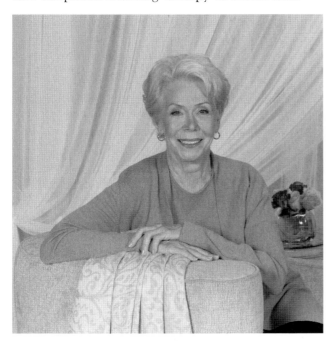

Louise Hay has had an enormous influence on a variety of CAM practitioners

How CAM therapists impose their views on users

As most people do not have a wide knowledge of complementary perspectives and philosophies, the therapeutic relationship can break down because of a mismatch between what the practitioner offers and what the user of the service wants. The practitioner's ideas about health, illness, mind and body may be at odds with the user's, which can lead the user to find another therapist who offers therapy that is more congruent with their beliefs.

The scholar Ursula Sharma argues that users of CAM most probably match themselves with practitioners who offer approaches that they can connect with and find palatable (Sharma, 1994). Conversely, when faced with a therapist or therapy that does not fit with their views on health, users will tend to fail to return. Sharma (1994, p. 20) notes that one area in which users of CAM may find that their views clash with particular therapists is the issue of personal change. For instance, users who attend for relief of symptoms may view the idea of changing their lifestyles or sense of self as intrusive or inappropriate.

Therefore, a CAM practitioner who promotes strict exclusion diets as being essential to healing may put off someone with a mechanistic view of their body who wants it 'fixed' with as little change to their lifestyle as possible. Similarly, practitioners who offer or promote New Age, spiritual or religious aspects to treatment may also find that some patients will leave the therapeutic relationship. However, others may be attracted by such approaches and actively seek practitioners who integrate ideas that fit with their own world views. The apparent need for congruence between practitioners and users makes it even more important for therapists to discuss their therapeutic orientation with users before starting a therapeutic relationship, so that users can make an informed choice about whether to invest their time, money and hope in such an approach.

9.5 The therapeutic relationship as a placebo

In Chapter 8, Mitchell and Cormack's proposition that the relationship aspect of a therapeutic encounter can be as important as the technical dimensions of healing was considered (Mitchell and Cormack, 1998). CAM practitioners argue that the therapeutic relationship itself may be an important tool in healing. Critics of CAM turn this argument on its head, suggesting that CAM is, in fact, no more than a powerful form of placebo. What they generally mean is that it is not the specific treatments used that evoke a healing response; rather, it is the combination of non-specific effects of the CAM therapeutic relationship which create **a belief** in the user that they are being healed. In other words, it is not the acupuncturist's needles, or the homoeopath's remedies, or the osteopath's manipulations that benefit the user, but the ritual, supportive relationship and powerful belief in the effectiveness of the therapy that makes users feel better. Obviously, CAM practitioners regard this assertion as contentious, and a denigration of their technical skills, which often have been learned over many years. Peters (2001, p. xi) notes that practitioners might find it demeaning having to accept that recovery might depend on responses they trigger. For many practitioners, calling CAM 'mere placebo' is a way of dismissing it as trickery or an elaborate sort of con. To call CAM a placebo is to infer that, if it heals users at all, the healing is all in the user's mind, and not a result of the treatment.

Placebo generally means an inert substance, given in place of an active drug or treatment. Over the centuries, physicians realised that some people felt better for taking a placebo, even if it was nothing more than water or sugar. The **placebo effect** refers to the phenomenon that, in certain conditions, including pain and depression, approximately 30 per cent of people will get better, even when they have been given a dummy pill or procedure. The placebo effect is not the same as spontaneous remission or the natural waxing and waning of symptoms over the course of a disease.

To understand why this is such a contentious debate, remember that orthodox medicine (not to mention pharmaceutical companies) has much invested in the idea of 'magic bullets', or specific interventions to cure specific diseases. Much clinical research is dedicated to proving that drug X works for condition Y. Drug trials are carefully designed to prove whether the drug (or procedure, or device) can demonstrate a desired specific effect beyond any possible placebo effect. In order to prove this, potential biases and variables are taken out of the equation as far as possible, so that the only aspect being tested is the intervention with the specific effect. This form of scientific method led to the development of the double-blind, **randomised controlled trial** (or RCT).

RCTs represent the scientific gold standard for assessing the effectiveness of any new treatment. They eliminate the very factors that exert a powerful effect in the CAM therapeutic relationship: the practitioner's time and interest in the user; the formation of a close, empathetic relationship; the giving of hope; and the practitioner's enthusiasm for the therapy. This represents a clash of systems and values. Some scientific scholars argue that the only definitive way to prove that a CAM therapy works is to subject it to the same scientific processes as conventional medicine (that is, the RCT), whereas other scholars (and many CAM therapists) argue that it is pointless to consider the specific effects of their therapy in isolation, since it is a combination of the specific and non-specific effects, acting together, that creates the power of the healing effect. They also argue that it is unfair and unrealistic to be expected to test their therapies in a way that fails to capture the holistic nature of the interaction.

This argument is not simply about research methodology. As with so many other dimensions of CAM, it has political overtones. The future integration of CAM requires more evidence of its efficacy and cost-effectiveness. Sustained consumer enthusiasm for CAM similarly depends increasingly on evidence to support its claims. Many practitioners appreciate that developing a stronger evidence base is essential to maintaining their increasing credibility and professionalisation, and they accept that research must be done. Compromises will have to be sought, which may include innovative research design for testing specific and non-specific effects (for example, the use of pragmatic RCTs, which test the intervention as a whole, as it is delivered in practice) and sufficient research funding in CAM, so that any placebo effect can be rigorously and scientifically tested (for example, by comparing an active CAM treatment with a placebo and no treatment whatsoever).

Regarding the claim that orthodox medicine is becoming more patient-centred, doctors may also want to explore how the non-specific effects of treatment might make patients feel better. Whether or not specific effects are caused by evoking a placebo response, or through chemical processes in the body (as PNI might suggest), anything that improves a patient's subjective experience of suffering is worth investigating.

Placebo might work through psychoneuroimmunology (Armstrong, 1993); that is, the complex interrelationship between the mind or psychology, the brain, the immune system and general health. A psychoneuroimmunological approach tries to take all these facets of a person into account in understanding a symptom, an illness or a disease. Thinking about and treating the whole person could evoke a stronger placebo effect. As Evans (2003) notes, rather than dismissing CAM practitioners as frauds or quacks, if their healing abilities are 'just' about placebo then orthodoxy could learn a great deal from them.

Without further research, the question of whether CAM is a placebo will continue to generate controversy and polarise CAM practitioners and scientists.

9.6 The failure of CAM therapeutic relationships

In Chapter 8 some of the various ways in which the therapeutic relationship can bring about healing were discussed. It was noted that, although therapeutic relationships have the capacity to heal, they can also harm. In reality, the outcome of most therapeutic encounters and relationships lies somewhere on a continuum between good and harm. Few therapeutic relationships are a complete success but, judging by the number of complaints, even fewer are a complete disaster. Studies of therapeutic encounters invariably show high levels of patient satisfaction (see, for example, Sharma, 1992; Kelner et al., 2000). None the less, it is important to consider the ways in which the therapeutic relationship can be unsuccessful or even counter-therapeutic. This can be considered in the following areas.

- **Clinical failure:** the therapy either does not help the user or makes them worse. This may be seen as a failure of the practitioner's ethical duty of beneficence and non-maleficence (see Chapter 4).
- **Failure in interaction or communication:** sometimes users fail to 'connect' with the practitioner, either personally or with the philosophy or ideas involved with their particular CAM. Sometimes a practitioner's style of interaction and questioning is not acceptable to the user. This can also be seen as a failure both of the practitioner's ethical duty of beneficence and non-maleficence and of the practitioner's duty to respect the person's autonomy.
- **Mismatch of expectations:** the user might have different ideas about how soon to expect results from the form of treatment they seek, or what kind of results to expect.
- **Breach of boundaries:** failure by the user, the practitioner or both to manage appropriate boundaries in the therapeutic encounter (for example, the patient or practitioner makes suggestive or judgemental comments, or the practitioner performs an examination that seems unnecessary). This can be seen as a failure of the practitioner's ethical duty of non-maleficence, in that they are actively harming the patient.

Of course, separating relationship failures in this way may be rather artificial. In practice, a therapeutic relationship flounders for several different reasons. As discussed earlier, the components of the therapeutic relationship operate synergistically. Thus, a clinical failure may result from failed communication or an inability to form a supportive, empathetic relationship with a user. A breach of boundaries may be detrimental to healing, even when the practitioner has been technically proficient. The most likely outcome of failure in communication or interaction is that the user will not return to that practitioner. Failed encounters of this sort are detrimental in that they may inhibit the patient from seeking further treatment that may be of benefit. Also, remember that users who pay for their CAM treatment may simply not have the resources to shop around indefinitely. However, it is failures of the final type that cause most concern, since they have the greatest capacity to harm patients directly. Although, stereotypically, people tend to associate breach of boundaries with practitioners acting in a sexually inappropriate way, the scope of failures is considerably broader.

Breach of boundaries

In this section, failures caused by breach of boundaries are discussed under the following headings:

- 'wounded healers'

- creating dependency to satisfy practitioners' emotional and financial needs
- sexual abuse and exploitation.

To reiterate a point made earlier, breaches of the therapeutic relationship cover a spectrum. Some breaches invariably thwart a successful therapeutic outcome (for example, when a therapist is physically aggressive and intimidating towards a patient). Other breaches may inhibit a maximally effective therapeutic outcome, but do not necessarily destroy the entire foundation of the relationship (for example, a therapist who tells the user more about their personal circumstances than the user cares to know). The most unacceptable sorts of breach tend to be expressly prohibited within practitioners' codes of conduct. Professional bodies in CAM prohibit sexual relationships between practitioners and users or former users, or direct financial relationships, such as borrowing or lending money. (For example, see the codes of ethics for osteopaths and chiropractors: General Chiropractic Council, 2004; General Osteopathic Council, 2004). Other breaches are more subtle and less well documented. While the focus here is on CAM relationships, it is important to remember that breaches of boundary occur in all health and caring professions (POPAN, 2000).

Wounded healers

Sometimes, practitioners allow their personal life and personal issues to become central to the therapeutic relationship. In a range of therapies, the practitioner is assumed to bring not only their skills but also their experiences to the therapeutic relationship. This has led to the concept of the 'wounded healer' (Nouwen, 1977): that is, a practitioner who, in experiencing physical, psychological or emotional pain, develops a greater understanding and empathy with other people's pain. The debates about whether practitioners can draw positively on their own negative past experience and their ways of getting over negative life events in their work are in the literature on pastoral care, counselling and psychoanalysis. The Catholic spiritual writer Henri Nouwen first developed the idea of the wounded healer and argued the need for all 'people workers' to recognise how their own experiences of abuse and pain can contribute towards a greater awareness of the needs of other people (Nouwen, 1977). The CAM movement took up this term, and in many therapies the idea of understanding one's own pain and personal coping mechanisms is central to being a practitioner.

Although there is no reason why personal experience may not provide a useful reservoir of insight into some users' experiences for a reflective practitioner, it can lead to therapeutic failure if practitioners cannot manage their own feelings adequately. If not properly understood, the notion of the 'wounded healer' could appear to excuse or support some of the following unhelpful assumptions.

1   'Wounded healers' are the most able practitioners to help users (having experienced pain themselves).

2   Inevitably there are ongoing issues with pain or personal distress.

3   It is appropriate to divulge this to users who have attended for treatment in an attempt to cope with their own pain and symptoms.

The concept also seems to imply that healers who are not 'wounded' are less able to be good, competent and caring practitioners. Clearly this is false. A practitioner need not have experienced the same pain as the user to be able to empathise. It would be like saying that only people who have experienced house fires can comfort others whose houses have burned down, or that only people who have explored their own capacity for deviance should become forensic psychotherapists. Many experiences can give an insight into another person's wish for healing or change. Also, people's ability to learn and use skills such as rapport, empathy and listening means that practitioners do not necessarily have to experience a difficult life to understand another person's difficult life.

The main problem with the wounded healer concept is that it can be used as an excuse for practitioners not to establish and maintain clear boundaries between themselves and the users. In the extreme case, the practitioner may feel it is all right to emotionally 'open up' to clients or users about their life experiences at inappropriate times or in inappropriate ways. For instance, a shiatsu practitioner who spends much of the initial interview before treatment regaling their clients with details of their failed marriage is unlikely to add to the client's sense of wellbeing or to inspire the sort of confidence in the practitioner that forges a good therapeutic relationship. Indeed, the relationship may change so that the client almost becomes the practitioner's counsellor or supporter. The alternative course of action is for the client to leave either immediately or at the end of the treatment and not return. Either way, it is difficult to see the interaction between such practitioners and their clients as being particularly therapeutic. Using the therapeutic relationship to fulfil the practitioner's own psychological or emotional needs can be seen as a form of abuse.

Creating dependency to satisfy practitioners' emotional and financial needs

Although a failed therapeutic relationship is often assumed to involve a patient not returning, the case of a patient who attends repeatedly can also be highly problematic. This phenomenon can be seen as a breach of boundaries in that an inappropriately extended therapeutic relationship changes from being a healing encounter into a dependency relationship or friendship. Unlike the timescale contracts that may be negotiated in counselling and psychotherapy, there are no fixed timescales for most CAM

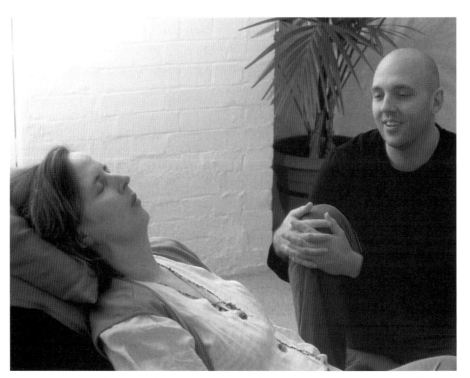

It is inappropriate for hypnotherapists to abuse their therapeutic privilege by telling the user about their own private affairs

therapies. Some CAM users will continue to attend as and when they feel like it, especially when the CAM therapies have a strong leisure or relaxation component, such as massage or aromatherapy. In the more 'medicalised' therapies, practitioners usually indicate to users the timescale in which they hope to see some improvement. Negotiating an appropriate timeframe helps patients to feel in control, and gives a realistic period in which to judge whether the treatment is beneficial.

Other CAM therapies are based on the notion of minimum intervention. For example, in osteopathy the general aim of the treatment is that patients are not long term. Once a lack of improvement or a levelling off is observed then the practitioner is expected to help the patient end the treatment. Of course, some patients will return for 'top-up' sessions, or when a condition flares up. However, research by the British School of Osteopathy suggests that returning patients are quite common (Pringle and Tyreman, 1993).

Practitioners are often at a loss to know where to send patients who report they are not getting better. In some cases, practitioners think these patients have no one else to turn to and that they have an ongoing duty to relieve the patients' distress, even though they cannot offer a cure. This raises interesting issues about what therapy is really for, and how attendance may be affected by lack of support or care for particular patient groups in orthodox services. Continually returning patients are the subject of a considerable literature in orthodox health care and they are often called 'heart sink' patients (for example, Pietroni and Chase, 1993; O'Rourke, 2000). The 'returnee' may be CAM's equivalent.

Sexual abuse and exploitation

Another issue that can cause a therapeutic relationship to break down is the failure to maintain appropriate personal or professional boundaries, to the extent that it constitutes serious abuse. A broad spectrum of activities can be called abuse. The term 'abuse' originates from the Latin meaning 'a departure from the purpose (use)' (Rutter, 1990, p. 41). Given this meaning, clearly some of the boundary issues mentioned above are on the fringes of the category of abuse within CAM. Much of the literature on abuse in one-to-one healing encounters is from counselling and psychotherapy and focuses on the issue of sexual abuse and exploitation within the therapeutic relationship (for example, Pope and Vetter, 1991; Jehu, 1994).

Perhaps the most easily identifiable abuse within CAM relationships is where a practitioner makes sexual moves towards a user or engages in a sexual relationship. Such behaviour constitutes a gross breach of trust. Such boundary violations are invariably counter-therapeutic, whatever the practitioner and the user may feel about it. As with all boundary violations, sexual exploitation is no more likely in CAM therapeutic relationships than in other healing encounters. However, factors which might increase the likelihood of abuse in CAM include working from home, or in other informal settings (including the user's home), lack of knowledge about what the therapy is supposed to involve, and lack of formal regulation (Stone, 2002).

Sometimes a breach of boundaries starts when a patient or user attempts to change the nature of the relationship. Oerton's research (2004) on therapeutic massage indicates that it is very common for practitioners (often, but not always, female) to have problems with clients (often, but not always, male) misinterpreting massage as sexual. Massage practitioners have the added problem of being incorrectly associated with sexual massage services. Oerton found that practitioners often sanitise the encounter to minimise the possibility of misinterpretation by wearing white tunics or robes (mimicking the dress of medical personnel); adopting a professional attitude to the massage encounter; and demonstrating boundaries by leaving the room while the patient or user is undressing and dressing. Working in a group practice of CAM practitioners can also help deter people or their therapists from trying to breach acceptable boundaries.

The processes of **transference** and **counter-transference** make it natural and normal for attraction and desire to arise for both user and practitioner throughout the therapeutic relationship. Transference is the way in which a user's feelings and actions towards their therapist are influenced by early childhood experiences, especially relationships with parents. Therapists, in turn, exhibit counter-transference: their own unconscious fantasies and wishes about their patients. Practitioners need to be aware of these forces and use them constructively in the professional relationship (Stone, 2002). The onus is always on the practitioner to manage and maintain appropriate boundaries, however the user behaves. Mitchell and Cormack (1998, p. 102) note that users are most likely to be abused sexually: where the practitioner's general behaviour is anti-social or domineering; if the practitioner works alone; if there are drug and/or alcohol problems and/or other sources of distress in the practitioner's life; and if the practitioner can rationalise that it is acceptable to use the therapeutic relationship for intimacy. Clients who are 'excessively dependent' are the most likely to be sexually abused by practitioners, as are clients who feel sorry for the practitioner or who have a need to please the practitioner. People who have suffered sexual, physical or emotional abuse at other times in their lives are particularly vulnerable to an abusive dynamic in the therapeutic relationship (Mitchell and Cormack, 1998, p. 103).

Complaints

The issue of complaints is uncomfortable for any health practitioner. CAM practitioners may be particularly reluctant to accept that their actions may give rise to complaints. Since many therapists do not perceive their therapy to be intrinsically harmful, they are unlikely to make provision for when it goes wrong. Moreover, the comparative absence of litigation against CAM practitioners may give a false sense of security, whereby therapists do not consider themselves above the law but see the law as of little concern to them. Similarly, the lack of power of many professional bodies in CAM means that practitioners may not believe they will be dealt with harshly, even if they are subjected to a formal complaint by a patient (Stone, 2002, p. 199).

Many therapists are reluctant to accept the idea that there can ever be failed therapeutic relationships. When a person consults a therapist only once and returns, the practitioner may assume this is a testament to their therapeutic skills. In the absence of a widespread audit of practice, few practitioners follow up why a patient has not returned. Although the comparative lack of complaints against CAM practitioners is encouraging, the following reasons may constrain dissatisfied individuals from expressing their concerns.

- The person may not know where or to whom to complain.
- The professional organisation of which the practitioner is a member may not have formal complaint procedures or the procedures may be very weak.

- The practitioner may not be a member of a professional organisation. Remember, there are very few 'protected titles' in CAM, so anyone can call themselves a 'masseur' or 'healer', and they do not need training to use such titles.
- The person may not be able to verbalise their complaint; for example, perhaps they felt threatened or uncomfortable. Therefore, it would be hard for them to present a firm case against the practitioner. Instead they may choose to 'vote with their feet' and not return for more treatment.
- The person may be embarrassed, especially if their concern is of a sexual nature or involves humiliation or threats.
- The amount of time and emotional energy a complaint takes may put people off following it through.
- Lack of expertise or knowledge may mean the person does not realise they are being treated in an incompetent or unprofessional way. This issue is very important in the diverse world of CAM where, with over 200 modalities available, few people know precisely what to expect from treatment.
- People may not want to initiate a complaint against someone they get on well with. Even when the therapy fails to deliver results or causes harm, people may be less likely to complain when they believe the therapist is fundamentally a good person.

The statutory bodies regulating osteopathy and chiropractic spend a considerable amount of their energy facilitating complaints from the public and investigating alleged practitioner abuses. The websites of some CAM professional organisations explicitly advise people how to bring a complaint (see, for example, General Chiropractic Council, 2004; General Osteopathic Council, 2004). In these professions, most complaints are about lack of communication and poor interaction between the practitioner and the user. However, note that, even in well organised complaint systems such as these, many users are unlikely to complain when they are unhappy because of the reasons outlined above.

9.7   The future of the therapeutic relationship

As discussed earlier in this chapter and in Chapter 8, therapeutic relationships are subject to constant review and reinterpretation. As the culture changed, the predominant shift in health care was away from paternalistic forms of relationships based on professional expertise towards partnership models in which the patient has more rights but also more responsibilities. This final section looks to the future and considers some of the factors that can impact on therapeutic relationships in CAM.

Integration

One factor which is already influencing the nature of the therapeutic relationship is the move towards greater **integration** with orthodox medicine. Whether or not CAM practitioners welcome this development, it is inevitable. The impetus for this is partly about providing health care that gives patient satisfaction, and also stemming the tide of the spiralling costs of hi-tech, orthodox medicine and medical litigation. Stacey (1988) points out that, when the state funds parts of the nation's health care, it has interests in the accountability of the practitioners in terms of costs as well as outcomes of treatment. Therefore, the structural and organisational changes within the NHS will impact much more directly on CAM, including:

- the introduction of auditing and risk management procedures
- the development of more effective complaints mechanisms
- improvements in accreditation
- moves to enhance the public protection functions of self-regulatory bodies
- a commitment to evidence-based practice.

How will this affect the therapeutic relationship? There could be a far greater emphasis on the safety and effectiveness of CAM than is currently the case. Integration is already prompting more funding for research into CAM. This will, in turn, influence training and practice, so that those aspects of practice which enhance good therapeutic outcomes are maximised, and those aspects which place patients in jeopardy are minimised.

Litigation

The level of litigation against CAM therapists is currently very low, particularly compared with corresponding actions being brought against doctors and other health care professionals. This, in turn, is reflected by the low annual indemnity insurance paid by most CAM practitioners. CAM therapists tend to attribute this to CAM's safety profile compared with orthodox medicine, together with CAM practitioners' ability to forge better therapeutic relationships with users. However, other commentators argue that the lack of litigation, as with the lack of formal complaints, is more indicative of shortcomings in the legal system (Stone and Matthews, 1996). As suggested above, psychological and institutional barriers may prohibit a patient from complaining. An additional reason that may currently make people disinclined to sue a practitioner is their unwillingness to litigate against a person with whom they have had a close relationship. Yet people seem to have fewer qualms about suing the NHS, which is a more remote bureaucracy. Paradoxically, litigation rates may increase if CAM is provided by conventionally trained practitioners or on the NHS.

Fear of litigation has already altered the nature of the therapeutic relationship in medicine. Two ways in which this happens is through 'defensive medicine' and a highly legalistic approach to information giving and obtaining informed consent. The nature of the CAM relationship could similarly change if litigation rates increased.

Scientific advances

Advances in science may have dramatic effects on future therapeutic relationships. As specific funding becomes available for testing CAM, and as CAM practitioners start accepting the idea that their future sustainability may depend on them citing scientific research to establish their claims, more information will become available about which aspects of the therapeutic relationship are more, or less, beneficial. This may include research testing the hypothesis that elements of the CAM therapeutic relationship evoke a particularly powerful placebo response in certain conditions. In this case, both CAM practitioners and orthodox practitioners could learn how to harness the placebo effect in addition to the specific effects of treatment. Similarly, developments in psychoneuroimmunology and quantum physics may begin to provide answers to questions which, until now, have been elusive. They could explain how energy-based practices work, or provide a basis for explanatory models for CAM that oppose conventional scientific thinking (for example, providing a theoretical basis for homoeopathy).

9.8   Conclusion

All therapeutic relationships can harm as well as heal. In orthodox medicine, the bulk of the responsibility is placed on the doctor, because healing is attributed to specific effects brought about through the doctor's diagnostic and technical expertise. In CAM relationships, where users are expected to exercise self-responsibility, it may be inappropriate to focus solely on the shortcomings of the therapist (even though the law is unlikely to recognise mutual responsibilities when therapy goes wrong). That said, it is the therapist's responsibility to create the necessary conditions and boundaries for healing to occur. Despite CAM's user-centred rhetoric, holism can be as disempowering for users as reductionism. Dominant ideas link healing with the removal of physical symptoms. Conversely, harmful treatments tend to be associated with direct physical harm. However, harm can take several forms and be emotional as well as physical. While total failures of the therapeutic relationship are comparatively rare, therapeutic relationships can fail to achieve their potential in several ways. Despite the high levels of satisfaction in CAM, the absence of complaints is no cause for complacency; it may indicate that existing regulatory frameworks are ill suited to respond to the holistic relationship. It remains to be seen how shifts towards more integrated patterns of delivery, and scientific advances in understanding the link between mind and body, will affect the therapeutic relationship in the future.

KEY POINTS

- CAM practitioners are not equally successful in forming healing therapeutic relationships. This can be because of personality and temperament but also through lack of training.

- Despite a professed commitment to holism, practitioners may impose their own world views on patients. Being holistic is not synonymous with being user-centred, and practising holistically does not guarantee that practitioners will consider users' views of their bodies and illnesses.

- CAM theories may offer new ways of understanding the body, which may or may not be helpful to users.

- Therapeutic relationships that heal can also harm. The ways in which therapeutic relationships fail include: failing to deliver a desired outcome; failing to achieve the conditions in which healing can occur; and abusing trust.

- Debates about placebo will continue to divide the supporters and detractors of CAM. Advances in psychoneuroimmunology will increasingly shed light on the ways in which the mind can directly influence the body.

References

Armstrong, D. (1987) 'Silence and truth in death and dying', *Social Science and Medicine*, Vol. 24, No. 8, pp. 651–7.

Armstrong, D. (1993) 'Public health spaces and the fabrication of identity', *Sociology*, Vol. 27, No. 3, pp. 393–410.

Budd, S. and Sharma, U. (1994) *The Healing Bond: The Patient–Practitioner Relationship and Therapeutic Responsibility*, London, Routledge.

Busby, H. (1996) 'Alternative medicines/alternative knowledges: putting flesh on the bones using traditional Chinese approaches to healing', in Cant, S. and Sharma, U. (eds) *Complementary and Alternative Medicines: Knowledge in Practice*, pp. 135–50, London, Free Association Books.

Coulter, A. (1999) 'Paternalism or partnership?', *British Medical Journal*, Vol. 319, pp. 719–20.

Coward, R. (1990) *The Whole Truth*, London, Faber and Faber.

Department of Health (DoH) (1999) *Mental Health National Service Frameworks*, London, DoH.

Department of Health (DoH) (2001) *The Expert Patient: A New Approach to Chronic Disease Management for the 21st Century*, London, DoH.

Doyal, L. and Pennell, I. (1979) *The Political Economy of Health*, London, Pluto Press.

Engels, G. (1980) 'The clinical application of the biopsychosocial model', *American Journal of Psychiatry*, Vol. 137, pp. 535–44.

Evans, D. (2003) *Placebo, The Belief Effect*, London, HarperCollins.

Fitzpatrick, M. (2000) *The Tyranny of Health: Doctors and the Regulation of Lifestyle*, London, Routledge.

Foucault, M. (1973) *The Birth of the Clinic: An Archaeology of Medical Perception*, New York, Vintage Books.

General Chiropractic Council (2004) website: www.gcc.org/page.cfm [accessed 18 September 2004].

General Osteopathic Council (2004) website: www.osteopathy.org.uk [accessed 18 September 2004].

Greenhalgh, T. and Hurwitz, B. (1998) *Narrative-based Medicine: Dialogue and Discourse in Clinical Practice*, London, BMJ Books.

Hay, L. (1984) *You Can Health Your Life*, Karlsbad, Hay House.

Jehu, D. (1994) *Patients as Victims: Sexual Abuse in Psychotherapy and Counselling*, London, Wiley.

Kelner, M., Wellman, B., Pescosolido, B. and Saks, M. (eds) (2000) *Complementary and Alternative Medicine: Challenge and Change*, Amsterdam, Harwood Academic Publishers.

Lee-Treweek, G. (2003) *Explaining and Managing the Body in Complementary and Alternative Medicine*, Paper given at the second Global Conference on Health and Disease, St Hilda's, University of Oxford, July 2003.

Mitchell, A. and Cormack, M. (1998) *The Therapeutic Relationship in Complementary Health Care*, Edinburgh, Churchill Livingstone.

Nouwen, H. (1977) *The Wounded Healer: Ministry in Contemporary Society*, New York, Doubleday.

Oerton, S. (2004) 'Bodywork boundaries: power, politics and professionalism in therapeutic massage', *Gender, Work and Organization*, Vol. 11, No. 5, pp. 544–65.

O'Rourke, A. (2000) *Patient Satisfaction*, Sheffield, The Wisdom Centre. Available online: www.shef.ac.uk/uni/projects/wrp/cgptsat.htm.

Peters, D. (2001) *Understanding the Placebo Effect in Complementary Medicine*, Edinburgh, Churchill Livingstone.

Pietroni, P. and Chase, H. D. (1993) 'Partners or partisans?', *British Journal of General Practice*, Vol. 43, No. 373, pp. 341–4.

POPAN (Prevention of Professional Abuse Network) (2000) *Annual Report*, London, POPAN. Available online: www.popan.org.uk.

Pope, K. S. and Vetter, V. A. (1991) 'Prior therapist–patient sexual involvement among patients seen by psychologists', *Psychotherapy*, Vol. 28, pp. 429–38.

Pringle, M. and Tyreman, S. (1993) 'Study of 500 patients attending an osteopathic practice', *British Journal of General Practice*, Vol. 43, No. 366, pp. 15–18.

Rutter, P. (1990) *Sex in the Forbidden Zone*, London, Unwin.

Sharma, U. (1992, revised 1994) *Complementary Medicine Today: Practitioners and Patients*, London, Routledge.

Stacey (1988) *The Sociology of Health and Healing*, London, Unwin Hyman.

Stone, J. (2002) *An Ethical Framework for Complementary and Alternative Therapists*, London, Routledge.

Stone, J. and Matthews, J. (1996) *Complementary Medicine and the Law*, Oxford, Oxford University Press.

Zollman, C. and Vickers, A. (1999) 'ABC of complementary medicine. Complementary medicine and the patient', *British Medical Journal*, Vol. 319, pp. 1486–9.

Chapter 10   CAM in supportive and palliative cancer care

Jeanne Katz

Contents

AIMS

- To discuss the various ways in which complementary and alternative therapies are used by people with cancer.
- To debate the contested issues influencing the use and acceptance of CAM for people with cancer.
- To understand the ways in which 'holism' is embraced by palliative care and by CAM.
- To consider the research on the use of CAM in cancer and palliative care.

10.1   Introduction

Chapters 6 to 9 described the patterns of complementary and alternative medicine (CAM) use and some reasons why people consult CAM practitioners. This chapter investigates why CAM may appeal particularly to people with cancer and dying people. Cancer was chosen to exemplify some of the issues addressed in earlier chapters because it is a disease in which the biomedical response is sometimes dramatic and drastic (depending on the site and nature of the disease). People who are given orthodox cancer treatments (such as radiotherapy or chemotherapy) undergo major life changes: they may be unable to work; their appearance changes; and they may perceive a considerable reduction in their quality of life – they may feel ill or lack energy, and may experience psychological and emotional reactions. In some situations CAM purports to redress some of these symptoms and aims to improve quality of life and mood, and to reduce feelings of discomfort. The central questions explored in this chapter are:

■   What is it about CAM that may appeal to people with cancer?
■   What is it about cancer (or cancer treatment) that can stimulate some people with the condition to look for alternative or additional treatment to biomedicine?
■   Which CAM treatments are perceived as most beneficial by people with cancer?

10.2   CAM use by people with cancer

People consult CAM practitioners primarily for chronic conditions. However, studies from many countries have revealed that many cancer patients also access CAM – a higher proportion than people with other conditions (Ernst, 2004), and this is increasing (Cassileth et al., 2001). A systematic review of 13 countries indicated that 7 to 64 per cent of those surveyed had tried complementary therapies, an average of 31 per cent (Ernst and Cassileth, 1998; Burstein et al., 1999). In the UK, a study in Southampton showed that 32 per cent of people with cancer sought CAM treatment in a variety of settings (Lewith et al., 2002). Several studies note higher CAM use among people with cancer who have more physical discomfort and more progressive disease (Burstein et al., 1999; Paltiel et al., 2001), but also for palliative reasons when the cancer is no longer expected to be cured by conventional medicine.

     People with cancer use a variety of CAM modalities. Cassileth et al. (2001) note that the most commonly used therapies 'included dietary treatments, herbs, homeopathy, hypnotherapy, imagery/visualization, meditation, megavitamins, relaxation, and spiritual healing' (p. 1390). A study in the USA surveyed 356 patients with colon, breast or prostate cancer. It showed that most people with cancer used at least one type of alternative medicine (Patterson et al., 2002). Even though this study was in Washington State, where health insurance covers the expenses of licensed alternative providers, its findings are extremely interesting:

> Overall, 70.2% of patients used at least one type of alternative medicine, with 16.6% seeing alternative providers, 19.1% using mental/other therapy, and 64.6% taking dietary supplements. Compared to males, females were

five times more likely to see an alternative provider and about twice as likely to use mental therapies or supplements ... Older patients were less likely to use mental/other therapy. Higher education (but not income) was associated with use of all types of alternative medicine. Patients with multiple medical treatments were two times more likely to take dietary supplements compared to patients having only surgery ... Varying by the type of alternative therapy, 83%–97% of patients reported that they used alternative medicine for general health and well-being, while 8% to 56% reported use for treatment of cancer. Almost all patients reported that the alternative therapy improved their well-being. Expenditures for alternative medicine averages $68 per user per year, but ranged from $4 to $14,659.

(Patterson et al., 2002, p. 477)

A study in Israel which explored CAM use by people with cancer had similar results (Paltiel et al., 2001). Of 1000 cancer outpatients surveyed, 51.2 per cent had used CAM since cancer was diagnosed, while 35 per cent had accessed CAM in the previous three months. CAM use was positively associated with women, those between 35 and 59 years old with advanced disease, those who had received higher education, and those attending support groups or individual counselling. Oneschuk et al. (1998), in their first Canadian study, also found that more women and more highly educated people use CAM. The most commonly used CAM products were herbs, shark cartilage and vitamins. In their second, smaller study (2000) they noted that only two non-ingested therapies were accessed: reiki and acupuncture.

The diagnosis of particular types of cancer may predispose people to turn to CAM. For example, several studies document high CAM usage by women with breast cancer (Lengacher et al., 2003) and men with prostate cancer (Salmenpera, 2002). In Finland, 33 per cent of women with breast cancer and 28 per cent of men with prostate cancer were reported to use CAM after diagnosis (Salmenpera, 2002). The figure for men is surprisingly high, bearing in mind that other studies suggest that men with cancer are five times less likely than women to access CAM (Patterson et al., 2002). In the UK, Rees et al. (2000) sent a postal questionnaire to over 1000 women diagnosed with breast cancer in the previous seven years to ascertain the prevalence and costs of complementary therapy. They found that nearly 33 per cent of their respondents had consulted a CAM practitioner since diagnosis, compared with 22.4 per cent in the previous year. The women with breast cancer used massage, aromatherapy, osteopathy, chiropractic, relaxation, meditation, and spiritual and faith healing.

The studies cited above provide evidence that people with cancer frequently consult CAM practitioners. The next section examines the reasons why people with cancer may choose CAM. It is important to remember that there are different kinds of cancer: some respond well to minimally invasive treatment (for example, some skin cancers); some respond well to targeted chemotherapy; others require radical treatment or sometimes extensive surgery (for example, breast and oral cancers). This chapter focuses mostly on the more serious, life-threatening types of cancer.

10.3   Why do people with cancer turn to CAM?

This section explores why people with cancer are attracted to CAM. You will consider your own views, then explore those proposed by a palliative care physician, and then examine research evidence. But first, it is important to differentiate between 'complementary' and 'alternative' medicine and possible differences in how they relate to cancer therapies. Vickers and Cassileth note that:

> 'Alternative' therapies typically are invasive and biologically active and are commonly promoted for use instead of, rather than as an adjunct to, mainstream therapy. Conversely, 'complementary' therapies are used together with mainstream care for management of symptoms and to improve quality of life. This distinction is especially important in oncology [cancer care], in which alternative methods are promoted as literal alternatives to conventional care.
>
> (Vickers and Cassileth, 2001, p. 226)

Throughout the literature, alternative therapies that purport to cure cancer are differentiated from complementary therapies that aim to relieve symptoms and work alongside orthodox medicine (for example, Tavares, 2003).

ACTIVITY   WHAT IS THE APPEAL OF CAM TO PEOPLE WITH CANCER?

Allow 10 minutes

In your opinion, why do many people with cancer use CAM? (You could draw on some factors described in earlier chapters.)

Comment

Your response may have included some of the following points.

- People with cancer may think that conventional medical treatment is not fast enough and want to do something immediately.
- CAM appears to offer comfort and symptom relief, whereas orthodox cancer treatment can be invasive, painful and cause side effects such as nausea, tiredness, anxiety or stress.
- People with cancer may be undergoing therapies with very unpleasant side effects and may choose to complement these therapies with something to enhance their quality of life.

- They may reject what biomedicine offers in terms of treatment and choose an alternative modality instead, which may concur more with their own beliefs about health and healing.

- People who have had radiotherapy or chemotherapy which did not cure their cancer may choose to try another route in the hope of a cure.

- Some alternative therapies may offer the hope of a cure.

- People with cancer may be frustrated with their relationships with orthodox health care providers and seek treatments where they hope their voice will be heard.

- They may be encouraged by friends and relatives, who have had positive experiences with particular modalities, to turn to CAM.

- The philosophy of CAM is perceived to be holistic (it relies on the body's ability to heal itself) and allows individuals some autonomy over the disease and its treatment.

Cancer physicians (oncologists) recognise the limitations, and possibly the drastic impact, of some forms of orthodox treatment for people with cancer. Many also recognise that such people are attracted to CAM. For example, Irene Higginson, a professor of palliative care, maintains:

- That patients experience symptoms of distress which conventional medicine is failing to recognize and treat.

- That practitioners of complementary medicine prey on individuals at a time when they are vulnerable, advocating untested therapies and taking the scarce resources (time and money) that patients and families have left to them.

- That complementary therapies offer important hope to individuals who have exhausted the resources of conventional medicine: 'at worst they do no harm, so why not give them a go'.

- Perhaps patients are seeking therapies whose effectiveness, though not proven is also **not disproven**, offering new hope when the 'magic' of conventional medicine has faded.

(Higginson, 2003, p. 427)

Higginson illustrates a rather mixed view of CAM. She alludes, as do many other physicians, to the potential monetary exploitation of people with cancer by those promising 'curative treatments'. However, she, like others, acknowledges that conventional health care providers may not address some symptoms of distress which people with cancer have. Michelle Kohn's report (1999) about CAM use in cancer care extends some of Higginson's assumptions, proposing an explanatory model around 'pull' and 'push' factors to explain why people may resort to using CAM (see Box 10.1).

BOX 10.1   REASONS FOR CHOOSING CAM

Orthodox medicine – 'push' factors

- Failure to produce curative treatments
- Adverse effects of orthodox medicine, e.g. chemotherapy side effects
- Lack of time with practitioner, loss of bedside skills
- Dissatisfaction with the technical approach
- Fragmentation of care due to specialisation

Complementary therapies – 'pull' factors

- Media reports of dramatic improvements produced by complementary therapies
- Belief that these therapies are natural
- Empowerment of patient through lifestyle and psychological equilibrium
- Focus on spiritual and emotional well-being
- Provision by therapist of 'touch, talk and time'

(Source: Kohn, 1999, p. 6)

The three different sets of explanations described in this chapter overlap and many resemble those for overall CAM use, described in Chapter 7. Most studies of CAM use among people with cancer reveal that **complementary health care is used alongside conventional medicine** in the same way as with other conditions (see Chapter 7).

Researchers suggest that cancer patients access CAM for three main reasons:

1 for symptom relief (Oneschuk et al., 1998; Pan et al., 2000; Cassileth et al., 2001)

2 to improve quality of life (Cassileth et al., 2001)

3 to lengthen their lives (Oneschuk et al., 1998).

CAM therapy (for example, relaxation and massage) may be used for any or all of these reasons. Before exploring the main reasons, there are three important additional reasons to consider: congruence of belief systems, searching for a cure, and seeking good therapeutic relationships.

Congruence of belief systems

The implications of post-modern values for health behaviour and different aspects of health beliefs were considered in earlier chapters. O'Callaghan and Jordan (2003) suggest that people who subscribe to post-modern values may be attracted to CAM because of the congruence of their belief systems with the underlying philosophies of many therapies. In their study, while post-modern values as a whole were associated with positive attitudes towards

CAM, natural remedies, rejection of authority and age contributed significantly to whether people could be predicted to use CAM. 'Natural remedies' involve the belief that CAM products are safer and more effective than prescribed drugs, which had negative side effects. 'Rejection of authority' implies that users should have some input to their care and participate actively in the healing process (O'Callaghan and Jordan, 2003).

Searching for a cure

Some people with cancer turn to alternative therapies instead of conventional medicine, or even in addition to it, in the hope of being cured. Yates et al. (1993) studied 152 patients with metastatic cancer (that is, cancer which has spread from the primary tumour) and reported that those using alternative therapies differed in some of their social attitudes, primarily in that they scored higher on the 'will to live' scale than those who did not seek alternative treatments.

Barrie Cassileth and her colleagues (2001) conducted an international survey in 33 countries to establish which alternative therapies people with cancer turned to for a cure (see Table 10.1).

TABLE 10.1 ALTERNATIVE THERAPIES FOR CANCER				
Diets and supplements	**Botanicals**	**Unconventional agents**	**Traditional medicine**	**Energy healing and other**
Gerson diet	Sun herbal compound	Shark cartilage, aleta de tiburon (shark fin)	Acupuncture	Magnetic fields
Macrobiotic diet	Bitter cucumber	Chelation	Curanderos	Homoeopathy
The Bristol diet	Traditional Chinese herbs	Autologous-targeted cytokines	Brujos	Naturopathy
High dose vitamins	Aloe vera	714X (Gaston Naessens)	Qi gong	Alevizatos treatment
Selenium	Reishi mushroom	Hasumi vaccine (made from patient's urine)	–	Kamateros spring water
Trace minerals	Rodent tuber	Di Bella therapy (somatostatin, bromocriptine, cyclophosphamide, and multi-vitamins)	–	Detoxification with diets and enemas

(Source: adapted from Cassileth et al., 2001, p. 1392)

The most frequently used therapies were dietary therapies, vitamins, botanical drugs and shark products. The authors explain why these were used:

> Alternative therapies (such as the regimen developed at the Gerson Clinic in Tijuana, laetrile, shark cartilage, or the Di Bella therapy) are active biologically, often invasive, and typically promoted as cancer treatment to be used **instead** of mainstream therapy.
>
> (Cassileth et al., 2001, p. 1390)

A more caring relationship

Many people use CAM because it is an opportunity to discuss their health problems in depth. Undoubtedly, the time given in CAM often exceeds that available in biomedical clinics. This mirrors the situation in consultations in the private sector where the attraction of time spent with the practitioner is also cited as an important reason for choosing to pay (Calnan et al., 1993). This reason for choosing CAM applies particularly to people with cancer who may feel they have disjointed relationships with health care providers as a result of having to attend several centres for different kinds of investigation and treatment. Health workers and people with cancer alike may complain that there is not enough time for proper interactions. However, the issue of whether the therapeutic relationship has a different or special meaning when the patient has a life-threatening illness raises the following questions.

- What does 'therapeutic' mean in the cancer context?
- Is cancer different from other health contexts (that is, does the fact that the illness may be life-threatening affect the nature of the relationship)?
- What are the ingredients of a therapeutic relationship for a person with cancer?

The answers to these questions may include:

- protected space and time, being heard, quality of ambience or surroundings
- unconditional, non-judgemental approach
- equality, respect and acceptance
- clarity, awareness of and transparency of agenda(s)
- having a particular need addressed
- clear boundaries.

The next section briefly explores the meanings of cancer in western societies, in order to understand why people with cancer may seek a more intense relationship with their health providers.

10.4   Experiences of cancer and health care

Media reports suggest that most people respond to a diagnosis of cancer with more alarm than to other conditions. A diagnosis of cancer for many people can seem like a death sentence, regardless of the stage (the extent to which it has developed or spread) or where it is in the body. The impact on the person and their family can disrupt normal dynamics and create new barriers as well as open up opportunities to consider their lives and relationships.

ACTIVITY   RESPONSES TO A DIAGNOSIS OF CANCER

Allow 1 hour

Reactions to a cancer diagnosis may be different from reactions to diagnoses of other diseases. Ask your friends, family or colleagues to describe how they think people respond to hearing that they have cancer. You need to be careful about who you ask, as cancer may be a reality for them. Ask them to differentiate between life-threatening and curable cancers. Make a list of their responses.

Comment

Your list might include the following responses.

- Cancer can be curable and, in that respect, is no different from some other diseases or illnesses.
- Cancer can be life-threatening.
- Cancer has a tendency to recur, sometimes in another part of the body.
- Cancer itself, or the treatment for it, could affect people's normal functioning (for example, chemotherapy can affect fertility).
- People with cancer may feel stigmatised.
- Cancer equals uncertainty in many spheres of people's lives.
- Cancer could have a destructive impact on personal relationships; alternatively, it could have a positive effect.
- Cancer treatment can be painful and/or sick-making.
- Becoming a cancer 'patient' can be infantilising.
- A diagnosis of cancer can precipitate many difficult emotions, such as anger.

Although many types of cancer are curable and not necessarily painful, the media frequently focus on pain, discomfort and even mutilation, intimating that physical degeneration and possibly loss of control over bodily functions are usually followed by death. For people diagnosed with cancer and with some other life-threatening diseases, life as an indefinite given becomes uncertain and a variety of fears and concerns enter their lives. Profound physical and emotional difficulties and stress may arise from both the illness and its treatment, which can be episodic or ongoing.

Cancer remains a dominant fear in western societies, where many fatal infectious diseases such as smallpox have been almost eradicated (although not, for example, HIV or the 'superbug' MRSA). Helman (2001) notes that people's experiences, as well as their cultural background, suggest that different diseases hold different symbolic meanings for them. Beliefs about what causes cancer are wide-ranging and include inhaling bad air and many other rational, as well as what may seem irrational, explanations (rationality being individually defined) (Sontag, 1978; Helman, 2001). Views about the origins of cancer vary enormously between different cultures, and people who live in English-speaking countries but originate from elsewhere may hold different views from people from the host societies.

Many studies demonstrate that how people are told that they have a disease, particularly cancer, affects interpersonal interactions with health workers thereafter (for example, Seale et al., 1997). In the mid-20th century the paternalistic model of the doctor–patient relationship predominated. Doctors used euphemisms such as 'warts' and 'cysts' when 'breaking the news' that people had cancer. Many people were unaware of the correct diagnosis, sometimes even until they died. Physicians believed that telling people they had cancer would eliminate hope, which might demotivate them from having the treatment that physicians were certain they needed. Revealing the diagnosis to patients is now standard practice in the UK, following the trend set in the USA. However, there are still reports of diagnosis and/or prognosis being withheld.

10.5 What do people with cancer need?

ACTIVITY THE NEEDS OF PEOPLE WITH CANCER

Allow 30 minutes

You may know someone who has or had cancer. Considering the different needs of the 'patient' and his or her 'carers':

- Who, apart from the 'patient', has needs?
- How may these needs be met?

Comment

There are many people who may have needs, including the main family carer, other family members and, in particular, dependent family members (elderly parents or children).

Constructive care planning is one way of meeting these needs, which might include any or all of the following factors.

- **Time** to talk about their illness and to be heard, especially by someone who is not personally involved and who will not be hurt or upset.

- **Physical concerns**, including pain, nausea, constipation, menopausal symptoms, and lack of energy.
- **Mental or emotional concerns**, including, most commonly, tension and anxiety but also depression, unresolved guilt, anger and loneliness.
- **Stress management**, including the need for relaxation, and the fear of needles or hospital.
- **Advice**, for example about self-help strategies.
- **Relationship difficulties** are common, including issues about sex.
- **Body image problems.**

(Source: Andrew Manasse, Cavendish Centre, personal communication)

For many people diagnosed with cancer the initial goal is to seek curative treatment. The information about what is wrong with them may be delivered by a variety of people, from the hospital specialist (for example, surgeon), who may refer them to a specialist radiotherapist or oncologist, or back to their GP, who has received some test results.

A diagnosis of cancer can cause confusion and distress and there are often conflicting suggestions and advice from family members, colleagues and acquaintances. These may include consulting a particular specialist, possibly in another area; seeing a consultant privately to expedite care; going to a holistic practitioner; and so on. Sometimes self-help support groups or alternative therapists are contacted, often by a well-meaning friend, and the plethora of information to absorb can be overwhelming.

Some physicians ask the person with cancer to decide or make choices at the point of diagnosis, most often about whether to have treatment once the implications have been explained. Cancer is often described as a journey, possibly because there are many stopping-off points and changes of direction. Also, as each cycle of treatment is completed there may be another barrage of tests, as further information is revealed about the success or failure of the last treatment regime. Treatments may vary considerably, even for the same diagnostic category: depending on where the tumour is and how far it has spread, a person may be offered radiotherapy or chemotherapy or both, at different times.

Therefore, people with cancer may have many hurdles to jump and sometimes a choice of treatment options. Increasingly, one option is whether to consider complementary and/or alternative therapies, either instead of or alongside conventional treatment. These could be options at any stage in the process, from first diagnosis to the final stages of terminal illness, and may address several concerns.

The world of cancer treatment is partly populated by physicians whose primary goal is to cure and for whom the main, but not the only, success factor is 'markers' and other scientific indicators that the treatment has arrested the disease. Increasingly, however, oncologists acknowledge the importance of quality of life issues and patient choice and refer people with cancer to CAM practitioners for a variety of treatments: for example, relaxation or touch therapies.

Table 10.2 lists the concerns of 157 people with cancer, according to several categories, who were seen at the Cavendish Centre in Sheffield.

TABLE 10.2   PATIENTS' EXPRESSED CONCERNS

Group	Concern	Number	Total	%
Physical	Pain	17	53	29
	Poor sleep	11		
	Menopausal symptoms	9		
	Exhaustion	9		
	Various physical	4		
	Lymphoedema	1		
	Nausea/vomiting	1		
Emotional	Anxiety, fear, panic, uncertainty	32	59	33
	Relationship problems	9		
	Depression, unhappiness	7		
	Unresolved feelings: guilt, anger, loss of dignity	7		
	Loneliness, isolation	2		
	Bereavement	1		
	Body image	1		
Stress management	Need for relaxation	20	34	19
	Stress	12		
	Needle phobia	1		
General support	General coping	7	12	7
	Need to be listened to	2		
	Coming to terms with the experience of cancer	2		
	Need to keep going	1		
Hospital treatment related	Worry related to hospital treatment including physical and emotional effects	12	12	7
Help with positive outlook	Self-help strategies	9	9	5
Total*			179	100

*Total = 179; that is, more than 157 because some patients voiced more than one concern.

(Source: Andrew Manasse, Cavendish Centre, personal communication)

While agreeing that some **complementary** therapies could provide relief, the medical establishment traditionally has been sceptical about 'unproven and unscientific' claims of **alternative** therapies (for example, Barnett, 2001). There is concern that people with cancer are hoodwinked, by 'quacks' practising alternative therapies, into believing that certain non-conventional treatments might 'cure' their cancer. These people may be persuaded to use their life savings to buy 'cures' and thus be financially exploited. Examples of 'non-proven' treatments include colonic irrigation and laetrile (see Section 10.7). The concern is about (a) the lack of regulation of complementary therapists; (b) the potential 'dangers' of these therapies, particularly when combined with conventional therapies; and, as noted above, (c) the potential economic exploitation of people with cancer.

The CancerBACUP information service acknowledges these tensions and advises patients:

> Some treatments included in alternative therapies have caused a conflict of views between doctors and alternative therapists. In general, doctors do not believe that there is valid scientific evidence available that these alternative treatments can cure cancer or slow its growth. They are concerned that certain therapies may give patients false hope and occasionally may even be harmful. Doctors also worry that patients may turn away from conventional treatments that could help them. People with cancer can be very vulnerable and there have been cases when people have been misled by promises of a miracle cure.
>
> (CancerBACUP, 2004)

Some people with cancer choose not to inform their medical practitioners of CAM use because they fear being labelled 'bad' or 'non-cooperative' patients. Sometimes they withhold information from the CAM practitioners about the conventional medicine they are taking. Clearly, it is the user's right to decide who to tell what, but a lack of openness could lead to medical complications with the orthodox medication they are taking.

It is important to note that complementary or alternative therapies for cancer are not available everywhere. Therefore, patient choice can be limited not only by financial factors but also by availability of a particular modality in a geographical area.

The next section considers the development of palliative care in the UK. This arose precisely because of a perception that people with cancer, and particularly those nearing death, were receiving poor health care and were isolated and their needs were not being met.

10.6   What is palliative care?

Palliative care is a relatively new health speciality. It emerged in the second half of the 20th century, initially in the voluntary sector. It was subsequently mainstreamed into the National Health Service (NHS). It was developed for people with cancer and, to a large extent, this disease category still dominates palliative care provision. In the NHS, supportive and palliative cancer care is offered in several settings, including tertiary centres, acute hospitals and in the community. The people providing the services include oncologists, specialists in palliative care, psychologists, GPs, counsellors in primary care, specialist nurses and community nurses.

Dame Cecily Saunders pioneered palliative care in the UK. Having seen the poor conditions in which people died of cancer in London hospitals, she strove to ensure not only that dying people received adequate pain relief but also that their social and emotional needs were addressed. She coined the phrase **total pain**, which encompasses physical, social, emotional, practical and spiritual needs (see Figure 10.1). She founded the modern hospice movement with the opening of St Christopher's Hospice in Sydenham, Kent, England in 1967. St Christopher's was designed to integrate research, teaching and inpatient care and became a flagship for the rapidly developing international hospice movement.

The terms 'hospice' and 'palliative care' are used in different ways in different countries. In the UK, hospice usually implies a building or a dedicated unit, and a palliative care service could be domiciliary or sited in another organisation (such as a hospital). In the USA, there are few

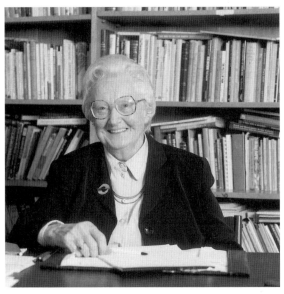

Dame Cecily Saunders, the pioneer of palliative care as a medical speciality

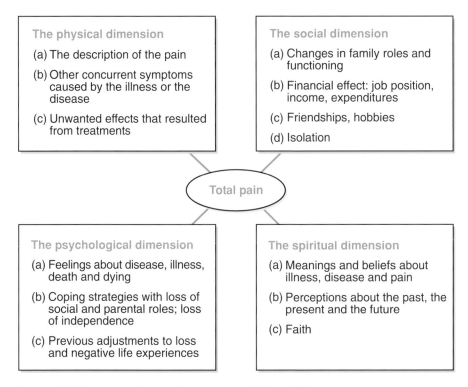

Figure 10.1 Total pain (Source: Payne et al., 2004, p. 279)

dedicated hospice inpatient units: hospice usually means a domiciliary service run by a multidisciplinary team.

Most hospice services in the UK started as – and have remained – domiciliary services; some developed into purpose-built facilities providing other services such as day care (Katz and Peace, 2003, p. 4). Fundraising for palliative care services was initially spearheaded by dedicated volunteers, many of whom had themselves observed painful deaths from cancer. Like CAM, palliative care services developed in an unplanned way (often through voluntary action). This is why the range of services is not evenly spread throughout the UK. The NHS has attempted to redress inequities in service provision, primarily with the help of Macmillan Cancer Relief, which has helped finance the building of many hospices. This charity also funds a variety of services, the most well-known being the Macmillan nurse (a specialist nurse who cares exclusively for people with cancer).

Palliative care services range from the multidisciplinary team staffed by combinations of palliative care physicians, specialist nurses, social workers, volunteers, physiotherapists, religious ministers and complementary therapists, to Macmillan nurses working on their own in community or hospital settings. Each service plans its workload and approach. Many services include CAM therapies, which are often provided by external staff or volunteers. The Hospice Information Service produces an annual guide to services, detailing the therapies or services that are available for palliative care provision in the UK. This gives contact details for the National Association of Complementary Therapists in Hospice and Palliative Care. Macmillan Cancer Relief has produced a guide to complementary therapies in palliative care (Kohn, 1999).

Definitions of palliative care are dynamic and regularly updated. The following one is suggested by the National Council for Hospice and Specialist Palliative Care Services.

> Palliative care is the active holistic care of patients with advanced, progressive illness. Management of pain and other symptoms and provision of psychological, social and spiritual support is paramount. The goal of palliative care is achievement of the best quality of life for patients and their families. Many aspects of palliative care are also applicable earlier in the course of the illness in conjunction with other treatments.
>
> (Tavares, 2003, p. 13)

Most palliative care organisations have the following aims.

1 To provide symptom control and pain relief for the dying person, avoiding inappropriate treatment.

2 To create a support system for dying people, providing social, emotional, spiritual and practical care in an individualised way, enabling them to exert control, independence and choice, an opportunity to live as actively as possible and participate in decisions relating to managing problems. This might include negotiating the most appropriate place to die (home, hospice or hospital).

3 To provide emotional, spiritual and practical care for the dying person's family and friends during the illness and after death (bereavement care).

4 To establish a team, with good communication between its members, including the dying person and his or her family.

5 To provide support and expert advice to those caring for dying people (the hospital team, GP, social worker, psychologist, district nurse, religious minister, dietician, complementary therapist, volunteer, chiropodist or physiotherapist), irrespective of whether the care is at home or in a hospital, residential home or hospice.

6 To research and provide education for those caring for dying people.

Similarities in status between palliative care and CAM

Dame Cecily's aim was to integrate palliative care into orthodox medical establishments but this was hard to achieve. In the same way as the contemporary medical establishment views CAM, much of what palliative care originally attempted to achieve was seen as 'soft' and not scientifically provable.

Eventually, however, it became a legitimate speciality in its own right. Even today, it is extremely difficult to undertake 'scientific' trials in palliative care (Grande and Todd, 2000). Some of the ethical problems, such as whether to start particular respondents on drug trials, resemble those of research in CAM.

There are other similarities between the approach of palliative care and many CAM therapies. For example, like CAM, palliative care recognises the principle of patient autonomy and strives to enable people to achieve the goals they set, improve their quality of life and respect their right to 'die with dignity'. Palliative care also strives to help people with cancer come to terms with the illness by enabling them to voice their concerns. This is also central to much of CAM practice. Palliative care, like CAM, uses the term 'holistic', the importance of which is increasingly being recognised (Chumpus and Hill, 1999; Grande and Todd, 2000). However, the perceptions of the term 'holism' differ somewhat when the total pain diagram (Figure 10.1) is compared with the much broader conceptual approach in CAM (Figure 10.2).

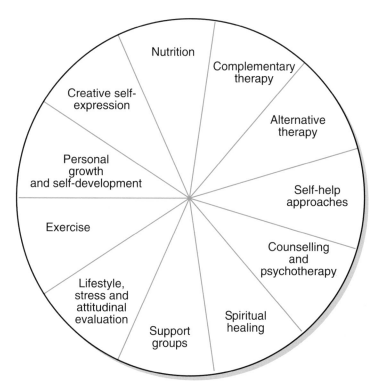

Figure 10.2 The holistic approach in complementary therapy
(Source: Daniel, 2001, p. 24)

Supportive and palliative care

The term 'supportive care' is enshrined in the NHS cancer plan (DoH, 2000) and demonstrates the government's stated commitment to seamless care and patient choice. It is intended to provide care for people with cancer and their families from the point of diagnosis, throughout the treatment programmes, and to include the terminal phase as well as bereavement care for informal carers. Basically, it encompasses the 'total care' that proponents of palliative care have striven to provide since the 1970s. It also positively embraces 'other' modes of health care in addition to traditional allopathic medicine.

Supportive care is a positive concept, which includes complementary therapies as one of nine services that can empower people with cancer and their carers to develop strategies for living with their cancer, and support them in the process. The following definition was developed by the National Council for Hospice and Specialist Palliative Care Services and is also proposed in the National Institute for Clinical Excellence consultation document (2002).

> Supportive care is that which helps the patient and their family to cope with cancer and the treatment of it – from pre-diagnosis through the process of diagnosis and treatment, to cure, continuing illness or death and into bereavement. It helps the patient to maximise the benefits of treatment and to live as well as possible with the effects of the disease. It is given equal priority alongside diagnosis and treatment.
>
> (Tavares, 2003, p. 14)

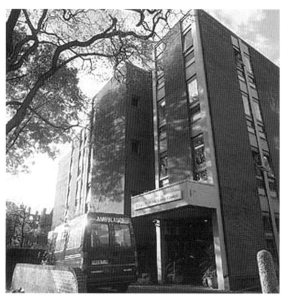

Edenhall Marie Curie Home is a hospice in north-west London where dying people can have a variety of complementary therapies to improve the quality of their final days

Many oncology units in general hospitals as well as hospices now provide CAM therapies for inpatients, outpatients and relatives (Kohn, 1999). Substantial numbers of hospice staff are trained in a variety of CAM therapies and use them when appropriate. Increasingly, health workers are interested in CAM as a way to provide symptomatic and emotional relief to people experiencing physical as well as mental distress.

10.7   Do CAM treatments meet users' expectations?

Section 10.3 explored why people with cancer turn to CAM. This section explores the evidence of whether their reasons for using CAM are addressed. The focus is on two aspects of meeting the needs of people with cancer. The first concerns those who use CAM to cure their cancer. The second is whether CAM use gives people with cancer relief from their symptoms and whether their quality of life is demonstrably improved.

Since the 1990s many studies have followed how people with cancer use CAM. Most included only small numbers in their research, therefore it is hard to draw conclusions (Barraclough, 2001). However, since 2000, several longitudinal studies have begun in the USA, funded by a variety of organisations, including the National Center for Complementary and Alternative Medicine (NCCAM), which is associated with the prestigious National Institutes for Health (NIH). These should, in time, produce evidence of whether specific CAM therapies produce the desired effect in people with cancer. Many of these trials are run at the Memorial Sloan-Kettering Hospital in New York City, one of the foremost cancer research centres in the world. It has a large, integrated, cancer care research centre where different therapies are used and followed scientifically in longitudinal studies (Zappa and Cassileth, 2003).

Where most orthodox cancer settings offer complementary therapies, the primary intention is to relieve physical symptoms and/or provide emotional comfort. Hence there is a clear division between providing therapies which offer 'care' as opposed to 'cure':

> These benefits – now supported by a considerable body of evidence – may be due partly to a specific effect of a particular therapy, and partly to general features: providing extra time and attention, offering more opportunity for active participation and choice, bringing positive meaning to the illness experience. The comparatively low costs of the therapies, and their relative freedom from toxic effects if correctly applied, would further support their use for improving 'quality of life'.
>
> (Barraclough, 2001, p. vi)

The rest of this section explores the evidence for the effectiveness of CAM in relation to (a) cure and (b) relief from symptoms in people with cancer.

CAM as a cure

Some people seek alternative treatments at the time of diagnosis or when orthodox treatments fail to cure them. Designing studies to examine the effectiveness of these treatments is methodologically difficult for many reasons: some relate to the different types of treatment using similar names and the different stages of disease in the people being studied. Kimby et al. (2003) carried out a study in Denmark, which highlights some of these issues and, in particular, notes that even unconventional treatments can be subcategorised into standardised and individualised treatments. Standardised treatments are offered to all people with cancer, whereas individualised treatment is offered on the basis of the therapist's more precise analysis of the person's needs.

Another Scandinavian study was a national multi-centre trial in Norway (Risberg and Jacobsen, 2003). This looked at the association between long-term survival and alternative medicine and found that people with cancer who took alternative medicines had shorter survival times than those who did not. In addition, people who used alternative medicine reported 'less hope and more mental distress' than those who did not. Indeed, users of CAM seemed to have a poorer quality of life than those who did not use CAM (Risberg et al., 2003). In contrast, Oneschuk et al. (1998, 2000) found that people with cancer had a high degree of faith in the anti-cancer effect of some therapies.

Using alternative medicines for curative purposes raises several concerns, for example:

> There are a multitude of potential interactions between conventional cancer treatments and UMT [unconventional medical therapies]. Many of these are just beginning to be recognized by the medical establishment and reported in reputable scientific journals. There is evidence that both renal and hepatic function can be impaired by various UMT. Multiple biochemical pathways can be affected. ... These effects could have an impact on drug concentrations in the body, resulting in increased toxicity and/or changes in effectiveness of chemotherapy and radiation therapy. Antioxidants may decrease the effectiveness of radiation therapy due to the scavenging of free radicals, which can damage DNA and result in cell death.
>
> (Metz et al., 2001, pp. 149–50)

The two alternative therapies most commonly used for curative reasons are herbal and shark products.

Herbal products

For many years one of the most popular alternative therapies purporting to provide a cure for cancer was **laetrile**, an extract of apricot stones or almonds. The anti-cancer properties of laetrile are advertised by several organisations, including World Without Cancer (2004) and Healing Daily (2004). Laetrile is expensive and hard to acquire in the UK and USA. It is promoted as a natural vitamin (B17) and proponents suggest that it could cure cancer. After a research trial showed that laetrile has little effect and that it could be harmful, it became less popular. However, 'it was revived recently by new promoters who dismiss the study, along with the general efforts of conventional regulatory bodies, as the result of pressure exerted by vested interests trying to protect their profits in the cancer industry' (Vickers and Cassileth, 2001, p. 229).

Another 'herbal' preparation is PC-SPES, which is used for prostate cancer (PC is prostate cancer and SPES is Latin for 'hope') (Weiger et al., 2002). The unconvincing evidence of its efficacy and concerns about its dangers prompted the American Food and Drug Administration to advise patients to stop taking it. This provoked considerable doubts about adequate quality control over herbal preparations, particularly about interactions with orthodox forms of treatment and the difficulties associated with assuring the potency of active natural compounds.

Several long-term trials are exploring the potential benefit of different CAM herbal preparations. One is researching the effectiveness of mistletoe lectin in treating people with refractory advanced solid tumours and for whom standard therapy has been unsuccessful. Another is studying the use of the Chinese herb Huang Lian in treating patients with advanced solid tumours.

Shark products

Shark cartilage is commonly used by people with cancer in search of a cure. Metz et al. (2001) note that CAM patients take shark cartilage because they believe sharks do not get cancer. However, there is evidence that sharks do develop malignant tumours. Shark cartilage can increase the chances of liver malfunction, which has implications for people having radiotherapy, chemotherapy or hormonal therapy.

In contrast to the findings cited by Metz et al. (2001):

> Despite the popularity of shark cartilage, there is currently insufficient evidence to support its efficacy in cancer treatment. However, adverse effects generally seem to be minor. Until the ongoing clinical trials provide further evidence, it seems reasonable for physicians to accept the use of shark cartilage in the absence of specific contraindications. It seems prudent to discourage the use of shark cartilage in patients with [certain medical histories].
>
> (Weiger et al., 2002, p. 895)

The curative potential of many CAM therapies is still unproven using orthodox scientific research methods, which many CAM promoters discount as at best irrelevant and at worst reflecting government and pharmaceutical company control over health issues. Many cancer treatments, which also do not necessarily guarantee a cure, are very unpleasant, which is why some people with cancer opt for treatments they perceive as being less toxic. The different aspects of manufactured risk were considered in previous chapters. A person with cancer weighs up one kind of risk against another when choosing either biomedical treatment for cancer or a CAM therapy that may avoid some of the unpleasant side effects of chemotherapy or radiotherapy.

Symptom relief and improvement in wellbeing

One of the primary reasons why people with cancer use CAM is for symptom relief (for example, Oneschuk et al., 1998). It is hard to separate out symptom relief and an improved quality of life as they are so interlinked: lack of pain for many people means the ability to move about, sleep better, etc.

Despite the popularity of CAM for symptom relief, the scientific evidence for its effectiveness remains limited. Pan et al. (2000) searched for evidence relating to pain management, breathlessness and nausea and vomiting and found that certain CAM therapies – for example, acupressure or acupuncture – could be used effectively alongside retraining to help people with breathlessness.

Other studies have found that people derive considerable benefit from CAM, more than that assessed using conventional scientific methods; for example, men with prostate cancer who have progressive disease or have had many treatments (Wilkinson et al., 1999). However, Kwekkeboom (2001) explored the use of CAM preparations for post-operative pain and could not show that CAM was more effective than conventional painkillers, although Metz et al. (2001) note the increasing evidence that some treatments are beneficial, particularly when used at the same time as orthodox treatments. The treatments which have attracted the most research attention are as follows.

Acupuncture

Many studies have demonstrated the potential of acupuncture to improve chemotherapy-induced nausea and vomiting (Weiger et al., 2002). Others suggest acupuncture causes the release of endorphins within the central nervous system, which may reduce people's perception of pain (Metz et al., 2001).

A study in San Diego in the USA explored the use of acupuncture in an oncology clinic. The results were inconclusive but suggested that acupuncture might help control symptoms for people with cancer, particularly nausea for those having chemotherapy for head and neck cancer (Johnstone et al., 2002). Despite the lack of scientific evidence, the authors concluded that acupuncture is safe, inexpensive and effective for pain control.

Acupuncture has also been used for cancer-related breathlessness with some success, but the authors note that some of the reduced symptoms might relate more to the placebo effect in the therapeutic relationship (Filshie et al., 1996; and see Chapter 9).

A large-scale randomised controlled trial is under way at the Memorial Sloan-Kettering Hospital to assess the effectiveness of acupuncture in the treatment of hot flashes (or flushes in the UK) for people with breast cancer.

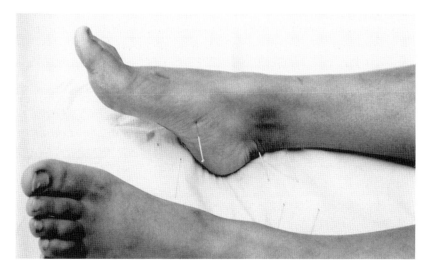

Acupuncture may relieve pain

Homoeopathy

Thompson and Reilly (2002) carried out a prospective observational study of homoeopathy for symptomatic control of 100 people with cancer. Most of those completing the study found the homoeopathic approach helpful for a range of symptoms.

If a patient makes a connection between life events and the onset of their disease, the homoeopathic approach allows for this connection within the consultation and emphasises it in the analysis of the narrative, which is then reflected in the prescription itself.

The investigators could not draw conclusions about the clinical effectiveness of the approach in symptom control, but they did note improvements in patient mood and quality of life. In particular, they noted CAM's role in engendering hope. Working with hope and expectation may be one way to maintain quality of life and using medications with minimal side effects has clear advantages.

Mind-body therapies

Different mind–body therapies have long been used to relieve emotional distress in people with cancer. For example, meditation is used to 'address some of the pervasive psychosocial difficulties associated with the disease' (Tacon, 2003). However, the most popular mind–body therapies used for pain relief by people with cancer are **hypnotherapy** and **visualisation** (Cancer Research UK, 2004).

Visualisation, although not considered one of the major complementary therapies, has been used, along with dietary measures, at the Bristol Cancer Centre with some success for many years, to help people with cancer live with their disease (Pietroni, 2000; Daniel, 2001). **Guided imagery** is one form of visualisation.

Metz et al. (2001) cite studies which demonstrate that guided imagery helps women having radiotherapy for early stages of breast cancer. They also note that **biofeedback**, when combined with relaxation training, helps reduce anxiety as well as nausea during chemotherapy. Similarly, Walker et al. (2003) demonstrate that relaxation therapy plus guided imagery (visualising

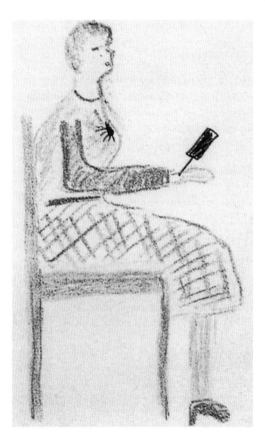

Visualising cancer

host defences attacking the cancer) improves quality of life, enhances coping and alters host defences in women with locally advanced breast cancer. Kwekkeboom (2001) also used guided imagery techniques, such as positioning, distraction, relaxation, heat, and eating and drinking. Although some patients saw them as effective, there was no difference in the pain-related outcomes for people who used only analgesia and those who used analgesia and non-pharmacological strategies.

Aromatherapy and massage

Aromatherapy is used extensively for stress relief in cancer and palliative care and is used frequently by palliative care teams and in hospices. It has also been shown to help lymph drainage in women with breast cancer (Weiger et al., 2002).

Kite et al. (1998), when developing an aromatherapy service in a cancer centre, noted that the main reasons for referral were tension, stress, anxiety and fear. They conclude that aromatherapy can help to reduce psychological distress and alleviate symptoms.

A study by Wilkinson et al. (1999) explored the effects of massage and aromatherapy on 103 people with cancer in a palliative care setting. Patients were randomly allocated to receive massage using either a carrier oil (massage) or a carrier oil plus the Roman chamomile essential oil (aromatherapy massage). The results, like those of Kite et al. (1998), demonstrate a statistically significant reduction in anxiety after each massage, and those receiving aromatherapy massages also noted improvements in their disposition, physical comfort and quality of life. The authors conclude that massage, with or without essential oils, appears to reduce levels of anxiety. They suggest that the addition of Roman chamomile essential oil may improve physical and psychological symptoms, as well as the person's overall quality of life.

Other forms of massage are being explored in clinical trials in the USA, particularly to confirm previous evidence that massage therapy not only helps with stress and anxiety but also may offer other forms of symptom relief (Weiger et al., 2002).

10.8 Moving towards integrated cancer care

Integrated cancer care is increasingly common in the UK and in the USA in both cancer and palliative care research and services. In the UK, the National Guidelines for the Use of Complementary Therapies in Supportive and Palliative Care were launched at the Houses of Parliament in 2003 (Tavares, 2003). While focusing only on complementary (not alternative) therapies, these guidelines cover areas such as service development and management and practice development. The document guides conventional and CAM practitioners through the morass of issues facing them when caring for people with cancer. The guidelines reflect a reality that acknowledges the limitations of orthodox medicine in addressing the wide-ranging consequences of cancer diagnosis and treatment, as well as concerns about the difficulty in assessing the effectiveness of CAM treatments. They also move towards some sense of integration and collaboration and recognise that the use of CAM by people with cancer is widespread and needs to be acknowledged by all parties.

10.9   Conclusion

This chapter explored the ways in which people with cancer and those needing palliative care have, to a certain extent, embraced CAM. This is a contentious area, not least because of the scientific community's concerns about the ways in which evidence is gathered on the effectiveness of CAM and the CAM community's scepticism about the values and ethos underlying the conventional scientific collection of evidence. However, official documents acknowledge the ways in which some CAMs can enhance the quality of life of both cancer patients and those needing palliative care (for example, Tavares, 2003). The alliance between CAM and palliative care organisations has resulted in considerable collaboration over the development of guidelines for CAM use in cancer and palliative care. What is essential is openness:

> When a patient with cancer seeks CAM therapy, the physician has an obligation to provide evidence-based advice in a manner that shows respect for the patient's beliefs and choices. ... The physician may begin by explaining that CAM therapies offer no 'magic bullets' and that current evidence supporting CAM is stronger for alleviation of cancer-related symptoms than for slowing of disease progression.
>
> (Weiger et al., 2002, p. 898)

Although this statement may seem 'paternalistic', as mentioned earlier many users do not disclose to their physicians that they use CAM, nor do they disclose their orthodox medications to CAM practitioners. This can lead to serious medical consequences. Therefore, it is essential that trusting, open and respectful relationships are developed so that the person with cancer is not endangered by interactions between the medical and CAM preparations:

> By becoming aware of what patients are taking, physicians can help patients to make more informed decisions. As physicians, we are trained to give patients all the information available so that they can make informed decisions on their treatment course. For the appropriate recommendations to be made, physicians must be aware of all other treatments in which a

patient may be participating ... Providing a non-threatening environment for discussion about these therapies is the first step in dealing with the utilization of UMT [unconventional medical therapies]. Directed questioning at the time of history and physical examination significantly increases the physician's ability to identify patients using UMT.

(Metz et al., 2001, p. 153)

In conclusion, it is important to note that not only has the effectiveness of many CAM therapies still to be demonstrated but also the costs of delivering these therapies needs to be evaluated.

KEY POINTS

- There are many different types of cancer with a variety of potential health outcomes.
- CAM is often used in conjunction with conventional medicine in cancer care.
- People differ in their perceptions of what cancer means to them and also in their definitions of quality of life.
- People with cancer are vulnerable and can be financially exploited by alternative therapists promising them a cure.
- CAM is used by people with cancer primarily for emotional and psychological support.
- No CAM preparation has yet been proven by scientific methods to be an effective cure for any cancer.
- Both palliative care and CAM embrace holism to enable users to exercise choice and control and to improve their quality of life.

References

Barnett, M. (2001) 'Overview of complementary therapies in cancer care', in Barraclough, J. (ed.) *Integrated Cancer Care: Holistic, Complementary, and Creative Approaches*, Oxford, Oxford University Press.

Barraclough, J. (ed.) (2001) *Integrated Cancer Care: Holistic, Complementary and Creative Approaches*, Oxford, Oxford University Press.

Burstein, H. J., Gelber, S., Guadagnoli, E. and Weeks, J. C. (1999) 'Use of alternative medicine by women with early-stage breast cancer', *New England Journal of Medicine*, Vol. 340, pp. 1733–9.

Calnan, M., Cant, S. and Gabe, J. (1993) *Going Private: Why People Pay for Their Health Care*, Buckingham, Open University Press.

Cancer Research UK (2004) 'Hypnotherapy, visualisation and cancer' [online], www.cancerhelp.org.uk/help/default.asp?page=5406 [accessed 9 July 2004].

CancerBACUP (2004) 'Cancer and complementary therapies' [online], www.cancerbacup.org.uk/info/complementary.htm [accessed 4 July 2004].

Cassileth, B. R., Schraub, S., Robinson, E. and Vickers, A. (2001) 'Alternative medicine use worldwide: the International Union Against Cancer survey', *Cancer*, Vol. 91, No. 7, pp. 1390–3.

Chumpus, L. and Hill, A. (1999) 'Exploring the views of carers of cancer patients in an inner city locality', *International Journal of Palliative Nursing*, Vol. 5, No. 3, pp. 116–23.

Daniel, R. (2001) 'Holistic approaches to cancer: general principles and the assessment of the patient', in Barraclough, J. (ed.) *Integrated Cancer Care: Holistic, Complementary, and Creative Approaches*, Oxford, Oxford University Press.

DoH (Department of Health) (2000) *The NHS Cancer Plan: A Plan for Investment, A Plan for Reform*, London, The Stationery Office.

Ernst, E. (2004) 'Complementary treatments may not cure your cancer – but they can make you feel better', *The Guardian*, 23 March, G2, p. 11.

Ernst, E. and Cassileth, B. (1998) 'Use of complementary/alternative medicine in cancer: a systematic review', *Cancer*, Vol. 83, pp. 777–82.

Filshie, J., Penn, K., Ashley, S. and Davis, C. L. (1996) 'Acupuncture for the relief of cancer-related breathlessness', *Palliative Medicine*, Vol. 10, pp. 145–50.

Grande, G. E. and Todd, C. J. (2000) 'Why are trials in palliative care so difficult?', *Palliative Medicine*, Vol. 14, pp. 69–74.

Healing Daily (2004) Website: www.healingdaily.com/detoxification-diet/vitamine-b-17-laetrile [accessed 18 May 2004].

Helman, C. (2001) *Culture, Health and Illness*, London, Arnold.

Higginson, I. J. (2003) 'Complementary evidence?', *Journal of the Royal Society of Medicine*, Vol. 96, No. 9, pp. 427–8.

Johnstone, P. A. S., Polston, G. R., Niemtzow, R. C. and Martin, P. J. (2002) 'Integration of acupuncture into the oncology clinic', *Palliative Medicine*, Vol. 16, pp. 235–9.

Katz, J. and Peace, S. (2003) 'Introduction', in Katz, J. S. and Peace, S. (eds) *End of Life in Care Homes: A Palliative Care Approach*, Oxford, Oxford University Press.

Kimby, C. K., Launso, L., Henningsen, I. and Langgaard, H. (2003) 'Choice of unconventional treatment by patients with cancer', *The Journal of Alternative and Complementary Medicine*, Vol. 9, No. 4. pp. 549–61.

Kite, S. M., Maher, E. J., Anderson, K., Young, T., Young, J., Wood, J., Howells, N. and Bradburn, J. (1998) 'Development of an aromatherapy service at a cancer centre', *Palliative Medicine*, Vol. 12, pp. 171–80.

Kohn, M. (1999) *Complementary Therapies in Cancer Care*, London, Macmillan Cancer Relief.

Kwekkeboom, K. L. (2001) 'Pain management strategies used by breast and gynaecologic cancer patients with post-operative pain', *Cancer Nursing*, Vol. 24, No. 5, pp. 378–86.

Lengacher, C. A., Bennett, M. P., Kip, K. E., Berarducci, A. and Cox, C. E. (2003) 'Design and testing of the use of a complementary and alternative therapies survey in women with breast cancer', *Oncology Nursing Forum*, Vol. 30, No. 2, pp. 811–21.

Lewith, G. T., Broomfield, J. and Prescott, P. (2002) 'Complementary cancer care in Southampton: a survey of staff and patients', *Complementary Therapies in Medicine*, Vol. 10, No. 2, pp. 100–6.

Metz, J. M., Jones, H., Devine, P., Hahn, S. and Glatstein, E. (2001) 'Cancer patients use unconventional medical therapies far more frequently than standard history and physical examination suggest', *The Cancer Journal*, Vol. 7, No. 2, pp. 149–54.

National Institute for Clinical Excellence (2002) *Guidance on Cancer Services – Improving Supportive and Palliative Care for Adults with Cancer*, London, NICE.

O'Callaghan, F. V. and Jordan, N. (2003) 'Postmodern values, attitudes and the use of complementary medicine', *Complementary Therapies in Medicine*, Vol. 11, pp. 28–32.

Oneschuk, D., Fennell, L., Hanson, J. and Bruera, E. (1998) 'The use of complementary medications in cancer patients attending an outpatient pain and symptom clinic', *Journal of Palliative Care*, Vol. 14, No. 4, pp. 21–6.

Oneschuk, D., Hanson, J. and Bruera, E. (2000) 'Complementary therapy use: a survey of community- and hospital-based patients with advanced cancer', *Palliative Medicine*, Vol. 14, pp. 432–4.

Paltiel, O., Avitzour, M., Peretz, T., Cherny, N., Kaduri, L., Pfeffer, R. M. et al. (2001) 'Determinants of the use of complementary therapies by patients with cancer', *Oncology*, Vol. 19, No. 9, pp. 2439–48.

Pan, C. X., Morrison, R. S., Ness, J., Fugh-Berman, A. and Leipzig, R. M. (2000) 'Complementary and alternative medicine in the management of pain, dyspnea, and nausea and vomiting near the end of life: a systematic review', *Journal of Pain and Symptom Management*, Vol. 20, No. 5, pp. 374–87.

Patterson, R. E., Neuhouser, M. L., Hedderson, M. M., Schwartz, S. M., Standish, L. J., Bowen, D. J. and Marshall, L. M. (2002) 'Types of alternative medicine used by patients with breast, colon, or prostate cancer: predictors, motives, and costs', *The Journal of Alternative and Complementary Medicine*, Vol. 8, No. 4, pp. 477–85.

Payne, S., Seymour, J. and Ingleton, C. (eds) (2004) *Palliative Care Nursing: Principles and Evidence for Practice*, Buckingham, Open University Press.

Pietroni, P. (2000) 'Complementary medicine – its place in the care of dying people', in Dickenson, D., Johnson, M. and Katz, J. S. (eds) *Death, Dying and Bereavement*, London, Sage/The Open University (K260 Reader).

Rees, R. W., Feigel, I., Vickers, A., Zollman, C., McGurk, R. and Smith, C. (2000) 'Prevalence of complementary therapy use by women with breast cancer: a population-based survey', *European Journal of Cancer*, Vol. 36, pp. 1359–64.

Risberg, T. and Jacobsen, B. K. (2003) 'The association between mental distress and the use of alternative medicine among cancer patients in North Norway', *Quality of Life Research*, Vol. 12, No. 4, pp. 539–44.

Risberg, T., Vickers, A., Bremnes, R. M., Wist, E. A., Kassa, S. and Cassileth, B. R. (2003) 'Does use of alternative medicine predict survival from cancer?', *European Journal of Cancer*, Vol. 39, No. 3, pp. 372–7.

Salmenpera, L. (2002) 'The use of complementary therapies among breast and prostate cancer patients in Finland', *European Journal of Cancer Care*, Vol. 11, No. 1, pp. 44–50.

Seale, C., Addington-Hall, J. and McCarthy, M. (1997) 'Awareness of dying: prevalence, causes and consequences', *Social Science and Medicine*, Vol. 45, No. 6, pp. 551–9.

Sontag, S. (1978) *Illness as Metaphor*, New York, Vantage Books.

Tacon, A. M. (2003) 'Meditation as a complementary therapy in cancer', *Family and Community Health*, Vol. 26, pp. 64–73.

Tavares, M. (2003) *National Guidelines for the Use of Complementary Therapies in Supportive and Palliative Care*, London, NCHSPCS/PoWFIH.

Thompson, E. A. and Reilly, D. (2002) 'The homeopathic approach to symptom control in the cancer patient: a prospective observational study', *Palliative Medicine*, Vol. 16, No. 3, pp. 227–33.

Vickers, A. J. and Cassileth, B. R. (2001) 'Unconventional therapies for cancer and cancer-related symptoms', *The Lancet Oncology*, Vol. 2, pp. 226–32.

Walker, L. G., Walker, M. B. and Sharp, D. M. (2003) 'Psychosocial oncology services for women with breast cancer', *Update in Urology, Gynaecology and Sexual Health*, Vol. 8, pp. 25–32.

Weiger, W. A., Smith, M., Boon, H., Richardson, M. A., Kaptchuk, T. J. and Eisenberg, D. M. (2002) 'Advising patients who seek complementary and alternative medical therapies for cancer', *Annals of Internal Medicine*, Vol. 137, No. 11, pp. 889–905.

Wilkinson, S., Aldridge, J., Salmon, I., Cain, E. and Wilson, B. (1999) 'An evaluation of aromatherapy massage in palliative care', *Palliative Medicine*, Vol. 13, pp. 409–17.

World Without Cancer (2004) Website: www.worldwithoutcancer.org.uk/laetrileandcyanide.html [accessed 18 May 2004].

Yates, P. M., Beadle, G., Clavarino, A., Najman, J. M., Thomson, D., Williams, G., Kenny, L., Roberts, S., Mason, B. and Schlect, D. (1993) 'Patients with terminal cancer who use alternative therapies: their beliefs and practices', *Sociology of Health and Illness*, Vol. 15, No. 2, pp. 199–216.

Zappa, S. and Cassileth, B. (2003) 'Complementary approaches to palliative oncological care', *Journal of Nursing Care Quality*, Vol. 18, pp. 22–6.

Complementary and Alternative Medicine in Different Settings

Edited by Tom Heller

Chapter 11 Traditional, folk and cultural perspectives of CAM

Andrew Vickers and Tom Heller

Contents

AIMS

- To widen the focus and consider CAM within its cultural contexts.
- To explore the relationships between CAM and traditional and folk practices.

11.1 Introduction

This chapter considers complementary and alternative medicine (CAM) within an international and a cultural context. This will illustrate the point that what makes a practice 'complementary' or 'alternative' is how it relates to, and possibly contrasts with, the dominant 'orthodox' or 'conventional' system of medicine. Of course, biomedical 'orthodox' medical approaches are not 'clean' of culture: although they have a different relationship with local cultures from systems such as ayurveda, they do have a rich cultural seam running through them.

However, considering a wider global and cultural picture will increase your insight into and understanding of CAM as it is practised in the UK.

The relationship between CAM and 'traditional' and 'folk' forms of health care is also a major theme of this chapter.

Many CAM practices are derived from 'traditional' healing practices: for example, acupuncture and herbal medicine. However, not all traditional healing practices can be described as CAM, which is a western concept that probably has little meaning in, say, sub-Saharan Africa. This chapter outlines the important distinctions between CAMs that are culturally specific (for example, shamanic healing), and those that are not (for example, beliefs about which herbs are effective for particular conditions). The effectiveness of a herb depends on its pharmacologically active ingredients; it is potentially usable worldwide; and its use does not normally rely on cultural beliefs or practices. A good example is the use of artemesinin (*Artemisia annua*) in the treatment of malaria (Trevett and Lalloo, 1992). Many other culturally determined health-related practices remain specific to their own culture, or are only transferable in exceptional circumstances.

CAM is often conceptualised in terms of particular therapies: acupuncture and herbal medicine are considered to be CAM, surgery is not, and so on. However, whether a particular therapy is seen as CAM, or as traditional medicine, or as part of current 'orthodox' practice is not always obvious or stable. For example, whether a therapy is defined as CAM varies from place to place: acupuncture is currently considered a form of CAM in the UK but is clearly an integral part of orthodox medicine in China (Hesketh and Zhu, 1997). Whether a practice is defined as CAM also varies from time to time: some CAM therapies become 'proven' and are accepted as part of and incorporated into conventional medicine. A good example is a high-fibre diet: at the end of the 19th century, this was associated with cranky health theories, such as those of Dr John Kellogg (1852–1943), while conventional nutritional advice emphasised a diet that typically contained just meat and potatoes. Similarly, treatments fall out of favour and become CAM: for example, certain types of herbal medicine for heart disease. In the 1930s, doctors often used *Digitalis* in its leaf form to treat heart disease: now it would probably be considered to be CAM.

In the mid-1990s, the National Institutes of Health, which oversee medical research in the USA, convened a panel to develop a definition of CAM. Their deliberations led to the publication of the following definition, which was also adopted by the Cochrane Collaboration in the UK.

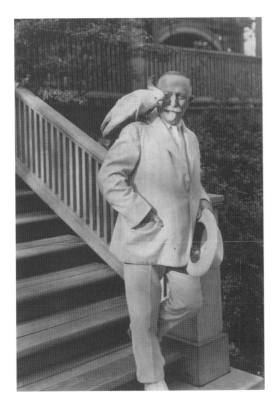

Preaching a lifestyle of exercise, fresh air and an astounding number of enemas, Dr John Harvey Kellogg pioneered many good ideas used in modern health care but accompanied them with other less helpful theories. Now that these theories have largely fallen out of favour with the medical establishment, would they be considered to be CAM?

Complementary and alternative medicine (CAM) is a broad domain of healing resources that encompasses all health systems, modalities, and practices and their accompanying theories and beliefs, other than those intrinsic to the politically dominant health system of a particular society or culture in a given historical period. CAM includes all such practices and ideas self-defined by their users as preventing or treating illness or promoting health and well-being. Boundaries within CAM and between the CAM domain and that of the dominant system are not always sharp or fixed.

(Zollman and Vickers, 1999, p. 693)

First, this definition defines CAM in terms of what it is not, rather than what it is. This seems to make sense: after all, there is little to connect iridology, chiropractic, the Alexander technique and herbal medicine, other than that they are not conventional or orthodox medicine as practised in the dominant health system in the UK.

Second, defining conventional medicine as that which is 'politically dominant' in 'a particular society or culture in a given historical period' allows CAM to vary with time and place because political systems are known to vary between countries and over time.

Third, this definition implies that CAM is more difficult to delineate where political systems are weaker. In contemporary Britain, where political and regulatory systems are strong, it is relatively straightforward to determine that, say, iridology is not part of officially sanctioned medicine. Such delineation would have been far more difficult 200 years ago in the UK or in, say, a rural Ugandan village today (see Box 11.1).

BOX 11.1   PERSPECTIVES ON INDIGENOUS HEALTH PRACTICES

It is important to recognise that there are widely different ways in which 'traditional' and 'folk' medicine are viewed by contemporary analysts (Johnston, 2003). For some people these historically based approaches to health seem to indicate, erroneously, that indigenous peoples throughout the world were previously living in perfect peace, prosperity, stability, health and environmental correctness before being brutally repressed by colonial powers that were bent only on commercial exploitation and profit. This doctrine largely ignores the benefits that orthodox 'western' medicine can bring and considers traditional medicines practised by indigenous peoples to have been effective at creating high levels of health and wellbeing before they were suppressed for reasons of cultural imperialism and capitalism. More balanced commentators both appreciate the contribution of modern medicine and recognise the significant benefits inherent in traditional medical systems and their practitioners (Struthers, 2003).

Chapters 3 and 6 have already considered how CAM is geographically and historically contingent: this means the definition is neither fixed nor stable, but varies with time and place, and is also subject to political influence. It is similarly important to consider 'traditional' approaches to health, healing and sickness in this context. Frank and Frank (1991) labelled traditional and indigenous forms of medicine as 'ethno-medical practices'. They identified three specific medical traditions covering the whole range of practice: **religio-magical**, such as shamanism; **rhetorical**, such as psychodrama; and **empirical**, which embraces a broadly scientific approach and is currently considered to be orthodox medicine in developed western societies.

11.2   CAM and folk medicine

Folk medicine is health advice dispensed by a person's friends and family who do not practise a recognised health profession. The way in which folk medicine is used usually has a strong relationship to a person's beliefs about what they can do for their own health and the health of their immediate family.

These folk medicine practices are strongly linked to the health beliefs and accounts of health described in Chapter 6. Everyone seems to have health beliefs, some of which, at least, are acted out in the practice of 'folk medicine' (see Box 11.2).

BOX 11.2   EUROPEAN FOLK HEALTH BELIEFS

Judith Hollis-Triantafillou, a general practitioner based in Athens, Greece, reported current Greek folk medicine practices based on the following beliefs.

- Diarrhoea is cured by a rigid diet consisting of tea without milk, overboiled rice, apple, boiled carrots and chicken breast.

- Tummy aches are relieved by an abdominal compress of cotton wool soaked in spirit.

- A feverish patient feels much better after a vigorous body rub with spirit or alcohol.

- The ancient practice of cupping and scarifying the thorax also reduces the fever and draws out poisonous vapours, although in unskilled hands it can result in full thickness burns and haemorrhage.

- Onion poultices reduce swelling and inflammation, and locally applied mustard plasters relieve aches and pains.

- Sea urchin spines can be removed by soaking the affected part in a weak solution of vinegar or, in an emergency, urine. The latter can also be used for jellyfish stings.

- Eating garlic in May keeps you healthy all year.

- Blood pressure can be measured by using a wedding ring suspended from a cotton thread and moved slowly above the extended forearm from wrist to elbow; the point at which the rotation changes from clockwise to anticlockwise measured in centimetres from the pulse gives the systolic pressure.

- Ouzo rubbed on a teething baby's gums gives everyone a good night's sleep.

(Source: adapted from Hollis-Triantafillou, 1995)

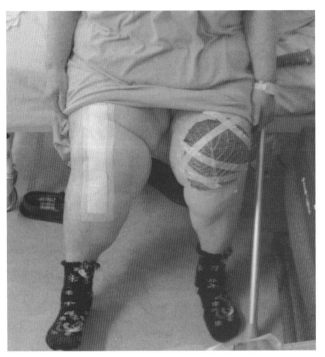

A 72-year-old woman with bilateral knee osteoarthritis was admitted to hospital for a total knee replacement. Post-operatively she was seen on the ward with the outer leaf of a cabbage taped to her non-operated knee. She said this was the only measure that provided relief from the symptoms of her osteoarthritis and that the outer cabbage leaves fitted well with the shape of her knee (Source: BMJ, 2003)

Differences between CAM and folk medicine

CAM is generally associated with defined groups of health practitioners: individuals who identify themselves as herbalists, chiropractors, Alexander teachers, and so on. Currently, folk medicine in developed western societies is generally not associated with health professionals. As mentioned earlier, it is usually considered to be the advice given by friends and family. In some cases, certain individuals do practise a form of folk medicine as a profession, but they are not organised into recognised professional bodies. For example, during the 19th and 20th centuries there were practitioners, such as bone-setters and the 'wise women' who attended women during childbirth, who followed certain therapeutic pathways.

CAM therapies comprise codified and recognised bodies of knowledge and expertise. The ways in which these can be classified were discussed in Chapter 2. A set of core principles can usually be deduced for a typical CAM therapy (such as, within homoeopathy, 'let like be treated by like'), as well as other more specific beliefs that are systematically related (such as arnica for treating bruising). CAM knowledge is documented in texts that seek to guide practice. Folk medicine beliefs exist in vernacular (usually oral) culture, do not usually have established core principles, and are neither systematically interrelated nor codified (see Box 11.3).

BOX 11.3 FOLK MEDICINE IN HISTORY

Many folk medicine concepts from historical times would be viewed with horror today. The following were collected from Cornish folklore.

- To cure goitre, go before sunrise on the first day of May to the grave of the last young man buried in the churchyard, pass your hand three times from head to foot of the grave and apply the dew collected to the part affected.

- To cure a sick woman, cut a live pigeon in half and put the bleeding parts on her feet.

- To cure thrush in a child, take it fasting on three mornings following to have its mouth blown into by a person who never knew its father, or take three rushes from a running stream and pass them separately through the mouth of the infant. Then plunge the rushes in the stream, and as the current bears them away the thrush will leave the child. Reading the eighth psalm three times a day for three days following will also cure thrush.

- To cure hiccups, wet the forefinger of the right hand with spittle and cross the front of the left shoe three times, saying the Lord's Prayer backwards. Frightening the affected person is another remedy.

(Source: adapted from Hawke, 1973)

It can be difficult to distinguish between traditional medicine and CAM in some contexts, partly because they are distinguishable not so much as separate types of medicine but rather as representative categories derived from different modes of classification. There may also be considerable continuity among various traditional systems. For example, in South Asia ideas about hot and cold foods are fairly consistently present in most communities and inform much day-to-day practice in the kitchen as well as in the treatment of sickness. These concepts are, likewise, present in the ayurvedic system practised by qualified doctors or vaids, although in a much more elaborate form. Even some biomedical doctors may base dietary advice to patients on this system of knowledge.

If many CAMs are considered to incorporate key concepts of the culture from which they grew, and can therefore be called 'traditional medicine', surely the same applies to the dominant biomedical 'culture', with its ideas well grounded in certain aspects of western culture (the mind–body divide and notions of the individual, etc.).

The Ethnomedica project, based in Kew Gardens near London, aims to collect and preserve a fast-disappearing aspect of British heritage – its medicinal plant traditions. Herbalists, and other suitably qualified people, are trained to collect information from an older generation of people – those who remember using local plants for medicinal and other purposes when they were younger:

> My grandfather always gathered the petals from Madonna lilies when in full bloom; these were packed lightly in a small wide-necked jar and covered with brandy. Any cuts were bound with one of these petals and held in place by a bandage (which would be a piece of clean cotton material) [M. E. H., Norfolk].

> Raspberry tea was used for inflamed eyes [R.C., London, aged 88].

> Beetroot was made into a tonic with sugar, carbonate of iron and stout [G. W., Bolton, aged 91].

> Unsalted hog's lard and oaten straw was made into a poultice for shingles [G. O'D., Tipperary, aged 69].

> Blackberry mould was applied to cuts and sores [C. F., London, aged 76].

> Cabbage leaves were used to poultice breast abscesses, boils and to remove splinters [L. B., London, aged 80].

> Onions boiled with milk were used to treat colds, and a hot onion was placed in the ear for earache [H. B.].

> Tea made from Purple Dead Nettle prevents spots [H. B.].

> (Ethnomedica, 2004)

ACTIVITY   COMPARING CURANDERISMO AND ACUPUNCTURE

Allow 20 minutes

Read the descriptions of curanderismo and acupuncture in Boxes 11.4 and 11.5. Curanderismo is traditional Hispanic healing, and acupuncture is part of traditional Chinese medicine.

What are the underlying differences between these two forms of culturally specific medicine?

Comment

Curanderismo and acupuncture appear to depend on culturally specific beliefs that are quite unlike those of most citizens in the UK: witchcraft and spirits in curanderismo; yin and yang in acupuncture. However, whereas in curanderismo belief in the underlying principles of the therapy is essential to treatment, this does not appear to be the case for acupuncture. Yin and yang, for example, are a class of explanation for the effects of acupuncture; concepts such as magical harm are an inherent component of curanderismo itself. Acupuncture, therefore, would appear to be more widely applicable than curanderismo.

Little research has been published that compares the effectiveness of various forms of therapy within the relevant culture with, for example, acupuncture practised in a European setting.

BOX 11.4   CURANDERISMO

Curanderismo is the art of folk healing by a *curandero*, the healer par excellence in the folk medicine practiced by Texas Hispanics. Healers can be either male or female and may even specialize in their practice. The three most common types of *curanderos* are the *yerbero* (herbalist), the *partera* (midwife), and the *sobador* (masseur). Though the *curandero* has the skill to treat a wide variety of illnesses, he is the only healer in the culture who can treat *mal puesto*, illnesses caused by witchcraft. He is thought to have been given a *don de Dios* (a gift from God) to heal the sick, and he learns his healing art through apprenticeship under another *curandero* or a spiritual manifestation. His chief adversary in the struggle between good and evil is Satan and those who have made secret pacts with him – the *brujos* or *brujas* (witches). Along with the treatment of *mal puesto*, *curanderos* also treat *mal de ojo* (the evil eye) and *susto* (loss of spirit). Typically, the *curandero* works on three levels, the material, the spiritual, and the mental. He may prescribe a herbal remedy or conduct a religious ritual. Quite often, a practitioner is called upon to treat the physical symptoms that patients believe come from supernatural causes.

(Source: Texas State Historical Association, 2004)

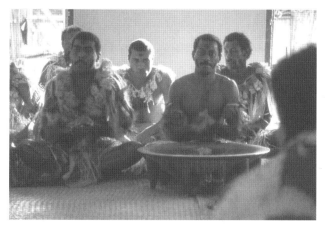

Despite the cultural differences, many elements of a traditional curanderismo ceremony would be familiar to people following more orthodox western religious practices

---

BOX 11.5   ACUPUNCTURE

Acupuncture, which means needle piercing, is an ancient treatment which originated in China, where it has traditionally been used for pain relief and the treatment of conditions such as arthritis, high blood pressure and various types of ulcers. Acupuncture involves inserting very fine metal needles into the skin at specially designated points of the body. When these needles are applied to the correct points a tingling feeling is experienced. It is said to work by manipulating the body's chi, or energy flow, allowing the body to regain its balance and heal itself. The chi travels along various routes in the body, known as meridians, and disease or other forms of ill health can arise if these meridians become blocked. A skilled practitioner of acupuncture can locate a weakness in a person's energy chain and effect treatment according to the symptoms displayed. These symptoms are known as a **pattern of disharmony.** The invisible meridians along which chi flows are named after organs of the body, and thus are thought to be related to these organs, which include the lungs, heart, spleen, kidneys and stomach. Every point along a meridian is affected by disharmony elsewhere on that meridian.

(Source: adapted from Alternative Health Directory, 2004)

How folk medicine becomes CAM

A consistent theme of this book is that medicine is dynamic and distinctions and boundaries between orthodox and complementary and alternative medicine are fluid. Similarly, historically there has been a rich interplay between folk medicine and CAM. Some folk medicine practices become professionalised and emerge as CAM therapies. The best examples are chiropractic and osteopathy. It has been argued that they developed from the folk medicine practice of bone-setting. D. D. Palmer (1907–1978) and Andrew Taylor Still (1828–1917) developed, respectively, chiropractic and osteopathy as autonomous professions in the late 19th century in the USA (see Box 11.6). They established schools, set out a coherent set of therapeutic principles, wrote textbooks and initiated a professional structure on the basis of techniques that until then were practised informally, often by barbers and such people.

BOX 11.6   THE BIRTH OF OSTEOPATHY

Andrew Taylor Still was born in Virginia in 1828, the son of an itinerant Methodist preacher who supported his family by farming and the practice of medicine. He assisted his father in both his ministerial and medical duties as well as assisting in the religious revival camp meetings his father held. It was during the time spent with his father tending to the religious and medical needs of Native Americans that Still decided to take up the practice of medicine under the guidance of his father. He studied the current texts on anatomy, physiology, pathology, surgery and materia medica. Early on, Still was well aware of the limitations of the materia medica of his day with the almost total preoccupation of allopathic medicine with symptoms and their suppression. The understanding of disease was crude at best and based on vague notions of 'physiological tension' which needed to be relieved by puking, purging, blood letting and heroic doses of morphine, opium, alcohol and mercury.

In 1874 he announced to the world the founding of his new medical science which he called Osteopathy. This new school of medical thought was conceived as a reformation or improvement of conventional medicine, not an alternative system. During the 1880s he continued to refine his science and made several attempts to train others. During this time patients flocked from all over America for his treatment. Hotels were built in the town of Kirksville to house the many hopeless patients who arrived daily for help, and several railroad companies advertised their train service to Kirksville. On 1 November 1892, the American School of Osteopathy was opened. This first class of eleven students consisted of former patients, family friends and five of Still's children. The forward-thinking Still admitted five women to the first class and was later reported to have said that he thought women made better osteopaths than men. By the late 1890s his school, infirmary and new surgical hospital were increasingly successful both academically and financially.

(Source: adapted from Masiello, 2004)

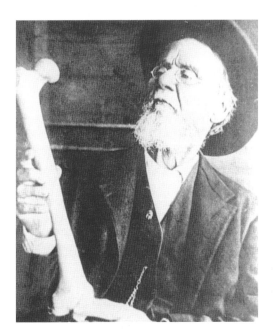

This rather grand photograph of Andrew Taylor Still is owned by the Still National Osteopathic Museum, Kirksville, Missouri, USA

CAM has also adopted elements of folk medicine piecemeal. A good example is homoeopathy. This was not derived from folk medicine: it was invented in the 18th century by Samuel Hahnemann based on his observations on the actions of drugs. Yet many homoeopathic medicines clearly derive from folk medicine. For example, the herb *Arnica montana* is a traditional treatment for bruising and muscle pain: indeed, mountain guides traditionally look for it on the hillsides during the first hike of spring. Today, homoeopathic textbooks list the homoeopathic form of arnica for treating bruising and muscle pain, despite it being paradoxical in homoeopathic terms: for like to treat like, herbal arnica should cause bruising and muscle pain if homoeopathic arnica is to treat it.

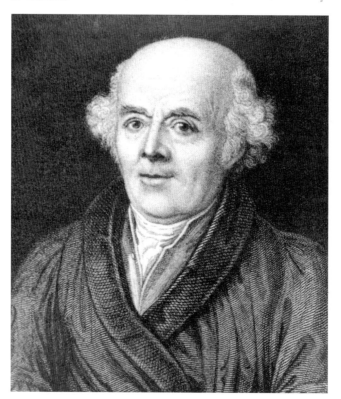

This image of Dr Samuel Hahnemann (1755-1843), the inventor of homoeopathy, was produced in Paris in 1841

How folk medicine becomes traditional medicine

Perhaps the most interesting link between folk medicine and CAM is when the former gradually became systematised and professionalised over the years. In such cases, the CAM therapy often incorporates key concepts of the original culture. Such therapies are sometimes called 'traditional' medicine. The most well known example is traditional Chinese medicine (TCM) and its associated therapies, such as acupuncture and herbal medicine (see Box 11.7). TCM is based on concepts such as yin and yang that are part of traditional Chinese philosophies and religion. When practised in the UK, it is generally accepted as a CAM. The dynamic nature of the relationship between traditional medicine and CAMs is illustrated by the way in which some oriental therapeutic practices have been adapted or transformed in the western cultural setting (Adams, 2002).

BOX 11.7   CHINESE MEDICAL SYSTEMS: ONE COUNTRY, TWO SYSTEMS

Overall, it is estimated that 40% of health care in China is based on traditional Chinese medicine, with a higher proportion in rural areas. This figure does not include the massive amount of self medication with traditional drugs, which are used not only to treat illness but also as health promoting drugs, ranging from nutritional supplements and tonics to aphrodisiacs.

Every city [in China] has a hospital practising traditional Chinese medicine, and there is a plan for every county to have one. In 95% of the hospitals practising Western medicine there are departments of traditional Chinese medicine, most with inpatient beds; when patients arrive at the outpatient department they can opt for Chinese or Western treatment. In Jiangsu province, one of the richer, more sophisticated eastern provinces, one quarter of all outpatients in one year (10 million) had opted for traditional treatment.

The collaboration between the two systems is well illustrated by the fact that in [Chinese] Western medicine hospitals around 40% of the medicines prescribed are traditional. Similarly, in the traditional hospitals 40% of all prescribed drugs are Western medicine. At township and village levels, doctors often prescribe both types of treatment simultaneously, without apparent contradiction. A survey carried out in two village health clinics in Zhejiang province showed that children with upper respiratory tract infections were being prescribed an average of four separate drugs, always a combination of Western and Chinese.

(Source: Hesketh and Zhu, 1997, p. 117)

Traditional medicines play an important and interesting symbolic role in CAM. Perhaps this is because closeness to a historical ideal is often a criterion for determining whether a particular technique (or practitioner) is valuable. This is in sharp contrast to conventional medicine where, in general, the latest advances and newest techniques are valued precisely because they are new. CAM practitioners often highly value historical and traditional forms of therapy, but appeals to historical ideals may distort their view of history in order to meet contemporary demands. The descriptions of traditional or historical CAM given by some CAM advocates may be unrealistically idealised.

11.3   Traditional medicine: locally available health or public health challenge?

Approximately 80 per cent of the world's population have only limited access to orthodox 'western' medicine and its associated drugs (WHO, 2002a). Instead, they rely primarily on locally available health practices, such as herbal medicine and traditional midwifery, or other forms of culturally specific health care that are known as 'traditional medicine'.

Traditional medicine covers a wide range of practices throughout the world. Attempts have been made to understand more about the features that are helpful and those that might be harmful, and to consider issues such as the efficacy of traditional approaches. James Waldram believes that notions of efficacy remain fluid and certainly cannot be considered simply from a scientific, biomedical standpoint. In his opinion, it is important to understand how indigenous peoples believe traditional medicine 'works' before rushing to a judgement:

> Medical anthropological inquiry needs to return to the field, to explore and comprehend how efficacy is understood within traditional medical systems themselves. The current propensity to employ biomedical concepts and methods, to search for apparent biomedical parallels within traditional medical systems, or to fixate on biomedical terminology that might have intruded into these systems often leads to a false sense of our ability to assess traditional medicine's efficacy.
>
> (Waldram, 2000, p. 619)

Johnston (2003) reviewed the recent literature on Native American traditional and alternative medicine and concluded, similarly, that some social scientists were guilty of using the dominant culture's philosophical approaches to construct categories of assessment and analysis. She also complains about the condescending attitude of biomedically trained practitioners towards native healers and healing.

Recent research has uncovered and celebrated the ways in which indigenous women healers from Native American cultures bring important skills to their work:

> It must be understood that indigenous culture is not like mainstream culture as it embodies a different perspective related to health and illness. Accordingly, the skills and tools utilized during healing encounters to correct imbalances and restore wholeness by indigenous women healers are quite different from those used in conventional medicine. For example, ceremony, ritual, and prayer [are] used during individual and group healing sessions. Also, the women commonly hold pipe ceremonies, sweat lodges, and rite of passage ceremonies, and they use herbs and medicinal plants for healing. ... Personal values may also be somewhat different as they contain

... components such as sharing, caring, kindness, respect, being humble, and a belief that all things are equal.

(Struthers, 2003, p. 352)

The positive and negative aspects of traditional medicine

In 2000, the World Health Organization (WHO, 2000a) produced a report on 'traditional medicine' (see Box 11.8). One view is that 'traditional' practices constitute a public health problem. Some traditional medicines are undoubtedly risky or even dangerous. For example, the misuse of traditional massage by Pacific islanders during pregnancy has led to brain damage and death, and traditional African bone-setting has allegedly led to cases of deformity and even amputation. In Papua New Guinea, cutting through the chest wall into the pleural cavity is believed to help relieve chest pain. In Pakistan, clarified butter is traditionally applied to the umbilical wound of newborns, which may lead to potentially fatal tetanus infection. Herbs taken as part of traditional medicine have also occasionally had adverse effects either directly or because they contain high levels of toxic metals.

BOX 11.8   OFFICIAL REGULATION AND CONTROL OF TRADITIONAL MEDICINE

The World Health Organization (WHO) has developed a strategy that provides a framework for policy to assist countries to regulate traditional or complementary/alternative medicine (TM/CAM) to make it safer, more accessible to their populations and sustainable (WHO, 2002a).

At the launch of the strategy in May 2002, officials of the World Health Organization were very concerned about the need to regulate and control traditional medicine and somehow contain the potential 'dangers' of traditional medicine, especially if its use was going to spread to the developed world:

> 'About 80% of the people in Africa use traditional medicine. It is for this reason that we must act quickly to evaluate its safety, efficacy, quality and standardization - to protect our heritage and to preserve our traditional knowledge. We must also institutionalize and integrate it into our national health systems,' says Ebrahim Samba, WHO's Regional Director for Africa.

> In wealthy countries, growing numbers of patients rely on alternative medicine for preventive or palliative care. In France, 75% of the population has used complementary medicine at least once; in Germany, 77% of pain clinics provide acupuncture; and in the United Kingdom, expenditure on complementary or alternative medicine stands at US$ 2300 million per year.

> But problems may arise out of incorrect use of traditional therapies. For instance, the herb Ma Huang (ephedra) is traditionally used in China to treat short-term respiratory congestion. In the United States, the herb was marketed as a dietary aid, whose long-term use led to at least a dozen deaths, heart attacks and strokes. In Belgium, at least 70 people required renal transplant or dialysis for interstitial fibrosis of the kidney after taking the wrong herb from the Aristolochiaceae family, again as a dietary aid.
>
> 'Traditional or complementary medicine is [a] victim of both uncritical enthusiasts and uninformed sceptics,' explains Dr Yasuhiro Suzuki, WHO Executive Director for Health Technology and Pharmaceuticals. 'This strategy is intended to tap into its real potential for people's health and well-being, while minimizing the risks of unproven or misused remedies.'
>
> (WHO, 2002b)

Some writers argue that traditional medicine offers important opportunities to improve health in developing nations (Puckree et al., 2002). While accepting that not all traditional health practices improve health, and indeed that some are dangerous, other writers argue that using locally available resources is a more expedient course of action than relying on modern medicine, whose provision is patchy at best (Bodeker, 2001).

The debate on the value of traditional medicines is not simply about efficacy. Another issue facing people in many developing countries is that of acceptability (leaving aside the huge issue of affordability!). Acceptability depends on many factors, one being the nature of social relationships involved in treatment. Thus some forms of biomedical treatment are popular in South Asia because they are considered very effective for infectious and acute diseases. However, the experience of being delivered in a modern health centre can be distressing for rural women because of the disrespectful way in which they may be treated. Traditional midwives offer a service that is less demeaning; but, although they may have useful skills and a fund of knowledge, they are often in a poor position to introduce new or improved practices because they are generally from a low 'caste' or 'class' too. Unfortunately, some biomedical services that are accessible to rural people in developing countries are even less respectful of their dignity than in developed countries. So, situations can arise where people prefer other kinds of healing. It is important to recognise that choices between traditional and other systems of healing depend on how systems are seen **in relation to each other**. People judge traditional medicine and biomedicine in terms of both how they compare with each other and how they are represented in their locality (Sharma, 2004).

The history of many nations in the world is of indigenous, 'traditional' cultures being colonised or somehow dominated by invaders. In some cases entire indigenous populations and their cultures, including their traditional forms of medical care, have been virtually wiped out by the new regimes (Fulder, 2002). Where people from the indigenous culture continue to exist, their health status is usually very poor and often it is hard for them to access the full range of services and opportunities, including health services (Ring and Brown, 2003). Although the history of many countries colonised during the expansion of the British Empire involved the widespread domination and humiliation of indigenous peoples, their cultural traditions, including those relating to health, were retained to a certain extent. In the current, possibly more enlightened, social climate, many of these traditional, cultural health care practices are being treated more seriously and sensitively again (see Box 11.9). For example, in New Zealand, Durie (2003) gives examples where providing health services to indigenous people involves a combination of conventional services and indigenous programmes. Similarly, in China (Normile, 2003; Zhang et al., 2003) and Africa (Puckree et al., 2002), efforts are being made to integrate traditional forms of healing with western orthodox approaches.

BOX 11.9 NAMING PEOPLE FROM INDIGENOUS COMMUNITIES

'Indigenous' has a number of usages that differ from 'to be born in a specific place', which is how the *Concise Oxford Dictionary* defines it. These usages tend to define indigenous by the experiences shared by a group of people who have inhabited a country for thousands of years, which often contrast with those of other groups of people who reside in the same country for a few hundred years. A number of alternative terms are preferred to indigenous. For example, in Australia, Aboriginal and Torres Strait Islander is appropriate and acceptable. In Canada and the United States, the term First Nations is used to describe the Indian, Métis, and Inuit populations, whereas in Hawaii, native Hawaiian finds favour. Many groups prefer their own language. The Maori of New Zealand use 'Tangata Whenua' or 'people of the land' in preference to Maori used by the colonising Victorian English who, unaware of its meaning (ordinary or common), ironically deemed the indigenous population to be the ordinary inhabitants, rendering themselves extraordinary in the process.

(Source: Cunningham and Stanley, 2003, p. 403)

Bodeker (2001) makes a case for using traditional health systems alongside orthodox medicine (where available) in developing countries. He cites two basic policy models that have been followed in Asia: an integrated approach, where modern and traditional medicine are integrated through medical education and practice (for example, in China and Vietnam); and a parallel approach, where modern and traditional medicine are separate within the national health system (for example, in India and South Korea). Chaudhury (2001) claims that the possibility of integration is more complex because proof of efficacy for traditional approaches using the randomised controlled trial may not be totally appropriate where the Prakriti (ayurveda system) or Mijaj (unani system) of individuals determines the specific therapy to be used. Chaudhury also discusses the important problem of regulating the traditional systems of medicine, the products used in them, and the practitioners of them, which is weak in most countries. This leads to the potential misuse of medicines by unqualified practitioners and a loss of credibility in the system.

Is orthodox medicine a form of imperialism?

Although the 'side-by-side' development of orthodox and traditional forms of medicine is often held up as an ideal model, in reality there is a more competitive aspect to the spread of commercial, 'modern', western medicine. For example, Fulder (2002) reports how the development of western orthodox forms of medicine has led to the virtual extinction of traditional herbal medical practice in Israel and the Palestinian areas.

ACTIVITY   EXTINCTION AND DIVERSITY IN ALTERNATIVE MEDICINE

Allow 20 minutes

Read the extract in Box 11.10 and then write down some of the reasons why the extinction of traditional forms of medicine is damaging.

Comment

The extinction of traditional forms of medical practice is accompanied by the potential for significant loss of knowledge and practical experience. For example, in the situation Fulder describes in Israel and the Palestinian areas, the detailed description of the use of herbs that has developed over many centuries assists in knowing not simply about the actions of the herbs themselves, but also about the type of person who responds to them, the exact varieties and parts of plants that it is best to use, and the interactions between the herbs. In some cases, the modern herbal preparations that are commercially distributed are not the same as the herbs used throughout centuries of experience and empirical development. The loss of traditional and indigenous forms of practice also has serious implications for the cultural dimensions of health care and the sensitivity that practitioners need to understand the people who approach them for help.

> **BOX 11.10   THE EXTINCTION OF TRADITIONAL FORMS OF MEDICINE**
>
> [W]hile there has never been as much interest in natural medicine, and the Western world is flocking to the health shops to buy natural remedies, indigenous medicine, which is alternative medicine par excellence, is, in some areas, verging on extinction. In particular, where traditional medicine is a verbal rather than literate tradition, it has contracted severely in the face of modernization … In Israel and the Palestinian areas, modern medical services are widely available, and this has contributed to a virtual disappearance of local traditional medicine, which is Arabic/Hippocratic medicine. Arabic/Hippocratic medicine comprises a huge body of knowledge with much of it written down in traditional texts. These encompass diagnosis and treatment, using at least 600 medicinal plants. … The paradox lies in the fact that … CAM use in Israel itself has been growing dramatically and, in a relatively short time, has reached similar levels of usage and availability to those in Europe and the United States. The health product and herbal industry has grown to match. Therefore, the population is highly interested in purchasing and using CAM products and services, while the local indigenous medicine, probably the most authentic CAM in the region, is rapidly disappearing. … There is a poignant aspect to this. That is that Arabic/Hippocratic medicine is the theoretical and conceptual basis of both modern medicine and modern Western herbalism. The herbs on sale in the health shops were mostly discovered by the Greeks and Arabs and this knowledge was brought into Europe in the medieval times … Thus, people are going into health shops in Israel to buy American or European herbal products that are derived originally from a local Arabic medicine that is becoming extinct in the process.
>
> (Source: Fulder, 2002, pp. 395-6)

11.4   Traditional medicine as a source of commercial medicines

Many of the drugs currently used in modern medicine were originally derived from herbs and other plants (CITES, 2004). People throughout history knew several properties of these plants, either as part of local folk medicine or from being used in other traditional forms of medicine. By 1994, pharmacologist Norman Farnsworth had identified over 119 plant-derived substances that are used globally as drugs (Farnsworth, 1994). Many of the prescription drugs currently sold in developed countries contain compounds derived from, or modelled on, naturally occurring chemicals in plants, and many of these (including reserpine, digitalis and vincristine) are from plants used in traditional medicine. Other well known examples include aspirin, morphine and Taxol (a cancer drug), which are related to compounds found in willow bark, poppies and yew trees respectively. As a result, pharmaceutical companies routinely screen herbs used in traditional medicine to determine whether any have pharmacological activity. If so, attempts are made to determine an active constituent that can be developed as a drug. A recent well known example is artemesinin, a drug now used to treat malaria. It was discovered by chemists who analysed wormwood, a traditional Chinese herbal treatment for malaria (Trevett and Lalloo, 1992).

ACTIVITY   WHAT IS GREEN, PRICKLY AND SOUR AND MAY SAVE A TRADITIONAL CULTURE?

Allow 20 minutes

Read the newspaper article in Box 11.11 and make notes on the possible benefits that the development of a drug for obesity might have for the San bushmen of the Kalahari. What problems might it cause for their traditional way of life?

Comment

The development of pharmacologically active agents derived from traditional herbal or plant products has interested big pharmaceutical companies who want to transform indigenous therapies and practices into expensive drugs. While the process of collecting genetic resources, or **bio-prospecting**, is not new, it has increased exponentially in recent years, often driven by dramatic advances in genetic engineering that allow scientists to manipulate active compounds in plants, soils and fungi more easily. Scientists increasingly focus on jungles, tropical rainforests, deserts and farms to develop new products and modern medicines, while governments in developing countries are slowly realising the need to protect the right to benefit from their dwindling natural resources. Opponents say that, in the absence of national and international laws to regulate bio-prospecting, the practice is nothing more than bio-piracy: the expropriation of genetic materials with no fair return for the people they are taken from. The critics worry that companies may patent the genetic materials they discover, preventing local indigenous communities from using their own resources in the future. Whether indigenous people benefit from patents will depend on many factors, not least their capacity to organise, develop leadership and raise money for litigation and also to define their boundaries and membership. For example, who decides who can benefit from an agreement like the one described in Box 11.11?

BOX 11.11   IT'S GREEN, PRICKLY AND SOUR, BUT THIS PLANT COULD CURE OBESITY AND SAVE AN ANCIENT WAY OF LIFE

Hunting with bows and poisoned arrows over the bleached sands of the Kalahari, it was sometimes days before the San bushmen had food or water. So precarious was survival that some believed their god was a 'trickster' who played jokes with the land and their fate.

The San learned that in this arid wilderness of southern Africa they could trust one thing. Sprouting 6ft high amid the prehistoric vegetation, green, prickly and sour, it was a plant they called Xhoba.

Hunters would cut a slice, munch it, and within minutes hunger and thirst would evaporate, leaving a feeling of strength and alertness. They could travel for days eating nothing else.

The trickster god has played another joke, except this time it is to the benefit of the San. Xhoba, a member of the Asclepiadaceae family of plants, is known in English as hoodia, but is more likely to become better known as P57.

Dotting the Kalahari desert of South Africa, Botswana, Namibia and Angola, it is being hailed as a wonder plant whose qualities as an appetite-suppressant could revolutionise treatment of obesity for 100 million westerners.

Patented by a South African research institute and licensed to a British Buddhist entrepreneur, the plant is now being developed by the US drugs giant Pfizer, at the cost of hundreds of millions of dollars, with the objective of turning it into a pill which will zap food cravings.

For the San it could be the second time they have been saved by Xhoba. Their hunter-gatherer culture, stretching back 20,000 years, has been promised a share of the royalties from the drug.

After years of talks a deal between tribal leaders and the Pretoria-based Council for Scientific and Industrial Research (CSIR), which owns the patent, has just been clinched, raising hopes that the San will receive millions of dollars each year.

The solicitor representing South Africa's aboriginal people, Roger Chennels, said yesterday that both sides had reached an accord. 'In the last two weeks we have finalised the percentages. The deal has been struck. It means job opportunities, salaries, scholarships and the right to grow the plant.'

A council of elders who sit on the working group of indigenous minorities in southern Africa decided at a meeting in Windhoek, the capital of Namibia, to share the money equally between all the San scattered across southern Africa, said Mr Chennels.

'They felt very strongly that traditional knowledge was a heritage which had to be shared. The San in each country will set up an audited trust. The focus will be on education and training of leaders, though in some cases the funds will be used to buy land where the San are tenants.'

Mr Chennels would not say what proportion of the royalties will go to the impoverished bushmen but left no doubt it will add up to a meaningful sum for the estimated 100,000 people scattered across the Kalahari, whose culture was recently feared to be on the verge of extinction.

Under the accord it is expected that San youths will be given scholarships to study abroad and those left at home will be employed tending plantations and teaching scientists what they know about hoodia.

'The scale of the thing is mind-boggling,' said Nigel Crawhall, of the Cape Town-based South African San Institute. 'The San are riding a huge wave in the pharmaceutical industry which is catering for the body adjustment market. Profits from the drug should be in the tens of millions of dollars.'

The hunters who snacked on hoodia to ward off starvation would be amazed to know it might end up in a capsule for Americans and Europeans wanting to trim waistlines, he said.

Nuisance

'It is an affirmation of the value of traditional knowledge. The challenge for the San community leaders will be to harness these resources to bring real economic change to their people,' said Mr Crawhall.

A big challenge. In some ways today's San resemble certain communities of the aborigines of Australia and north America: depressed, unemployed, poor, prone to alcoholism. Optimists hope the San will use the windfall well.

'You could say it is grim here. There are no jobs and alcohol abuse is a problem. Children are told to study hard at school but there are very few opportunities after they graduate,' said Betta Steyn, speaking from a dust-blown craft shop in the Kalahari.

The San in Botswana and Namibia are often regarded as a nuisance by the authorities and herded into towns. Those in South Africa were persecuted by the apartheid regime and to redress that grievance Nelson Mandela's government granted them ownership of more than 40,000 hectares.

Yet they remain impoverished. Many of the Bushmen live in houses made of grass hundreds of miles from the nearest town, including one called Hotazel, otherwise known as Hot as Hell. The lucky ones have some goats. 'If this deal works out, the impact will be immense, it could transform our fortunes,' said Ms Steyn.

Some elders attribute aphrodisiac qualities to the plant, though Pfizer, which makes Viagra, has not marketed that angle. One elder told the Mail and Guardian in Johannesburg: 'When the grandfathers eat the Xhoba, the grandmothers can't let them out of their sight.'

After identifying the relevant bioactive compound the CSIR obtained a patent in 1997, which it licensed to a Cambridgeshire-based botanical pharmaceuticals company, Phytopharm, which was founded by Richard Dixey after he returned from the Himalayas with a passion for Buddhism and traditional healing.

'We called it P57 because it was the 57th product that we spent money on. It is the only true appetite suppressant and will help those who eat a lot of ice cream at 3am and still don't feel full.'

Clinical trials in the UK suggested it could reduce appetite by 2,000 calories a day, making it a potential runaway success in a multi-billion pound industry. Dr Dixey hopes it will be available on prescription by 2007 after further clinical trials overseen by Pfizer, which paid Phytopharm $32m for the right to develop the drug.

(Source: Carroll, 2003)

Some traditional medicines are already proving to have commercial uses, as described in Box 11.12.

BOX 11.12   EXAMPLES OF THE COMMERCIAL HARVESTING OF TRADITIONAL REMEDIES

Aids

Samoa has signed a landmark agreement with a US research group that will guarantee 20% of revenues received from the development of an anti-HIV/Aids compound called Prostratin, which is extracted from the bark of a Samoan tree called mamala. For centuries traditional healers in Samoa have ground up the stem of the plant and steeped it in hot water as a treatment for the yellow fever virus.

Psoriasis

The treatment Exorex was launched in the UK in 1998 after its developer discovered Zulu trackers rubbing banana skin on their bodies to soothe itchy skin.

Stress

Kava has become a popular herbal remedy for alleviating stress and an acceptable alternative to valium. [In Europe, however, it has been recently withdrawn because of fears about liver toxicity (Escher and Desmeules, 2001).] The plant is found throughout the Pacific and has been used for 3,000 years for its medicinal properties. Kava (*Piper methysticum*) plays a key role in Fijian, Samoan, and Tongan societies where it is drunk in ceremonies to honour visitors and unite participants.

Smoking/alcohol

Sceletium is a creeping, daisy-like plant that grows in arid conditions which has been taken by African bushmen for thousands of years. Doctors in South Africa say they have had remarkable results treating patients for tobacco and alcohol addiction using *Sceletium* tablets. The plant, which grows only in the Cape region of South Africa, has been used by the San people since prehistoric times to treat depression and alcohol and drug dependence.

> ### *Cancer*
>
> The drugs Velban and Oncovin are regularly used in [the] treatment of Hodgkin's disease. They were developed in the 1960s from Madagascar's rosy periwinkle plant, which was used in folk medicine for treating dysentery, menstrual disorders, toothache and diabetes.
>
> (Source: Carroll, 2003)

11.5 Cultural diversity

All communities in the UK comprise, to a greater or lesser extent, a diverse mix of people from a variety of backgrounds, each with their own cultural and ethnic histories (Social Trends, 2003). Throughout history a constant feature of the UK's demographic pattern has been the influx and exodus of people into and from other parts of the world. This has occurred as invaders, economic migrants and people fleeing repressive regimes elsewhere have settled in the UK and helped to create the nation state, its economy and its institutions. It is important not to reinforce the tendency to believe that 'other people' have cultures or cultural beliefs, and that only 'traditional' and folk beliefs relate to culture. There is also a danger of seeing 'cultures' as 'closed boxes', which people move between, ignoring the debate about the role of 'culture' in the health practices of British ethnic minority groups (Sharma, 2004). Social scientists studying ethnic groups in the UK emphasise the ways in which migrants adapt practices and construct new cultural formations rather than simply conserve the culture they brought with them (Reed, 2003).

ACTIVITY   CULTURAL AND ETHNIC DIVERSITY

Allow 15 minutes

Choose a person whose background is familiar to you. This could be yourself, or a close relative, or someone you know in another context. Quickly list what you know about their background. What different nationalities and cultural backgrounds have gone into creating this person?

Comment

One person who has done this activity said:

> I chose one of my sons. Although he has lived in England all his life he has come from eight great-grandparents representing very different cultural heritages. On one 'side' of the family four of his great-grandparents were central European, from various countries within the then Austro-Hungarian Empire. On the other 'side' one great-grandparent was from Belgium, one from the Home Counties, England, one from Northumberland and one from Scotland.

Other people were not convinced of the importance of the ethnicity or cultural background of their family, but were more concerned to concentrate on geographical diversity: for example, 'The fact that my son was brought up in Leicester is probably more significant in terms of understanding cultural differences than his family history.'

With such a potentially rich mix of people and cultural practices, it is important to try to understand the ways in which people from all groups in the community think about their own health. What happens when people import their own cultural practices, including medicine, into their new country as immigrants? One of the most influential studies in the UK looked at British Bangladeshi people and how their health beliefs and folk models affect their view of diabetes (Greenhalgh et al., 1998). This study used a range of qualitative methods to chart observable health-related behaviour and, more importantly, to discern the underlying attitudes and belief systems driving that behaviour. The anthropological analysis of this research accepted that there are three levels of cultural behaviour: what people say they do (for example, during an interview), what they actually do, and the underlying belief system driving that behaviour. However, in addition to the cultural issues, the researchers also commented on the wider context in which health-related behaviour takes place. The researchers found examples of structural and material barriers to improving the health of Bangladeshi people living in the UK. Poor housing, unsafe streets and financial hardship were at least as important in preventing certain outcomes (such as taking regular exercise) as religious restrictions or ethnic customs. Han (2000) reached the same conclusion when studying the sociopolitical context of the ways in which Korean immigrants used their traditional medicine after settling in Australia. Korean people living in Australia certainly used the available biomedical services when this was appropriate, but they also used traditional Korean herbal medicine and acupuncture and other informal remedies, despite their high cost, in order to stay fit for work.

There is surprisingly little research evidence about the use of CAM by ethnic minority groups in the UK. Cappuccio et al. (2001) studied the use of alternative medicines in a multi-ethnic population. They found that the regular use of non-prescribed medicines, cod-liver oil, primrose oil and garlic varied by ethnic group and gender, black people of African origin being significantly more likely to use them than either white people or people from South Asia. Ong (2003) found that, not surprisingly, high proportions of the Chinese population living in the UK are regular users of TCM. Johnston (2003) studied the children who attended a dermatology clinic in Leicester and found that they often used TCM, especially children from ethnic minority groups.

Kate Reed explored the health choices of British Asian mothers in Leicester. She found a highly fluid pattern of CAM use: British Asian women's use of western and non-western medicines changes according to many different parameters. For example, western approaches are used for certain types of illness, particularly if they are considered very serious. However, this might change if the western remedies are deemed to be ineffective:

> the women appeared to be moving toward drawing more on non-Western remedies advocated by their mothers, while at the same time they were being influenced by younger generations and other populations and communities.
>
> (Reed, 2003, p. 169)

11.6 Conclusion

This chapter discussed various aspects of folk and traditional medicine as well as their associated cultural heritages, beliefs and practices. Extending the scope of this study like this should further your understanding of how CAM fits into the wider picture of health care.

In every society there is an enormously wide range of health beliefs and practices. Although in western 'developed' societies the orthodox, or biomedical, approach seems to dominate, many other systems still exist. Even without government sanction, or financial support through statutory channels, many long-standing cultural practices and care systems remain in existence through folk heritage and within cultural 'memory' and, indeed, current practice. The recent resurgence of interest in these forms of health care and in developing certain elements of CAM in western societies could be considered a response to dissatisfaction with some of the more rigid elements of the biomedical model. The growth of interest in CAM may be part of a general search for a return to more traditional health care practices that are congruent with the philosophical values of multiracial, multicultural, post-modern societies (Astin, 2000).

In some cases, the development and spread of modern biomedical services has threatened long-standing 'traditional', culturally based systems with extinction (Fulder, 2002). In many developing countries culturally appropriate elements within traditional forms of health care are being eroded by the growth of commercially influenced, western, 'orthodox' medical practice. However, official recognition is belatedly coming to the defence of some forms of traditional and folk medicine (WHO, 2002a), and current progressive opinion, and even official policy in some countries, allows for 'the best of both worlds' to coexist and learn from each other (Durie, 2003).

A major theme of this chapter was how boundaries between the various forms of CAM and traditional, orthodox and folk medicine can overlap and that there is some scope for change from one to another. There are no clear demarcation lines between the various forms of health care practice, but societies change and populations move geographically in response to social and economic forces. People in transition between various cultures are particularly vulnerable to health problems and it may be especially important to recognise and develop their culturally specific forms of support and health care.

KEY POINTS

- Many CAM practices are derived from folk or 'traditional' forms of health care practice.

- Some CAM practices are culturally specific and are appropriate only within certain cultural parameters. Others may be more widely applicable and used in a broader setting.

- The definition of what is or is not CAM can change according to the social and cultural context.

- Folk medicine still exists throughout the world and is often related to the way in which people think about their own health and caring for others.

- Traditional forms of medicine are often viewed with suspicion by the orthodox medical system, but more enlightened policy allows for the development of both systems for the benefit of people in developing countries and post-colonial societies.

- Traditional medicine remains largely unregulated and uncontrolled and potential dangers are associated with some forms of its practice.

- Traditional medicines can be threatened by unscrupulous commercial exploitation and 'bio-prospecting', particularly biologically active herbal preparations.

- Migrant and immigrant people may be especially vulnerable at the time of their migration and they often bring their own health beliefs and practices to their new setting.

- Most 'modern' western societies comprise a wide range of people from diverse backgrounds and ethnic origins. Their use of CAM and traditional medicines is of particular interest in understanding more about culturally specific forms of CAM.

References

Adams, G. (2002) 'Shiatsu in Britain and Japan: personhood, holism and embodied aesthetics', *Anthropology and Medicine*, Vol. 9, No. 3, pp. 245–65.

Alternative Health Directory (2004) 'Acupuncture description and practitioners' [online], www.alternativehealthuk.ci.uk/acupuncture/page1.html [accessed 1 July 2004].

Astin, J. (2000) 'The characteristics of CAM users: a complex picture', in Kelner, M., Wellman, B., Pescosolido, B. and Saks, M. (eds) *Complementary and Alternative Medicine: Challenge and Change*, Amsterdam, Harwood Academic Publishers.

BMJ (2003) Letter in 'Minerva', *British Medical Journal*, Vol. 326, p. 1406.

Bodeker, G. (2001) 'Lessons on integration from the developing world's experience', *British Medical Journal*, Vol. 322, pp. 164–7.

Cappuccio, F., Duneclift, S., Atkinson, R. and Cook, D. (2001) 'Use of alternative medicines in a multi-ethnic population', *Ethnicity and Disease*, Vol. 11, No. 1, pp. 11–18.

Carroll, R. (2003) 'It's green, prickly and sour, but this plant could cure obesity and save an ancient way of life', *The Guardian*, 4 January. Available online at www.guardian.co.uk/print/0,3858, 4576633_103681,00.html [accessed 16 February 2004].

Chaudhury, R. (2001) 'Challenges in using traditional systems of medicine', *British Medical Journal*, Vol. 322, p. 167.

CITES (2004) Website: www.cites.org/eng/resols/10/10_19.html [accessed 16 February 2004].

Cunningham, C. and Stanley, F. (2003) 'Indigenous by definition, experience, or world view', *British Medical Journal*, Vol. 327, pp. 403–4.

Durie, M. (2003) 'Providing health services to indigenous peoples: a combination of conventional services and indigenous programmes is needed', *British Medical Journal*, Vol. 327, pp. 408–9.

Escher, M. and Desmeules, J. (2001) 'Hepatitis associated with Kava, a herbal remedy for anxiety', *British Medical Journal*, Vol. 322, p. 139.

Ethnomedica (2004) 'Aims and policy statement' [online], www.kew.org/ethnomedica/AimsPolicy.html [accessed 22 June 2004].

Farnsworth, N. (1994) 'Biodiversity and human health', *Ciba Foundation Symposium*, Vol. 185, pp. 42–51.

Frank, J. and Frank, J. (1991) *Persuasion and Healing*, Baltimore, MD, Johns Hopkins University Press.

Fulder, S. (2002) 'Extinction and diversity in alternative medicine', *The Journal of Alternative and Complementary Medicine*, Vol. 8, No. 4, pp. 395–7.

Greenhalgh, T., Helman, C. and Chowdhury, A. (1998) 'Health beliefs and folk models of diabetes in British Bangladeshis: a qualitative study', *British Medical Journal*, Vol. 316, pp. 978–83.

Han, G. (2000) 'Traditional herbal medicine in the Korean community in Australia: a strategy to cope with health demands of immigrant life', *Health*, Vol. 4, No. 4, pp. 426–54.

Hawke, K. (1973) *Cornish Sayings, Superstitions and Remedies*, Redruth, Dyllanson Truran.

Hesketh, T. and Zhu, W. (1997) 'Health in China: traditional Chinese medicine: one country, two systems', *British Medical Journal*, Vol. 315, pp. 115–7.

Hollis-Triantafillou, J. (1995) 'Folk wisdom', *British Medical Journal*, Vol. 311, p. 335.

Johnston, S. (2003) 'Native American traditional and alternative medicine', *The Annals of the American Academy*, Vol. 585, pp. 195–213.

Masiello, D. J. (2004) 'Osteopathy' [online], www.dr-dom.com/osteopathy_history.html [accessed 23 June 2004].

Normile, D. (2003) 'The new face of traditional Chinese medicine', *Science*, Vol. 299, pp. 188–99.

Ong, C. (2003) *Complementary and Alternative Medicine: The Consumer Perspective*, London, Prince of Wales's Foundation for Integrated Health.

Puckree, T., Mkhize, M., Mgobhozi, Z. and Lin, J. (2002) 'African traditional healers: what health care professionals need to know', *International Journal of Rehabilitation Research*, Vol. 25, pp. 247–51.

Reed, K. (2003) *Worlds of Health: Exploring the Health Choices of British Asian Mothers*, London, Praeger.

Ring, I. and Brown, N. (2003) 'The health status of indigenous people and others', *British Medical Journal*, Vol. 327, pp. 404–5.

Rudgley, R. (1998) *The Encylopedia of Psychoactive Substances*, New York, Little, Brown and Company.

Sharma, U. (2004) Personal communication.

Social Trends (2003) *Social Trends 33*, London, Office for National Statistics.

Struthers, R. (2003) 'The artistry and ability of traditional women healers', *Health Care for Women International*, Vol. 24, pp. 340–54.

Texas State Historical Association (2004) *The Handbook of Texas* [online], www.tsha.utexas.edu/handbook/online/articles/view/CC/sdc1.html [accessed 13 February 2004].

Trevett, A. and Lalloo, D. (1992) 'A new look at an old drug: artemesinin and qinghaosu', *PNG Medical Journal*, Vol. 35, No. 4, pp. 264–9.

Waldram, J. B. (2000) 'The efficacy of traditional medicine: current theoretical and methodological issues', *Medical Anthropology Quarterly*, Vol. 14, No. 4, pp. 603–25.

WHO (2002a) *WHO Traditional Medicine Strategy 2002–2005*, Geneva, World Health Organization.

WHO (2002b) 'WHO launches the first global strategy on traditional and alternative medicine', Press release, 16 May. Available online at www.who.int/inf/en/pr_2002_38.html [accessed 16 February 2004].

Zhang, G., Bausell, B., Lao, L., Handwerger, B. and Berman, B. (2003) 'Assessing the consistency of traditional Chinese medical diagnosis: an integrative approach', *Alternative Therapies*, Vol. 9, No. 1, pp. 66–71.

Zollman, C. and Vickers, A. (1999) 'What is complementary medicine?', *British Medical Journal*, Vol. 319, pp. 693–6.

Chapter 12   Investigating patterns of provision and use of CAM

Andrew Vickers, Tom Heller and Julie Stone

Contents

AIMS

- To understand ways of investigating the patterns of CAM provision and use within a geographical locality.
- To consider some of the geographical issues in the distribution and spread of contemporary CAM modalities.

12.1   Introduction

In Chapter 7 the question 'What do people want?' was considered and the decisions individuals make about who uses complementary and alternative medicine (CAM), and why, were studied. This chapter consolidates Chapter 7, focusing in more detail on the ways of investigating the choices people make about therapy. It also focuses on the practitioners who use CAM in their work and asks who they are and why they have become CAM therapists. The dynamic nature of the spread of CAM use within a community and among communities is also discussed. In addition, this chapter looks at some of the geographical patterns of CAM use and discusses the ways in which these patterns are determined.

12.2   Investigating CAM

How is it possible to discover who uses CAM, and why? To answer these questions usually means going behind the official statistics. It may even be necessary to do original research by interviewing people or distributing questionnaires. Such surveys are very common in CAM research. Two main methods are used. Researchers may take a random sample of people from the general population and either interview them by telephone or send them a questionnaire. Alternatively, researchers may approach a particular group (for example, people with rheumatoid arthritis or cancer) and interview them about their use of CAM. Different types of question are also used. Some surveys ask closed questions, such as 'Do you use any form of complementary medicine?' The answer to this can be recorded as either 'yes' or 'no'. Open questions ask, for example, 'What do you think about the use of complementary medicine?' The answer to this type of question can be much longer, more complex and certainly more difficult to record, interpret and report on.

Analysing survey results

Surveys of CAM use can be surprisingly disparate, with wide variations in the results. To understand this lack of conformity, it is necessary to analyse critically how a survey was designed and what the figures actually represent. This section considers some of the reasons why CAM surveys yield such different results. Two crucial issues might explain some of the inconsistencies in the results of surveys: first, the researchers might use different definitions of CAM; second, they might use different definitions of who is a CAM user.

Earlier chapters showed that there is no single, widely accepted definition of CAM. Rather, definitions of CAM are politically and historically contingent, and the boundaries of what is considered CAM are in a state of constant flux. In the absence of a single, overarching definition of CAM, researchers doing CAM surveys may have to generate their own definitions, which can potentially vary enormously. For example, in surveys of the US general public, Eisenberg et al. (1993, 1998) included prayer, physical fitness and dietary change as CAM practices. On the other hand, Paramore (1997) studied pain management specifically and included only four principal therapies, which might account for the substantial difference between the use of CAM found in the three surveys (34 per cent, 42 per cent and 10 per cent, respectively).

A population-based survey of England initially defined CAM as seeing a practitioner of one of five main therapies, namely acupuncture, chiropractic, homoeopathy, medical herbalism and osteopathy, but later included two further therapies – aromatherapy and reflexology – because of the high number of mentions from respondents (Thomas et al., 2001, 2003).

In a report of the BBC Radio 5 Live survey of CAM use in the UK, which ranked the popularity of certain therapies, chiropractic was not in the top seven (Ernst and White, 2000). This may seem surprising but remember that the survey was self-selecting: only listeners to Radio 5 completed the survey. This in itself is highly selective and excludes many sectors of the community. However, this finding could also indicate that consumers no longer define commonly available treatments such as chiropractic and osteopathy (ranked seventh) as complementary or alternative but rather as mainstream (Ong and Banks, 2003).

Some researchers gather together the results of many other surveys and produce a 'meta-analysis' or systematic review of the currently published research. For example, Harris and Rees (2000) reviewed 638 references to published surveys on CAM use and decided that only 12 of them could be included in their review because all the others had problems with their research methodology.

Most surveys encourage the idea of CAM being about visits to a practitioner. This excludes many practices which could also be interpreted as CAM. For example, several cultures follow diets that recommend a balance of 'hot' and 'cold' foods and the use of certain herbs to treat or prevent illness, or that advocate the routine use of exercise such as yoga or t'ai chi (for example, as part of ayurveda and traditional Chinese medicine or TCM). As Chapter 11 shows, these activities may be considered folk or informal traditions, possibly because they may fall outside the realm of financial transactions. Yet a person who pays someone else for advice about herbs, diet and exercise tends to be characterised as a CAM user. Should a culturally sanctioned therapy administered, for example, by a family member count as CAM or not? For instance, in Hawaii, a parent or grandparent might routinely administer traditional massage techniques to a child. In the UK, although increasing numbers of parents learn baby massage, most parents pay for such therapies for their child. Is the former folk medicine but the latter CAM? Perhaps in some situations the use of certain remedies or home-based practice is so well integrated and incorporated into the way people live that it is not seen as treatment or therapy. Should the exchange of money be considered the defining difference?

There is an interesting distinction between seeing a CAM practitioner (such as a chiropractor) and self-administering CAM, such as by taking herbs, changing diet or practising yoga, meditation, etc. For example, the BBC Radio 5 Live survey reported, in addition to the seven most popular, the use of 22 therapies or practices, including t'ai chi, qi gong and yoga, as well as over-the-counter (OTC) purchases (Ernst and White, 2000). Surveys that include self-administered CAM naturally tend to report a much larger prevalence of use than those reporting only practitioner-administered CAM. Whereas there are several surveys about why people consult practitioners, relatively little is known about who self-administers OTC CAM products, and why.

TABLE 12.1   RESULTS FROM A SELECTION OF SURVEYS INVESTIGATING CAM USE IN DIFFERENT SETTINGS

Author(s) and date	Country	Sample	Percentage of sample who use CAM
MacLennan et al. (1996)	Australia	General public	48
Norheim and Fonnebo (2000)	Norway	General public	20
Thomas et al. (1993)	UK	General public	8
Thomas et al. (2001)	UK	General public	12
Eisenberg et al. (1993)	USA	General public	34
Eisenberg et al. (1998)	USA	General public	42
Druss and Rosenheck (1999)	USA	General public	8
Ni et al. (2002)	USA	General public	29
Paramore (1997)	USA	General public	10
Malik et al. (2000)	Pakistan	Cancer patients	55
Ramsey et al. (2001)	USA	Arthritis patients	47
Wolsko et al. (2003)	USA	Back pain patients	54
Patterson et al. (2002)	USA	Cancer patients	70
van de Weg and Streuli (2003)	Switzerland	Cancer patients	39
Rees et al. (2001)	UK	Cancer patients	32

ACTIVITY   CAM SURVEY RESULTS

Allow 20 minutes

Table 12.1 shows the results from a selection of CAM surveys. Look carefully at these results and write some notes on your impression of them. For example, one feature is the widely differing proportion of people who are reported to use CAM. Make a list of the possible reasons why surveys give such inconsistent estimates of the proportion of the general public using CAM.

Comment

Table 12.1 shows that the proportion of people using CAM seems higher among groups with a particular medical problem than among the population in general. This is more important than it might seem: many sceptics have dismissed CAM as merely a placebo for the 'worried well', which infers that CAM's popularity is confined largely to people who are not really ill. This is not borne out by the surveys. The other noticeable feature of Table 12.1 is that estimates for the prevalence of CAM vary widely.

The differing results of surveys may reflect true differences in CAM use. For example, rates of CAM use may vary from country to country or from year to year. However, such true differences seem an unlikely explanation for the enormous variation in the surveys' results. Methodological differences between studies are a more plausible explanation.

Some of the surveys were 'face to face'; others were the result of a telephone survey; while others were self-administered. Some are reported single-time studies, while others are longitudinal surveys done at more than one time. These different methods of collecting statistics could affect the results obtained.

The subject of self-administered CAM also raises important issues about the definition of CAM. It is tempting to define CAM as any health-related action by a person that is not part of orthodox medicine. However, this would include many folk practices such as eating chicken soup for a cold, taking a hot bath and a glass of whisky for insomnia, or wearing a copper bracelet for arthritis. Perhaps one reason for the scant research on this topic is the sheer diversity of health practices that people adopt, which may be so ingrained that they do not even think of them as 'health practices', whether CAM or not.

The failure of surveys to differentiate between CAM delivered by a therapist and self-administered interventions or classes can also affect the reasons people cite for **why** they use CAM. For example, consider the results from the BBC Radio 5 Live survey in Table 12.2, in which people gave their reasons for using CAM.

TABLE 12.2 RESPONDENTS' REASONS FOR USING CAM*	
Reason	Percentage
Just like it	20.8
Find it relaxing	18.8
Good health/wellbeing	13.9
To find out about other ways of life	10.6
To meet other people/make new friends	0.8

*Total = 245 respondents

(Source: adapted from Ernst and White, 2000, p. 35, Table 4)

ACTIVITY   THE PURPOSES OF CAM SURVEYS

Allow 30 minutes

List some of the purposes for commissioning CAM surveys. Who wants this information and why? In what ways do you think the design and outcomes of a survey might be influenced by the reasons for commissioning it and the organisation funding the research?

Comment

There are numerous, diverse reasons for surveys of CAM usage. As with all health care research, it is necessary to look behind the statistics and critically evaluate why the research was designed in the way it was, and what the implications are for the results. The reasons for CAM surveys include:

■ estimating CAM use in the general population to determine the potential for NHS provision and future health policy

■ developing services or projects in a particular locality

■ developing a business plan, which may require a survey of a local area for CAM use to determine, for example, whether to open a TCM shop in the high street

■ preparing large-scale studies by market researchers to determine the levels of commercial use and the size of a market sector (for example, Mintel, 2003).

Surveys commissioned by different groups may have several more or less explicit objectives. For example, researchers trying to identify public safety issues might commission a survey to determine adverse effects of OTC CAM-related remedies. Researchers wanting to secure mainstream funding for CAM might opt for the widest possible inclusion criteria of what CAM is and who is a CAM user, to show the wide extent of its use. Finally, research objectives are determined largely by who funds the research. The commercial sector has spawned many surveys of CAM use that were specifically designed to do 'market research' on CAM, to help commercial decision makers determine investment potential for various geographical areas.

Are more people using CAM?

The public's use of CAM is said to be increasing. This seems plausible because, in the past 30 years or so, CAM has gone from being a fringe activity to a presence in nearly every high street, bookshop and hospital. However, it is difficult to find hard facts and figures: very few surveys are repeated a few years apart using the same methods on the same population. This makes it difficult to track any changes in CAM use, with two exceptions: the population survey of England by Thomas et al. in 1993 and 2001 and the US surveys by Eisenberg et al. in 1993 and 1998. Both sets of sequential surveys showed that each year approximately 5 per cent more people used CAM than in the previous year:

> A prior national survey of one in eight randomly selected general practices in England estimated that 39% of general practices ... provided some access to complementary or alternative medicine (CAM) therapies in 1995. A repeat survey, conducted in 2001, estimated that one in two practices in England now offer their patients some access to CAMs ... The change was due to increased provision in-house; the proportion of practices making NHS referrals remained unchanged. The proportion of services supported by patient payments rose from 26 to 42%.
>
> (Thomas et al., 2003, p. 575)

There is also evidence that each CAM user is having more CAM treatments and using more CAM products. For example, while the number of US citizens who used CAM in 1997 was 25 per cent higher than in 1993, the number of visits to practitioners increased by nearly 50 per cent (Eisenberg et al., 1998).

How much can be learned about CAM users' beliefs?

In an attempt to learn more about why people use CAM, sociologists and psychologists have compared the beliefs (not just health beliefs) of CAM users with those of people who have never used CAM (see for example, Sirious and Gick, 2002). Some of these 'push' and 'pull' beliefs were explored in Chapter 7. In general, CAM users are more likely to have some of the following characteristics:

- a holistic orientation to health
- less confidence in prescribed drugs
- a belief in the importance of a 'healthy mind'
- a commitment to environmentalism
- a commitment to feminism
- an interest in spirituality and personal growth psychology
- less confidence in medical science
- a belief that medical science and scientific methodology can be harmful.

However, studies examining the different beliefs of CAM users and non-users arguably do not explain **why** patients use CAM. One explanation for this is that people's beliefs after consulting a practitioner may differ from their beliefs before they went. What if particular health beliefs are not a cause of CAM use but a result of it? Perhaps the best way of knowing would be to interview many people who are yet to use CAM, monitor them for several years, and then see who started to use CAM. However, this would be impractical and such a study has not been attempted. Interesting areas for further research include whether certain health beliefs correlate with pursuing one form of CAM over another, and whether different beliefs can predict whether people become one-off or committed CAM users.

12.3   Wider considerations that may govern CAM use

Changes in the provision and uptake of complementary and alternative therapies do not happen in a vacuum but have a relationship with wider social and societal movements. This section explores some of these features and relates them to the changes in CAM described in this chapter and in Chapter 7.

The decline of organised religion

In the early 20th century the relative roles of medicine and religion were clear and distinct. Medicine treated the physical body and serious psychological disorders; religion dealt with the spirit, which often involved what might now be described as mild psychological illness. The decline of some conventional forms of religion throughout the UK during the 20th century, and the increasingly isolated way in which many people live, has left growing numbers of people looking for other forms of support and nurture, especially when serious illness raises issues about their role and meaning in life. Of course, not all forms of religion have declined: the Islamic faith and some types of evangelical Christianity have grown. However, orthodox medicine, broadly speaking, has not made up for this more general decline, which has been a source of criticism. For example, one of the most well known critiques of modern medicine is Ivan Illich's *Limits to Medicine* (1976). One of his main points is that medicine's desire to eradicate death, pain and sickness has compromised and undermined wider society's capacity to cope with the human reality of death, pain and sickness.

It is questionable whether orthodox medicine is 'wrong' to avoid direct involvement in spiritual and existential concerns. Doctors might argue that they do not downplay such issues because they consider them irrelevant; they just do not believe they are the best people to deal with them. CAM could be considered to address people's need for support and their search for meaning, replacing a role previously performed by priests and other spiritual advisers. A person who is feeling low might be told they are stressed or need to restore balance to their life. A person with a more serious illness might be given an explanation for the cause of their disease in readily understandable terms: an energy imbalance; pollution; stress; an allergy to a common food; a personality trait. Such explanations can give meaning to their illness: they provide a 'story to live by'. This is in distinct contrast to biomedical explanations, which rely on scientific veracity but may not resonate with people's everyday lives.

High tech, high touch

It is often said that modern societies have led to reduced social interaction (Putnam, 2000). Contrast the stereotypical image of a tribal woman cooking in a village, surrounded by her extended family, with the modern image of a family member cooking alone in an isolated western suburban home. Similarly, many folk-healing interventions are directed at whole families or communities, not just the individuals: for example, the Hawaiian problem-solving technique *ho'oponopono* is a type of family psychotherapy in which each family member has an opportunity to air their grievances in a supported environment (Shook, 2002). Orthodox medicine, in contrast, is usually targeted at the individual and only occasionally involves other family members. Although the same could be said about some CAM interventions, many CAM therapies provide individuals with an opportunity for social interaction, sometimes in the intimate form of physical touch, sometimes in the form of group activities such as yoga or relaxation classes.

A study in the UK of older people's use of CAM seems to confirm this social aspect (Andrews, 2003a). The respondents in this study were prepared to travel up to nine times further to visit a practitioner in a group setting. Interviewees perceived group practices as hubs, or centres, of therapeutic activity. One respondent described her visits to a therapist who worked in a group practice and said 'it's like a day out'. Almost all CAM therapies involve lengthy talks with the CAM practitioner; this social interaction may be one of the attractions.

Julie Burchill, writing rather provocatively in a newspaper article that could offend single people, alludes to altogether less salubrious motives:

> It may be crude and cruel to point this out, but the majority of pamperees are single women who are probably chronically deprived of the tactile exchanges that solo ladies, bless 'em, report missing much more than rough old sex itself. Whereas a man missing sex will go and pay a prostitute, a woman missing being touched will go and pay for a massage. I can't get my head around this – surely the groper should be paying the gropee, not the other way around?
>
> (Burchill, 2003, p. 46)

Prosperity

The average UK citizen is considerably more prosperous now than 25, 50 or 100 years ago. This affects CAM use in two ways. First, people have more disposable income to spend on health products or pursuits. Second, many of the conditions treated by CAM, for example fatigue or mild anxiety, only become significant once people have addressed more pressing concerns, such as feeding and clothing themselves and their children. The way in which Maslow (1971) characterised these needs was discussed in Chapter 1.

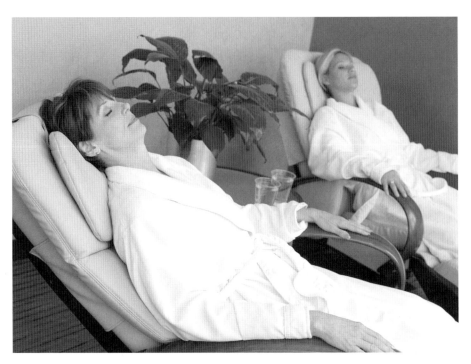

For some people, CAM is part of a lifestyle choice and has many features that are similar to beauty therapy

The use of CAM can be located in the study of the geography of consumption (Doel and Segrott, 2003). The increase in CAM use represents an increase in market-driven health care, in which 'smart consumers' draw on a variety of resources in search of better health (Kelner and Wellman, 2001). Wiles and Rosenberg (2001) suggest that the increased consumption of CAM might represent a form of consumption of culture, other cultures, and consumption of the past. There is certainly a greater surge of interest in the UK in TCM, shiatsu and ayurveda than, say, British folk remedies, which might indeed represent an ongoing fascination with 'the exotic'.

Surveying the evidence, Sharma (1992) found that the stereotype of CAM users being wealthy and better educated than non-users was borne out. However, recent UK-based surveys (for example, Ong et. al., 2002) found a great range of income groups represented by CAM users, not just wealthy people. Although, in various European studies, a larger proportion of patients are from a higher socioeconomic demographic group (Reilly, 2001), Sharma makes the important point that aggregated information can mask interesting differences: for example, the higher uptake of faith healing among poor people. As well as class and socioeconomic status, the availability of CAM services is also a significant predictor of use. A US survey found that states with more CAM providers per capita had a commensurately higher per capita visit rate (Cherkin et al., 2002). The issue is not as simplistic as it seems.

Wealthier people use CAM more, but they also live in wealthier neighbourhoods, stimulating a demand for various service industries and responding to the supply of them, including private CAM providers.

CAM and changes in medicine: cause or effect?

Some CAM practitioners claim that CAM is revolutionising medicine. However, it might be more accurate to say that a revolution in medicine is bringing about CAM. The dramatic increase in the use of and interest in CAM appears to stem from a set of wider social changes. Certainly, the previous distrust and separation of orthodox and complementary medicine that created such a barrier between them has been considerably eroded. George Lewith and his colleagues (2001) surveyed 12,068 members and fellows of the Royal College of Physicians, one of the most prestigious medical institutions, to determine their use of and attitudes to CAM. This group most commonly practised and referred people to acupuncture, aromatherapy and manipulative medicine:

> Of the group who responded, almost a third are using CAM either personally or within their clinical team, despite the fact that only 5.2% have had some form of formal or informal training in one or other of the CAM therapies. This is a cause for concern and justifies the criticisms made by many CAM professionals that conventional physicians may be undervaluing their training and expertise.
>
> (Lewith et al., 2001, p. 171)

12.4 The geography of CAM

The geography of CAM in this context means both the locational availability of CAM (that is, the geographical areas where CAM is practised) and the situational context of CAM (for example, the different settings where CAM is practised). Doel and Segrott (2003) describe their difficulty as geographers faced with the task of studying the phenomenon of CAM:

> What, then, are we as geographers to make of a mass-mediated space of CAM that is literally beyond belief and beyond finality? What are we to make of its ambivalent and risky action plans? What are we to make of its heterogeneous, incommensurate, and incompossible [cannot coexist] materials and practices?
>
> (Doel and Segrott, 2003, p. 754)

Where is CAM located?

Andrews (2002) comments that 'health geography' provides a comprehensive understanding of the dynamic relationship between people, health and place. Questions such as where CAM is situated, and what is offered where and by whom, are deeply entwined. For example, certain geographical areas attract more CAM use than others. The greater the consumer demand for CAM, the higher the CAM profile is likely to be in a given area. At the same time, the presence of many therapists in a relatively small geographical area can increase and induce demand (Andrews, 2003a). Other practical factors that may influence the location of CAM are the presence of large therapeutic training schools (which often have a reduced fee clinic attached), the relationship between CAM and mainstream health providers, and local regulatory provisions.

Demographic factors also affect the geography of use. Although CAM almost certainly flourishes in areas with a wealthier population, including higher proportions of people who already use private medicine, it is widespread throughout the UK. People who are more affluent may also be more willing and able to pay for non-conventional therapies. People with greater disposable income already use other service industries, and may thus feel more inclined to pay for therapy as a treat, for example regular aromatherapy sessions or massages. They are also more likely to buy, for instance, expensive nutritional supplements. A higher uptake of CAM might also be expected among populations with a higher concentration of alternative beliefs and lifestyles, which is borne out by some of the US literature:

> Levin and Coreil (1986) argue that in contemporary American society there is an emergent subculture that can be broadly defined in terms of involvement in various forms of esoteric, spiritual pursuits (e.g. meditation, eastern and western mystical traditions). They further note that these interests are often coupled with the belief in and use of various forms of holistic healthcare and alternative medical approaches. As McGuire (1988) reports, many of these people see health and physical well-being within the larger context of personal (psychological) or spiritual growth and development. Her findings also suggest that interest in CAM may be a reaction to and a way to counter what people experience as an overly rationalized life experience (of self, body, and emotions).
>
> (Astin, 2000, p. 104)

Despite the widespread increase in CAM in the UK, the geographical distribution of CAM services varies significantly. Because the NHS provides relatively little CAM, its uptake in the UK often depends on private CAM services in a given area. There is also little research on the precise distribution of CAM in the UK. Although CAM use is largely concentrated in and around big cities, this is not a strict rule; many small towns and rural areas also have high concentrations of therapists. Cities attract a higher proportion of single people and those with significant disposable incomes (although this is matched by a correspondingly higher proportion of people on very low incomes). Much of the current lifestyle coverage of CAM therapies presupposes a cosmopolitan user, and newer 'faddy' therapies, promoted in health magazines and the lifestyle sections of newspapers and women's magazines, seem to proliferate more in large cities than in other areas.

The higher profile of CAM in cities may also reflect the greater ethnic diversity of urban areas. The use of CAM by people from different ethnic backgrounds is generally under-researched, but evidence suggests the use of folk and culturally sanctioned healing alongside orthodox forms of treatment (Greenhalgh et al., 1998).

Anecdotally, in the UK a higher proportion of people are thought to use CAM in the south than in the north, although there are few statistics to substantiate this. The BBC Radio 5 Live survey was of a small sample of people in the catchment area of the radio station. Even so, the research showed significant differences in the following geographical regions: 22.5 per cent in 'the north' ($n = 95$), compared with 26.2 per cent in 'the midlands' ($n = 79$) and 29.9 per cent in 'the south' ($n = 144$) (Ernst and White, 2000). Of the respondents from London and the South East, 30 per cent said they or a member of their household used CAM in 1999, compared with 21.7 per cent of those from the north/north-west or Yorkshire (Ong and Banks, 2003).

However, beyond the north–south divide there are pockets of intense CAM activity in areas such as Totnes, Glastonbury and Hebden Bridge, which are all associated with green or left-of-centre politics and alternative lifestyles. Wiles and Rosenberg (2001) argue that regional identity is constructed around the kinds of consumption in a particular region. The nature of certain areas may make them ideally suited to the widespread provision and uptake of CAM. Their observations about British Columbia provide an interesting comparison with towns in the UK where CAM flourishes:

> British Columbia is often referred to by the Canadian media as 'lotus land' – a place of former laid back hippies, back-to-the landers, escapees from the capitalist east.
>
> (Wiles and Rosenberg, 2001, p. 221)

It is also worth considering the idea of certain locations being therapeutic in themselves:

> Individuals and groups form attachments to specific locations and territories as a result of experiences and memories associated with them. This territoriality evokes what is called a 'sense of place', a distinctiveness

associated with a specific area. Research on therapeutic landscapes and the reasons why some places are perceived as healthful highlight the role of place **as** therapy ... Specific physical features such as mountains, springs, rivers and caves are believed to have health promoting and curative properties in some cultures.

(Chacko, 2003, p. 1090)

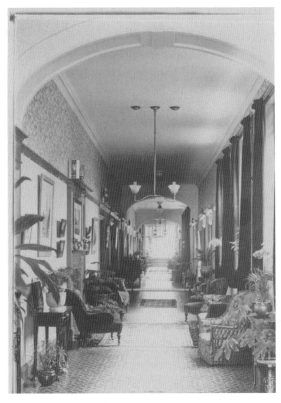

Some settings may feel as though they have calming or healing properties in themselves

ACTIVITY   TOTNES: A CASE STUDY

Allow 30 minutes

Andrews (2003a) identifies the link between CAM consumption and a strong 'sense of place', and highlights Totnes in Devon as an area of significant CAM usage.

Read the extract in Box 12.1 from Gavin Andrews' article about the geography of CAM, which is based on a study of the use of CAM by older people in Devon and Buckinghamshire. As you read it, make some notes on why CAM is so popular in this specific location.

Do you think these factors might be generalisable to other areas, including your own?

Comment

This case study vividly demonstrates how the increased presence and visibility can both supply and stimulate demand for CAM. What is striking is the extent to which CAM is an integral part of the alternative character of the town and many of its inhabitants. It is safe to assume that many people who live in, or move to, Totnes either subscribe to CAM beliefs themselves or are sympathetic to them. In effect, CAM use is normalised in this area: its use is both expected and encouraged among its inhabitants. This provides a level of peer expectation and acceptability in accessing CAM, which is why institutions such as Dartington College, as well as individuals, driven by a liberal and spiritual rationale, are attracted to this location.

People who choose to live in Totnes appear to have the strong sense of place described by Chacko (2003). Andrews refers to Totnes itself being a healing environment, which reinforces and is reinforced by the high level of therapeutic activities that go on there. This sense of place is associated with the perceived healing and spiritual nature of the environment (in the same way as, say, the city of Bath is associated with the healing properties of its water).

BOX 12.1   A THERAPEUTIC SETTING FOR CAM: THE CASE OF TOTNES

In certain cases, both the CM [complementary medicine] clinics and their host towns were found to be integral to the overall user experience. The most prominent example of a symbiotic relationship existing between clinics and their location was a range of practices in the small town of Totnes in Devon. The town was widely recognised for its tradition of alternative lifestyles and spiritualism and boasted many organic food shops, vegetarian cafés, health food shops, new age clothing and bookshops, and a wide variety of alternative lifestyle clubs and societies. This distinct local identity is acknowledged by older users, many of whom considered Totnes to be a spiritual landscape. An interviewee summarised this local image and culture:

> Lots of people either retire here or give up their careers and change their lifestyles. Therapies are only part of the total Totnes thing ... You've seen what it's like! The schoolchildren busk on the street, lots of people with funny clothes, all these rare shops. It makes a nice atmosphere, but it's hard for me to summarise it all for you. You just have to experience it.

Some users found it difficult to distinguish between the image of the town and their treatments because the two were considered to be very much interrelated. Nevertheless, they still acknowledged Totnes as a significant location for CAM. ... Some older users found the Town itself to have a particularly welcoming atmosphere for CM:

> People generally are more educated and informed about complementary medicine in this town, so you don't feel like you are doing something unusual ... Totnes is a very healing place and people feel safe here.

Given this image, the town itself may be described as one element of a therapeutic landscape, where to a degree, place, health and healthcare provision are interrelated. Arguably, in Totnes, the clinics themselves may be regarded as therapeutic places, however, they are also located within this wider therapeutic environment of the town. The two scales may be experienced as one, and together form a symbiotic and mutually supportive relationship. This finding supports Wiles and Rosenberg (2001) who argue that the consumption of CM may be a geographically constituted process, where both local and regional identity is important to the consumption of CM, and vice versa.

It may well be that, nationally, Totnes is a rare example of clinics being situated within a setting also known for its therapeutic qualities. However, it may be the case that elements of the Totnes case study exist elsewhere. Certainly, the dynamic highlighted between practice and locality was observed, albeit to a lesser extent, in certain towns in the other study county of Buckinghamshire. Further research is required to investigate this dynamic in greater detail, and to investigate the intricacies of the relationship between particular users, practices and their host localities.

(Source: Andrews, 2003a, pp. 342-3)

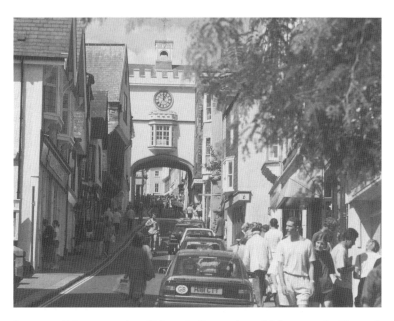

Some small towns, such as Totnes in Devon, have high concentrations of people involved with CAM therapies, both as practitioners and as clients

Wiles and Rosenberg (2001) discuss some of the factors affecting the geographical availability of CAM in North America. Some North American studies indicate that CAM is used more by people living in the western states or provinces. There is very little discussion about, or reflection on, **why** these patterns emerge. However, the patterns probably result from a variety of place-specific factors, each of which is highly complex. Other non-academic explanations can develop in the absence of established certainty. Thus certain communities or landscapes are thought to be therapeutic because they are west-facing and derive their energies from the sun setting into the western sea; others develop on ley lines or in places with special magical or mystical powers (see Box 12.2).

BOX 12.2   LEY LINES

Ley lines, or leys, are alignments of ancient sites stretching across the landscape. Ancient sites or holy places may be situated in a straight line ranging from one or two to several kilometres in length. A ley can be identified simply by the alignment of marker sites, or it might be visible on the ground for all or part of its length as the remnants of an old straight track.

Ley lines were 'rediscovered' on 30 June 1921 by Alfred Watkins (1855-1935), a well known Herefordshire businessman. While looking at a map for features of interest, he noticed a straight line that passed over hill tops through various points of interest, all of which were ancient. At the time of his discovery Watkins had no theory about alignments but on that June afternoon saw 'in a flash' a whole pattern of lines stretching across the landscape.

What are the settings for CAM delivery?

As Andrews (2003a) points out, there has been very little geographical research specifically on the practice and consumption of CAM. In the UK, little is known, for example, about local, regional and national distributions of CAM therapists; the spatial relationships with biomedical services; the migration and mobility of therapists; spatial referral networks; or the role of CAM in the community. Verheij et al. (1999) researched the geographical trends of CAM use in the Netherlands and found evidence of place variations associated with population characteristics and religious beliefs.

CAM is provided in an enormous variety of settings. Indeed, it is hard to think of places where it is not available. Wiles and Rosenberg (2001) talk about CAM as an example of **hidden consumption**, not least because of the 'diffuse spaces' in which CAM practitioners work.

In some settings, CAM practitioners work with other CAM practitioners as part of a team. Such environments might be seen as hubs of therapeutic activity, where people can access a range of mutually beneficial therapies. Patients attending natural health centres are more likely to try a variety of therapies: Sharma (1992) calls these 'eclectic users'. Depending on the relationships among practitioners (for example, the centre may operate as a legal partnership), therapists probably refer their patients to other practitioners working in the same clinic.

12.5   The practitioners of CAM

This section focuses on the people who become practitioners of complementary and alternative therapies. The extract in Box 12.3 discusses the growth in numbers of practitioners up to the end of the 1990s.

BOX 12.3   THE PROFILE OF CAM PRACTITIONERS

The number and profile of complementary practitioners is changing rapidly. In 1981 about 13 500 registered practitioners were working in the United Kingdom. By 1997 this figure had trebled to about 40 000, with three disciplines – healing, aromatherapy, and reflexology – accounting for over half of all registered complementary practitioners, with roughly 14 000, 7000, and 5000 members respectively. Although membership of these disciplines is high compared with other complementary disciplines (only 1118 chiropractors and 2325 osteopaths were registered at the time), very few practise full time.

Nearly 4000 conventional healthcare professionals also practise complementary medicine and are members of their own register (such as the British Medical Acupuncture Society for doctors and dentists). Of these, nearly half practise acupuncture (mainly doctors and physiotherapists), about a quarter practise reflexology (mainly nurses and midwives), and about one in seven practises homoeopathy (mainly doctors, chiropodists, and podiatrists). Many more conventional healthcare professionals, especially general practitioners, have attended basic training courses and provide limited forms of complementary medicine without official registration.

(Source: Zollman and Vickers, 1999, p. 838)

These statistics show there is a huge variation in the number of practitioners of different therapies. It can be difficult for many of these therapies to determine precisely the numbers in each therapeutic group because there may be several different professional bodies, each with their own registers.

There are many routes to becoming a CAM practitioner. The diversity of individuals' journeys to become therapists reflects the range and scope of the practice of complementary and alternative medicine itself. In addition, choosing a career in CAM seems to mirror many of the reasons why individuals decide to use CAM for their ailments. For some it is a move away from orthodox forms of medical treatment that they consider harmful or not in line with their general philosophical beliefs. Some practitioners may have strong ideas about health and healing, including the responsibility people have to lead healthier lives. For others, there may be more pragmatic financial considerations: becoming a CAM practitioner is a career path that can help meet personal financial needs. For many practitioners, working in CAM is a 'calling', in the nature of a spiritual quest. Sharma's research (1992) similarly identifies two broad reasons for people choosing to become therapists. The first is a desire to heal and help people and the second is a desire to work independently and relatively free from bureaucratic constraints.

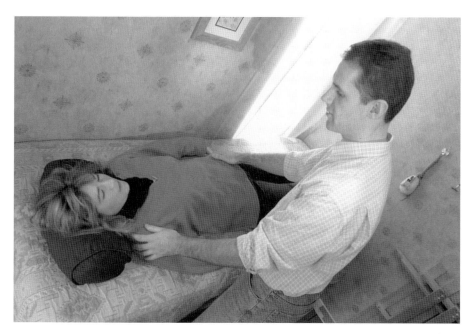

Chris Colgan from Croydon in Surrey had spent all his working life in IT and retail until he left his job to become a reiki healer. 'I'd rather be earning a fraction of what I was getting before, and do what I am doing now. It's much more satisfying.'

Orthodox health professionals practising CAM

CAM is often practised by orthodox health professionals who take additional training in particular methods. Some examples are given in Table 12.3 (overleaf). The number of practitioners is substantial: for example, currently in the UK more than 1000 doctors have qualifications in homoeopathy and several thousand are trained in acupuncture.

TABLE 12.3 ORTHODOX PRACTITIONERS AND THEIR CAM INTERESTS	
Profession	Typical therapy
General practitioner	Acupuncture, homoeopathy, hypnosis
Physiotherapist	Acupuncture, osteopathy, reflexology or chiropractic
Nurse	Massage, aromatherapy, reflexology, relaxation therapy
Clinical psychologist	Hypnosis
Occupational therapist	Relaxation techniques

Adams (2003) notes that an increasing number of general practitioners in the UK are personally practising CAM when treating their NHS patients. His research identifies several positive gains from the point of view of a selection of these 'GP therapists'. They believed the inclusion of complementary therapies in their repertoire had several functions. It filled gaps when treating conditions for which conventional practice was ineffective; it provided safer techniques in situations where there may be adverse or potential side effects from conventional treatments; and it helped to maintain job satisfaction and relieve boredom for the practitioners themselves.

Andrews (2003b) interviewed nurses in the UK who had left the NHS to pursue their careers in complementary medical practice (see Box 12.4). He found that nurse therapists were of a variety of ages, at different career stages, and had originated from a wide range of sub-disciplines of the nursing profession. Reflecting the complementary medicine private sector more generally, the ex-nurse therapists operated independent small businesses either from their own homes, or in dedicated rented accommodation, or in group practices with other therapists. Many practised more than one modality of complementary medicine and had gradually broadened their treatment portfolio over time. The majority practised part-time, but half of all therapists wanted to increase their client base and the hours they work.

Just as commentators argue that users adopt complementary medicine because of a complex interplay of 'push' factors from orthodox medicine and 'pull' factors from complementary medicine, Andrews argues that nurse therapists are motivated to leave or reduce their nursing commitments and go to private complementary medicine through a similar combination of factors. In the case of nurses, push factors are less associated with negative

> **BOX 12.4   NURSES' REASONS FOR LEAVING THE NHS AND TRAINING AS CAM THERAPISTS**
>
> The following nurses' statements are from Gavin Andrews' research into why nurses leave the NHS and become CAM practitioners.
>
> 'It's patient contact as in nursing but I gain more satisfaction as it is one-to-one contact and for longer periods.'
>
> 'Great satisfaction in helping people empower themselves by choosing their preferred type of healing as opposed to being limited to NHS services. Personally I also get satisfaction from them taking responsibility for their own health.'
>
> 'I can plan my timetable. I can work to my own set of high standards, I do not have to continually waste time and energy trying to please "the boss" or other work colleagues. Plus I don't have to listen to other colleagues moaning all the time.'
>
> (Source: Andrews, 2003b, p. 411)

experiences of orthodox medical treatment; rather, they are associated with their first-hand and negative experiences of orthodox medical provision. Respondents cited a wide range of factors: some were institutional, such as the continually changing organisational structures of the NHS and the scarcity of resources; some were work-related, such as long working hours, high pressure and stress; others were related to care issues, such as a lack of time with patients and experiences of poor patient outcomes.

Complementary medicine equally provides a wide-ranging set of pull factors. Some are experiential, such as being able to devote more time to each patient or nurses having witnessed or been given a successful treatment themselves; others are more conceptual and involve a belief in the alternative ways in which many CAM modalities understand and explain the body and the healing process. In this respect, the experiential and conceptual aspects of complementary medicine combine to present an attractive alternative paradigm of care.

12.6   Conclusion

This chapter focused on the patterns associated with the use and provision of CAM services. It described some of the ways of discovering who uses CAM and why. In addition, some of the wider societal features that might tend to affect the patterns of CAM use were considered. The decline of organised religion, the consumption of health care and new forms of spirituality were all discussed as possible forces affecting how people in contemporary society use CAM. Geographical factors impinge on the provision and uptake of CAM in a given locality. The study of 'health geography' is a way of understanding some features of the dynamic relationship between people, health and place.

Different patterns of people in their communities also generate and support different levels of CAM provision and use. Although it is hard to determine definitively how much CAM is 'out there', clearly CAM takes place in a multitude of settings, not all of which would traditionally be considered health-related. This highlights the extent to which CAM is increasingly a consumer phenomenon, concerned not only with treating illness but also with lifestyle and self-improvement issues. CAM is provided by a variety of practitioners, including growing numbers of conventionally trained ones. A significant number of them choose to leave the statutory health service, preferring to offer CAM in a setting which, to them, has greater opportunities for providing person-centred and holistic care.

KEY POINTS

- CAM is a general term that can describe a wide range of practices and approaches to health and health care.
- Discovering who uses CAM and why is open to problems of methodology.
- Some general patterns about the use of CAM are discernible, relating to the types of people who are most likely to use CAM, the therapies they use, and for what purposes.
- The number of people using CAM is growing and this is related to changes in wider society.
- The distribution of CAM in any geographical locality depends on a wide variety of factors, including demographics, the availability of services, and the 'sense of place' associated with certain therapeutic environments.
- The greater the number of CAM therapists in a geographical area, the greater the uptake of CAM.
- CAM practitioners represent a diverse group. Their characteristics and reasons for practising CAM vary and they may differ significantly in their approach.

References

Adams, J. (2003) 'The positive gains of integration: a qualitative study of GPs' perceptions of their complementary practice', *Primary Health Care Research and Development*, Vol. 4, pp. 155–62.

Andrews, G. (2002) 'Towards a more place-sensitive nursing research: an invitation to medical and health geography', *Nursing Inquiry*, Vol. 9, No. 4, p. 221.

Andrews, G. (2003a) 'Placing the consumption of private complementary medicine: everyday geographies of older people's use', *Health & Place*, Vol. 9, No. 4, pp. 337–49.

Andrews, G. (2003b) 'Nurses who left the British NHS for private complementary medical practice: why did they leave? Would they return?', *Journal of Advanced Nursing*, Vol. 41, No. 4, pp. 403–15.

Astin, J. A. (2000) 'The characteristics of CAM users: a complex picture', in Kelner, M., Wellman, B., Pescosolido, B. and Saks, M. (eds) *Complementary and Alternative Medicine: Challenge and Change*, Amsterdam, Harwood Academic Publishers.

Burchill, J. (2003) 'Trick or treat?', *The Guardian Weekend*, 22 November, pp. 46–7.

Chacko, E. (2003) 'Culture and therapy: complementary strategies for the treatment of type-2 diabetes in an urban setting in Kerala, India', *Social Science and Medicine*, Vol. 56, No. 5, pp. 1087–98.

Cherkin, D., Deyo, R., Sherman, K., Hart, G. L., Street, J., Hrbek, A., Cramer, E., Milliman, B., Booker, J., Mootz, R., Barassi, J., Kahn, J. R., Kaptchuk, T. and Eisenberg, D. (2002) 'Characteristics of licensed acupuncturists, chiropractors, massage therapists and naturopathic physicians', *Journal of the American Board of Family Practitioners*, September–October, Vol. 15, No. 5, pp. 378–90.

Doel, M. A. and Segrott, J. (2003) 'Beyond belief? Consumer culture, complementary medicine, and the dis-ease of everyday life', *Society and Space*, Vol. 21, pp. 739–59.

Druss, B. and Rosenheck, R. (1999) 'Association between use of unconventional therapies and conventional medical services', *Journal of the American Medical Association*, Vol. 282, No. 7, pp. 651–6.

Eisenberg, D., Kessler, R. and Foster, C. and others (1993) 'Unconventional medicine in the United States – prevalence, costs and patterns of use', *New England Journal of Medicine*, Vol. 328, pp. 246–52.

Eisenberg, D., Davis, R., Ettner, S., Appel, S., Wilkey, S., van Rompay, M. and Kessler, R. (1998) 'Trends in alternative medicine use in the United States, 1990–1997: results of a follow-up national survey', *Journal of the American Medical Association*, Vol. 280, No. 18, pp. 1569–75.

Ernst, E. and White, A. (2000) 'The BBC survey of complementary medicine use in the UK', *Complementary Therapies in Medicine*, Vol. 8, pp. 32–6.

Greenhalgh, T., Helman, C. and Chowdhury, A. M. (1998) 'Health beliefs and folk models of diabetes in British Bangladeshis: a qualitative study', *British Medical Journal*, Vol. 316, pp. 978–83.

Harris, P. and Rees, R. (2000) 'The prevalence of complementary and alternative medicine use among the general population: a systematic review of the literature', *Complementary Therapies in Medicine*, Vol. 8, No. 2, pp. 88–96.

Illich, I. (1976) *Limits to Medicine. Medical Nemesis: The Expropriation of Health*, London, Boyars.

Kelner, M. and Wellman, B. (2001) 'The therapeutic relationships of older adults: comparing medical and alternative patients', *Health and Canadian Society*, Vol. 6, No. 1, pp. 87–109.

Levin, J. and Coreil, J. (1986) '"New age" healing in the US', *Social Science and Medicine*, Vol. 23, pp. 889–97.

Lewith, G., Hyland, M. and Gray, S. F. (2001) 'Attitudes to and use of complementary medicine among physicians in the United Kingdom', *Complementary Therapies in Medicine*, Vol. 9, No. 3, pp. 167–72.

MacLennan, A., Wilson, D. and Taylor, A. (1996) 'Prevalence and cost of alternative medicine in Australia', *The Lancet*, Vol. 347, pp. 569–73.

Malik, I., Khan, N. and Khan, W. (2000) 'Use of unconventional methods of therapy by cancer patients in Pakistan', *European Journal of Epidemiology*, Vol. 16, No. 2, pp. 155–60.

Maslow, A. (1971) *Motivation and Personality*, New York, Harper and Row.

McGuire, M. (1988) *Ritual Healing in Suburban America*, New Brunswick, Rutgers University Press.

Mintel (2003) *Complementary Medicines in the UK*, London, Mintel.

Ni, H., Simile, C. and Hardy, A. (2002) 'Utilization of complementary and alternative medicine by United States adults: results from the 1999 national health interview survey', *Medical Care*, Vol. 40, No. 4, pp. 353–8.

Norheim, A. and Fonnebo, V. (2000) 'A survey of acupuncture patients: results from a questionnaire among a random sample in the general population in Norway', *Complementary Therapies in Medicine*, Vol. 8, No. 3, pp. 187–92.

Ong, C.-K. and Banks, B. (2003) *Complementary and Alternative Medicine: The Consumer Perspective*, London, The Prince of Wales's Foundation for Integrated Health.

Ong, C.-K., Peterson, S., Bodeker, G. and Stewart-Brown, S. (2002) 'Health status of people using complementary and alternative medical practitioner services in four English counties', *American Journal of Public Health*, Vol. 92, No. 10, pp. 1653–6.

Paramore, L. (1997) 'Use of alternative therapies: estimates from the 1994 Robert Wood Johnson Foundation National Access to Care Survey', *Journal of Pain Symptom Management*, Vol. 13, No. 2, pp. 83–9.

Patterson, R., Neuhouser, M., Hedderson, M., Schwartz, S., Standish, L., Bowen, D. and Marshall, L. (2002) 'Types of alternative medicine used by patients with breast, colon, or prostate cancer: predictors, motives, and costs', *The Journal of Alternative and Complementary Medicine*, Vol. 8, No. 4, pp. 477–85.

Putnam, R. (2000) *Bowling Alone: The Collapse and Revival of American Community*, New York, Simon and Schuster.

Ramsey, S., Spencer, A., Topolski, T., Belza, B. and Patrick, D. (2001) 'Use of alternative therapies by older adults with osteoarthritis', *Arthritis and Rheumatism*, Vol. 45, No. 3, pp. 222–7.

Rees, R., Feigel, I., Vickers, A., Zollman, C., McGurk, R. and Smith, C. (2001) 'Prevalence of complementary therapy use by women with breast cancer. A population-based survey', *European Journal of Cancer*, Vol. 36, No. 12, pp. 1359–64.

Reilly, D. (2001) 'Comments on complementary and alternative medicine in Europe', *The Journal of Alternative and Complementary Medicine*, Vol. 7, Supplement 1, pp. S23–S31.

Sharma, U. (1992) *Complementary Medicine Today. Practitioners and Patients*, London, Routledge.

Shook, E. V. (2002) *Ho'oponopono. Contemporary Uses of a Hawaiian Problem-Solving Process*, Hawai'i, University of Hawai'i Press.

Sirious, F. and Gick, M. (2002) 'An investigation of the health beliefs and motivations of complementary medicine clients', *Social Science and Medicine*, Vol. 55, pp. 1025–37.

Thomas, K., Fall, M. and Williams, B. (1993) *Methodological Study to Investigate the Feasibility of Conducting a Population-based Survey of the Use of Complementary Health Care*, Final report to the Research Council for Complementary Medicine, October 1993, London.

Thomas, K., Nicholl, J. and Coleman, P. (2001) 'Use and expenditure on complementary medicine in England – a population based survey', *Complementary Therapies in Medicine*, Vol. 9, pp. 2–12.

Thomas, K. J., Coleman, P. and Nicholl, J. P. (2003) 'Trends in access to complementary or alternative medicines via primary care in England: 1995–2001. Results from a follow-up national survey', *Family Practice*, Vol. 20, No. 5, pp. 575–7.

van der Weg, F. and Streuli, R. (2003) 'Use of alternative medicine by patients with cancer in a rural area of Switzerland', *Swiss Medicine Weekly*, Vol. 133, No. 15–16, pp. 233–40.

Verheij, R., de Bakker, D. and Groenewegen, P. (1999) 'Is there a geography of alternative medical treatment in the Netherlands?', *Health & Place*, Vol. 5, pp. 83–97.

Wiles, J. and Rosenberg, M. W. (2001) '"Gentle caring experience." Seeking alternative health care in Canada', *Health & Place*, Vol. 7, No. 3, pp. 209–24.

Wolsko, P., Eisenberg, D., Davis, R., Kessler, R. and Phillips, R. (2003) 'Patterns and perceptions of care for treatment of back and neck pain: results of a national survey', *Spine*, Vol. 28, No. 3, pp. 292–8.

Zollman C. and Vickers, A. (1999) 'ABC of complementary medicine. Users and practitioners of complementary medicine', *British Medical Journal*, Vol. 319, pp. 836–8.

Chapter 13   Cash and CAM: the private sector and CAM practice

Julie Stone and Tom Heller

Contents

AIMS

- To focus on the private provision of CAM and some of the financial and commercial aspects of its recent development.
- To consider the differences and similarities between private and statutory provision of CAM.

13.1   Introduction

This chapter focuses on the extent to which the development in the use of complementary and alternative medicine (CAM) in the UK over the last 30 years has been almost entirely within the private sector. Historically, CAM was forced to operate at the margins of orthodox medicine, while biomedically trained practitioners enjoyed almost monopoly status within the state-funded health care system (the NHS). This chapter reviews the reasons why people are prepared to pay for CAM, and considers the advantages and disadvantages of CAM being provided within the private sector. As with all social processes, the privatised use of CAM is not in a vacuum. To appreciate this phenomenon fully it is necessary to explore the social, economic, political and regulatory factors that shape the private provision of CAM and to consider the following major questions.

■ Are markets 'a good thing'? Can they deliver products of public value? Can they be successfully regulated?

■ What are the consequences of the liberalisation in trade of health care services?

■ What, if anything, makes private commercial health care (of any kind) offered in a market setting **different from** publicly provided health care?

■ Why do people use private health care **of any kind** when they can access biomedical services free at the point of delivery?

■ What factors in the UK have favoured the public health care system? What is this system supposed to deliver? How and why are these expectations changing or being challenged?

■ What is known about popular attitudes to paying for health care and how are these changing?

13.2   Provision of CAM in the private sector

Although CAM has always existed in a wide variety of forms, its recent history is one of development from a cottage industry into a multimillion pound market (Mintel, 2003). Within the last 30 years, there has been a huge growth in CAM (Stone, 2002). While many cultures around the globe have relied on traditional forms of healing, there are now high levels of use of alternative forms of health care in all developed nations. In the USA, more people are now thought to consult complementary and alternative therapists than primary health physicians (Eisenberg et al., 1998). Remarkably, this transition has occurred mostly in the private sector, with individuals seeking and often paying for the therapies themselves, even where there is free access to biomedical health care (unlike in the USA). Whereas in the past non-conventional approaches to health were dismissed by the medical establishment as a marginal activity, they are now part of mainstream culture and are seen and used by the public as a viable and accessible alternative to western orthodox medicine.

ACTIVITY   UNLIMITED ACCESS TO CAM?

Allow 15 minutes

Do you think that consumers should have unlimited access to any 'therapy' of their choice, as long as they pay for it themselves? For example, consider the case for and against colonic irrigation. Read the extracts in Boxes 13.1 and 13.2 (opposite) and make notes on whether you think that people should be able to purchase this form of therapy with their own money or that the NHS should provide this service.

BOX 13.1   THE CASE FOR COLONIC IRRIGATION

While the lungs, skin, kidneys and liver also serve to eliminate toxins, people have experienced throughout history that when they ensure that the colon is cleansed and healed, the well-being of the whole body is greatly enhanced. Colonic hydrotherapy has been found to be the most effective process available to accomplish this work quickly and easily. ... This condition [toxins in the body] is prevalent in all civilized societies, and particularly in the UK. Common signs include: headaches, backaches, constipation, fatigue, bad breath, body odour, irritability, confusion, skin problems, abdominal gas, bloating, diarrhoea, sciatic pain, and so forth. ...

Working with a skilled therapist a colonic can be a truly enlightening educational process. You will learn to expand your awareness of your body's functioning by including signals from your abdomen, your skin, your face and even from that most taboo of natural products, your eliminations. You will find that you can spot the beginnings of developing conditions through clues from these body regions and functions before they become serious. You can deal with them sooner and more easily than you otherwise might if you waited until they produce effects seen elsewhere in the body. Also, the solar plexus is the emotional centre of the body and the transverse colon passes right through it. If an emotional event is left uncompleted, it often results in physical tension being stored in the solar plexus, which affects all organs of the area, including the colon. This ongoing tightening of the colon muscle results in diminished movement of faecal material through the colon, which is experienced as constipation. Not only do colonics alleviate the constipation, they can assist you in creating a fully holistic view of your body's functioning, leading to a better quality of life. ...

Not infrequently, someone having their first colonic will remark that it was one of the most wonderful experiences of their life.

(Source: Association of Colonic Hydrotherapists, 2004)

BOX 13.2   THE CASE AGAINST COLONIC IRRIGATION

Colonics is popular as a health fetish. The ideas of 'cleansing' and 'detoxification' have no physiological significance, but these do have emotional meaning to people who believe themselves to be 'unclean' or 'impure' in some way. Just as the ancient Egyptians did, health neurotics may temporarily relieve their health anxieties by colonics, laxatives, and purges. Colonics also has erotic appeal to some. A substantial amount of colonic product marketing is aimed at male homosexuals. Colonics is often done in massage parlours that serve erotic desires. Colonics can be a kind of 'Dr Feelgood quackery' (i.e., a procedure that elicits a feeling in a patient which is interpreted as beneficial).

(Source: US National Council Against Health Fraud, 1995)

Comment

The reasons why people are attracted to colonic irrigation may well reflect a broader concept of health need than the functional model characterising most biomedical approaches. Certainly people's use of colonic irrigation does not appear to be based on an evaluation of the available clinical evidence. People seek CAM therapies for a variety of motives, not all of them 'health-related' in the strictest sense. This need not challenge the validity of these therapies, merely question the likelihood of their being integrated alongside more orthodox 'health' approaches.

Boxes 13.1 and 13.2 are both expressions of opinion, albeit directly opposed to each other. In an attempt to form an 'objective' opinion there have been attempts to assess the effectiveness of the treatment from a biomedical point of view (see for example, Ernst, 1997, and Harvard Medical School, 2004).

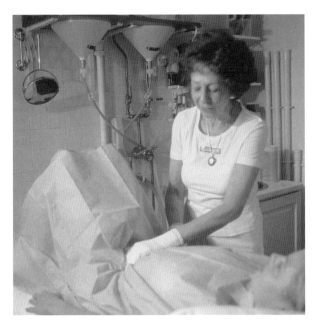

There are advocates for the use of colonic irrigation, and those who have strong opinions against it. Objective research into its effectiveness is ultimately hard to find

Colonic irrigation is a useful therapy to test the limits of the government's commitment to free choice. The question is: should the NHS pay for such treatments because of their growing popularity or should competent adults be free to pursue interventions of limited medical benefit, and with potentially serious side effects, as long as they pay for them?

In the UK, the NHS provides health care free at the point of delivery, funded centrally through taxation and national insurance contributions. Every adult and child is entitled to be registered with a general practitioner (GP), through whom they have access to NHS treatment as and when appropriate. Yet people spend millions of pounds each year by choosing to use CAM.

CAM is not cheap. Some practitioners offer a sliding scale, but the average rate for an hour-long consultation ranges from £20 to £60. A recent survey discovered that the average expenditure by respondents who use CAM was more than £13 a month (Ernst, 2000). The fact that people are prepared to pay this much suggests a high level of consumer confidence that CAM delivers results, together with a possibly significant level of dissatisfaction with the biomedical model. Of course, even treatment within the NHS can incur significant costs, such as paying for prescriptions and dental care, or the hidden costs of waiting for 'free' treatments. Users of CAM seem to value the freedom to select a form of health care that suits them, from the highly professional to the frankly outlandish, perhaps reckoning that how they treat their health and wellbeing is their own business. Often it seems that people choose CAM in addition to using orthodox services as a form of post-modern consumption, where 'pick and mix' dominates the health care scene as well as many other markets (Siahpush, 1999). Ironically, this more recent form of consuming health care services matches the way in which people could choose from a wide variety of therapies in the time before the inception of the NHS (Porter, 1989).

ACTIVITY   CHOOSING TO PAY FOR HEALTH SERVICES

Allow 10 minutes

Think for a few minutes about contact you have had with the health care system recently. This could involve you personally or someone you know.

- Did you pay directly for this service?

- Would you have been prepared to pay for it?

- Do you think exchanging money would affect how you felt about this service?

- Do you think there would be a difference between your attitude to paying for orthodox health care and a CAM service?

Comment

Health and health care systems are very important parts of everyone's lives. Paying directly for services can complicate how those services are perceived. Many people, even if they claim to disapprove of private forms of health care in principle, are prepared to pay for help for themselves or those close to them if the need arises.

Typical responses to this activity included the belief that waiting until NHS treatment is available is too much to contemplate: 'My aunt was in considerable pain with her hip and the local waiting list was over a year long. The whole family clubbed together so that she could go private and have the operation done within a month.' For other people there might be problems involved in the exchange of money: 'I did go to a private therapist for several months because of persistent back pain. I could never make out whether he was keeping me coming along because of the fee involved, or whether he really thought that he could make me better.' Yet others might put aside any scruples about the ability to pay for private attention: 'I paid for private treatment for my problem. I consider that I have earned the money for myself and that I could spend it on the extra comfort I got in the private hospital and also on the ability to have the operation at the time I wanted. All the staff were nice to me because they knew I was paying.'

However, does the exchange of money affect the way they feel about the service? Some said they wondered whether the therapist kept them coming back for all those sessions just to help her pay the mortgage and 'the exchange of money was a problem and neither of us felt comfortable either about asking or giving the fee. I felt that it spoilt one part at least of the relationship between us.'

Separating CAM from informal healing

Chapter 11 described how traditional and informal healing involves health care approaches that are congruent with, and embedded in, people's cultural belief systems. Every culture produces its own meanings and definitions of health and illness. In the UK, these exist alongside broad, general support for scientific methods and the biomedical model. People live constantly with a range of concepts of health (Greenhalgh et al., 1998). In contrast to the technological and possibly invasive procedures involved in orthodox medicine, folk practices may use healing foods and herbs, rituals involving hygiene and purification of the body, or ceremonies to ward off evil spirits or appease ancestors. These practices are often provided by members of a family, and may involve the patient's wider community. Sometimes folk healing uses professional folk healers, who may or may not expect the sick person to pay them for their services.

Unlike therapeutic encounters with a professional CAM practitioner, folk and informal healing practices are often an integral part of their user's everyday life and relationships. As such, they may be less likely to form the basis of a commercial transaction. Outside the dominant western orthodox systems, traditional healing rituals are more akin to religion than medicine, which is at odds with secular tradition or biomedical concepts of health and disease. The focus of this chapter is on professional or commercial CAM transactions. However, it is important to recognise at the outset that the boundaries between paid and unpaid healing, and formal and informal provision are not always clear cut, and some of what could be considered CAM interactions do not involve any money being transferred. Examples include a healer who offers her services to a church congregation, reiki practised by one friend on another, or a master leading a group of t'ai chi students through a dawn practice in a public park.

ACTIVITY   ADVANTAGES OF PRIVATE CAM USE

Allow 10 minutes

Think for a few minutes about the advantages of the availability and use of CAM in the private sector.

Note down the benefits that you think users or clients receive from using CAM within a private or fee-paying system.

Why do people access private health care **of any kind** when biomedical services are free at the point of delivery?

Comment

Positioning CAM within the private sector has advantages and disadvantages for users. One important advantage of private CAM practice is that people can self-refer to a practitioner, without necessarily having to be referred by a GP, as is the case for most other specialist services. Being able to seek and receive CAM treatment gives some patients a sense of autonomy and control, and may offer hope, particularly if their condition is not amenable to orthodox treatment. People's reasons for choosing to pay for health care might include the expectation of a speedier service without being subject to NHS waiting lists, a perceived better standard of care and individualised treatment. Some of these points are recognised by health insurance schemes, which will reimburse the costs of some CAM treatments.

The emphasis that CAM practitioners place on self-responsibility allows people to feel that they are actively engaging in a therapeutic partnership, rather than simply having something done to them. Private CAM gives people access to a variety of meanings and interpretations of their illness, and allows them to experiment with a range of healing approaches, the details of which will usually not form part of their official health records:

> However, it is also the case that many homoeopaths have a personal commitment to individual responsibility in health care. As one practitioner put it, '[I'm] realising that every thought, deed, action that you take, has an effect. So, therefore, your responsibility for who you are, and what you do, is much greater'.
>
> (Scott, 1998, p. 200)

The freedom to consult a therapist of their choosing extends to the freedom to negotiate terms with the practitioner over details such as price, or frequency and duration of treatment, without being tied to a centralised protocol, as may be the case for a user accessing therapy through their GP. In a free market, people can consult from a diverse array of practitioners offering a wide range of modalities, subject, of course, to being able to fund consultations themselves.

From the practitioner's perspective, the private sector may be thought to encourage diversity and creativity, allowing them to be as complementary or alternative to the medical model as they feel is appropriate. Significantly, working in the private sector gives practitioners great autonomy. Many practitioners choose CAM precisely because they enjoy being self-employed and working in an unsupervised, unregulated and independent fashion: 'I've the freedom to work with my own ideas, make my own decisions without the constraints of the NHS' (Andrews and Hammond, 2004, p. 49).

Of course, the work of CAM therapists is never entirely unregulated. For example, a nurse therapist working in private outside the NHS is still required to work according to nursing codes of practice. Also, many other practitioners work to codes of practice designated by their own professional bodies.

CAM therapists choose to work in this relatively unstructured way, even though it means handling the small business aspect of practice and not enjoying the statutory protections such as holiday pay, sickness benefit and maternity leave that is available when working within a more formal structure such as the NHS. Practitioners may also value the lack of interference in how they practise. This makes them wary about the thought of CAM moving out of the private sector into the NHS, where the nature and content of the treatment that could be offered may be more circumscribed. As Chapter 12 showed, a growing proportion of CAM practitioners also work in another capacity. For example, a nurse or midwife might also have a small private practice in reflexology or aromatherapy. These practitioners often view their private CAM work as a means of fulfilling their therapeutic potential and giving people more meaningful attention than they can within the NHS.

ACTIVITY   DISADVANTAGES OF PRIVATE CAM USE

Allow 15 minutes

Think for a few minutes about the disadvantages of CAM availability and use within the private sector. What disadvantages are there for people using the service and for the practitioners or therapists?

Make two lists. In one list, note down the disadvantages you think users or clients may experience from using CAM within a private or fee-paying system. In the other list, note any disadvantages you can think of for the practitioner or therapist.

Do you think that markets can deliver publicly valuable services such as health care?

Comment

The same factors which provide consumer freedom may also compromise consumer safety. As discussed in greater detail later, most private CAM practice is unregulated, which means people cannot assume that the practitioner they consult has the necessary and appropriate qualifications to treat them. Numerous private colleges and institutions offer 'professional' certification, but the standard of CAM training varies enormously. People are increasingly seeking practitioners who belong to a recognised professional body, since this implies the practitioner works within a code of ethics and has appropriate professional indemnity insurance. However, the standard of professional bodies varies, and limits of competence, boundary issues and complaints mechanisms may be problematic in this sector. There are also concerns about whether practitioners, particularly those working in sole private practice, keep sufficiently up to date with developments in their therapy or therapies or in CAM as a whole. This concern is not confined to CAM practice: practitioners in the orthodox sector may also struggle to keep in touch with rapidly changing advances in treatments.

CAM practitioners should also keep up to date with developments in orthodox medicine so they are aware of their own limitations and can communicate effectively with the client's general practitioner if this becomes necessary. People may have little comeback if something goes wrong. Although incidents of litigation and numbers of complaints are currently low, they are increasing (Stone, 2002).

There are other concerns about the potential for developing dependence. When 'clients' pay for a service, how can they be sure that the practitioner is not encouraging dependence to ensure themselves a steady income in the future? A whole area of concern may open up within private practice regarding the financial versus clinical reasons for the relationship between therapist and client. In addition, there may be problems about the continuity of care. People with a limited income may try a therapist but not complete the course of treatment for financial reasons.

The discipline of audit and research is usually less well developed within the private sector and it is particularly hard to gather 'evidence' of effectiveness in situations where the 'client' is free to pick and choose therapists and courses of treatment.

Opponents of the private provision of CAM routinely argue that the lack of regulation makes patients unduly vulnerable and open to exploitation (Beyerstein, 2001). CAM practitioners may overstate their claims (particularly on the internet) but there is little hard evidence to substantiate the claim that they are more likely to exploit patients' vulnerabilities than other health care workers. Although some experts feel that tighter regulatory controls will reduce the incidences of abuse, ultimately, whether a therapy is statutorily regulated or not will not determine whether individual practitioners act ethically (see Box 13.3 overleaf).

BOX 13.3   CHECKING OUT CAM THERAPISTS

How do users and consumers know whether a particular private CAM therapist is bona fide? One approach taken by an independent organisation called Dr Foster is published in the *Good Complementary Therapist Guide* (Dr Foster, 2002), which sets out their standards and criteria against which any therapists they list are measured. All therapists featured in the guide are registered either with statutory regulators or with professional organisations which maintain a register of members. They also set educational standards and require members to graduate from an accredited college, and run a continuing professional development programme. In addition, they require members to abide by codes of conduct, ethics and practice, run a complaints system and disciplinary procedure that is accessible to the public, and require members to take out professional indemnity insurance.

What are the potential disadvantages for CAM therapists? Although most practitioners enjoy the level of autonomy that private practice gives them, others feel isolated working in sole practice, without the support and collegiality of professional colleagues. For many practitioners, the excitement of generating a client base may be offset by the anxiety of how they will pay their bills. Arguing for greater integration of CAM into the NHS, Fox (2001) maintains that there are advantages for CAM therapists working more closely with the NHS, including the possibility of a more secure income, an opportunity to work with other health professionals, and a wider patient base. A further concern about CAM being located within the private sector is that access is limited to people who can afford to pay for it. Even when CAM is available through the NHS, the therapists may give their time for no payment, as a gesture of goodwill and in order to have at least a presence in that NHS unit. However, this arrangement raises issues about whether the therapies are really valued by the decision makers within the NHS.

A more general concern is whether a private health market can ever provide an adequate level of health care services. As noted in Chapter 12, the geographical distribution of CAM is patchy throughout the UK. Some areas have many CAM practitioners and commercial outlets, whereas other areas do not. If CAM is provided subject to market forces, there will always be a concentration of service provision in certain areas and a paucity in others. A market-led approach to health care provision in CAM as well as biomedical facilities will inevitably move towards providing the sorts of services that people demand and can pay for; they will not be distributed according to need. The range of services offered is unlikely to represent the full spectrum of health needs of any given population, and is less likely to cater to the health needs of more vulnerable members of society, who are least able to pay for private health care.

Sociologists, anthropologists and policy makers have all been fascinated by the popularity of CAM, especially when people have to pay the bill themselves (Andrews et al., 2003). The reasons for using CAM may give some clues about what patients think they are purchasing, and how they will judge whether they have had value for money.

The reasons why people consult CAM practitioners seem broader than the reasons for consulting orthodox doctors (Astin, 1998). The appeal of paying for these services is the ability to see a practitioner when the person wants (usually within a shorter timescale than waiting for specialist NHS care), and the sense of buying time: time to be heard and treated as an individual and time to consider therapeutic options – both of which may be rushed in a publicly funded health care environment.

13.3   Current patterns of private CAM provision

The high sickness levels and mortality rates characteristic of pre-modern Britain resulted in a strong demand for a wide variety of healers, including orthodox medical practitioners (Porter, 1989). In practice however, the majority of the population was precluded from seeking the attentions of a professional physician by the high cost of such treatment. Medicine was therefore primarily a domestic matter, and people resorted to lay and professional healers only out of necessity. In short, until well into the 19th century, there was a pronounced culture of medical pluralism: it was standard practice to go outside orthodox medicine in search of relief (Stone and Matthews, 1996).

In the 20th century, modern 'scientific' medicine took centre stage, and went to considerable lengths to stifle opposition. Historically, the strength of the medical establishment has been so great that doctors secured their position as the monopoly providers and determiners of medicine and health care, while negotiating provision free at the point of delivery through the NHS. Despite a softening towards CAM (BMA, 1993), some elements within the medical establishment still find it hard to accept the notion of integrating CAM with their orthodox approaches (Fitzpatrick, 2002).

ACTIVITY   THE ROLE OF GOVERNMENT

Allow 15 minutes

What do you think the government's role should be in the provision of health services? Do you think that everything a country's people request should be provided, or should each individual have to pay for the services that they and their family use? Consider the following list and make notes about each therapy and why you think it should either be included free, as part of NHS services, or be available only to those paying privately.

- Hip replacement
- Heart and lung transplant

- Chiropractic for back pain
- Cosmetic surgery for breast augmentation
- St John's Wort for depression
- Counselling for relationship problems
- Reflexology for stress
- IVF for infertility

Comment

Of course, each person has their own opinion about the free availability of services within the NHS. A list like this helps you to think about your own position as a member of society who is potentially in a situation where you or a member of your family may need one of these services. Also, each member of society is potentially in a position of paying taxes to fund the 'free' provision of these services. Does this make a difference to how you feel about this list of services? Ultimately, governments have to make the final judgement about which services should be made freely available.

The range of services to be provided by the NHS is not formally set out in a statute. Rather, Section 1 of the NHS Act 1977 imposes on the Secretary of State for Health a 'duty to continue the promotion in England and Wales of a comprehensive health service designed to secure improvement (a) in the physical and mental health of the people of those countries, and (b) in the prevention, diagnosis and treatment for illness, and for that purpose to provide or secure the effective provision of services in accordance with this Act.' Section 3 of the Act limits the Secretary of State's duty to provide listed services 'to such extent as he considers necessary'. Historically, the services provided by the NHS have fallen within the dominant biomedical model, and there is no statutory basis for including or excluding CAM as part of a comprehensive health service. The services that a government believes 'ought' to be provided as part of a comprehensive health service changes over time. Increasingly, service provision is tied to services that are shown to be effective according to criteria established within the practice of 'evidence-based medicine'. The National Institute for Clinical Excellence (NICE) is a quasi-independent body, which was established specifically to give advice about the effectiveness or ineffectiveness of certain treatments.

Governments have a vested interest in the nation's health. By 2006, the proportion of the GDP (gross domestic product) spent on health in the UK will be about 8 per cent, compared with a European average of 11 per cent (Boyle and Appleby, 2001). In industrialised societies, the interest in public health provision is based on social welfarism, but it also has economic underpinnings, tied in with the need to have a healthy workforce. It is probably no coincidence that a small amount of officially sanctioned research funding has been made available to establish the efficacy of chiropractic, given the number of working days lost each year through people suffering from lower back pain. The rising cost of health care is a major concern to all governments where hi-tech medicine is practised.

The scope in which CAM operates largely depends on how governments view non-orthodox therapies as fitting in with overall health strategies. Governments trying to reduce dependence on the state, and foster a sense of independence and self-reliance, may look favourably on complementary therapies that promote self-healing and people taking personal responsibility for their own health and wellbeing. This support at policy level usually falls short of the financial provision of sustainable local CAM services.

Although the stance of previous UK governments towards CAM was one of 'benevolent neutrality' (Stone and Matthews, 1996), recent official pronouncements have been more responsive to consumer pressure. However, CAM therapists should be under no illusions. Chapter 14 explores how working in the NHS could alter the way in which CAM practitioners practise. The government seems to support greater integration of CAM only if it can reconstitute itself in a way that is compatible with, and possibly under the control of, orthodox forms of medicine and medical power. Critically, this means establishing an evidence base demonstrating CAM's effectiveness. CAM is also expected to fit in with the NHS's commitment to quality assurance and accountability. Official policy insists that all regulatory bodies (whether within the NHS or not) act together and work towards these goals (Department of Health, 2000).

The government underpins the existing medical establishment and its power base in society both directly and indirectly. It does this by statute, restricting privileges to registered medical practitioners only (Department of Health, 1983) through its support for, and reliance on, revenue from the pharmaceutical industry; through its medical licensing policies, which operate against small natural health manufacturers; and through its slowness in centrally funding CAM research and provision. Although the government would like to be seen as responding to consumer demand, the likelihood of widespread CAM provision throughout the NHS is far from guaranteed. Despite paying lip service to the notion of equal access, the key question that will dominate widespread integration of CAM into the NHS is whether CAM will result in overall cost savings (Department of Health, 2000).

13.4   Economic aspects of CAM provision and use

How important is CAM within the overall economy? As previous chapters show, the definition of CAM can vary from survey to survey. The distinction between CAM and informal healing is not always obvious, which may distort the findings about CAM use. This aside, it is generally accepted that there is a substantial and growing use of CAM throughout the developed world.

ACTIVITY   CONSUMER SURVEYS

Allow 20 minutes

Read the following parts of a press release that accompanied the Mintel survey *Complementary Medicines in the UK 2003*.

What are the main features of the report that illuminate the growth of the private sector in CAM provision and the 'economics of demand' that have apparently fuelled this growth?

CONSUMERS PUT THEIR FAITH IN COMPLEMENTARY MEDICINES

Latest research from Mintel sees the complementary medicines market rising almost 60% in the last five years to reach £130 million. Despite this rapid rate of growth, the market slowed somewhat in 2002, held back by the manufacturers' need to invest only in products that would meet new legislative requirements and a related decline in promotion as brands were consolidated. In addition, some negative publicity regarding either the strength of herbal remedies, or the lack of efficacy of homeopathic remedies and aromatherapy oils discouraged some consumers from entering the market. However, this is likely to only be a temporary lull, as many new companies are looking to expand into the category once the new legislative framework is in place. Mintel is forecasting that [the] total market will grow by 45% over the next five years to reach £188 million. Market growth will pick up in 2003 and 2004, although manufacturers may have to work harder to persuade more cynical consumers of the efficacy of their products. "Taking a more 'scientific' approach could be a double-edged sword in that it will bring them into competition and perhaps conflict with highly researched conventional medicines which have far greater financial backing and are used to investing heavily in research, NPD and advertising" comments Amanda Lintott, Consumer Analyst.

HERBAL MEDICINE LEADS THE WAY

Herbal medicines dominate the market accounting for almost 60% of the sector value. Homeopathic remedies retained a static market share in 2000 and 2003, as they have failed to move into the mainstream as quickly as herbal remedies. Nevertheless, the sector has successfully drawn in new consumers, especially for products to treat ailments associated with stress and modern lifestyles. Aromatherapy essential oils have a declining sector share, as consumers take up the benefits of aromatherapy in toiletry products rather than in oil form. If anything has held back the sales of essential oils, it has been the success of toiletry and other products based on aromatherapy principles, which offer the pleasant fragrances without the potential mess and difficulty of dealing with oils.

(Source: Mintel, 2003)

Comment

The Mintel survey demonstrates the enormous growth in the commercial sector that is associated with CAM products and services. Many commercial organisations are aware of rapid market growth and attempt to tap into the market potential. Once significant numbers of commercial organisations are interested in the sector, they will create additional pressure on consumer demand through advertising and also through the greater availability of CAM-related products. In this way, the sales of CAM products and services will continue to grow.

Further surveys

Other surveys have found similar results to the Mintel survey, often from an academic rather than a commercial base. Thomas et al. (2001) found that in 1998 there were an estimated 22 million visits to practitioners of the more established therapies (compared with 14 million visits to accident and emergency departments). The survey asked whether respondents had purchased any over-the-counter (OTC), herbal or homoeopathic remedies. The results showed that 13.6 per cent of respondents had visited a practitioner of one of the eight named therapies in the preceding 12 months, and overall 28.3 per cent of respondents had either visited a CAM therapist or purchased an OTC remedy. The most commonly consulted CAM therapists were osteopaths (4.3 per cent of respondents), chiropractors (3.6 per cent), aromatherapists (3.5 per cent), reflexologists (2.4 per cent) and acupuncturists (1.6 per cent). Of the respondents, 8.6 per cent had bought an OTC homeopathic remedy and 19.8 per cent had bought an OTC herbal remedy. The NHS paid for an estimated 10 per cent of the visits to practitioners but the authors estimate that £450 million of people's own money was spent on six of the principal therapies (excluding aromatherapy and reflexology) during the preceding year.

In 1999, the Department of Health commissioned a study of the professional organisation of CAM bodies in the UK. This was a follow-up to a study on the same subject three years earlier. It looked at how many people were working as CAM practitioners. The results suggest there are approximately 50,000 CAM practitioners in the UK, there are approximately 10,000 statutory registered health professionals who practise some form of CAM in the UK, and up to 5 million people have consulted a CAM practitioner in the last year (Budd and Mills, 2000).

Also in 1999, the BBC commissioned a telephone survey of 1204 randomly selected British adults. This survey did not specify which therapies it classed as CAM; instead respondents were asked whether they had used 'alternative or complementary medicines or therapies' within the last year. This survey also found that each CAM user spent approximately £14 per month on CAM, a large proportion (37 per cent) spending less than £5 per month. The authors extrapolated this information to the whole nation and estimated that the UK has an annual expenditure of £1.6 billion on CAM (Ernst and White, 2000).

The situation in other countries

The global market for CAM is huge and growing all the time. Some aspects of this are detailed in Box 13.4. In the most frequently cited US survey, Eisenberg et al. (1998) conducted two national telephone surveys of two randomly selected sets of adults, surveying levels of CAM usage in 1990 and 1997 respectively. They questioned respondents on their use of 16 'alternative therapies' and defined accessing alternative medicine as having used at least one of the 16 therapies (either as an OTC preparation or through a professional consultation) within the previous year. The 16 therapies included mega-vitamins, self-help groups, imagery, and commercial and lifestyle diets. Their remit did not include osteopathy, which is generally regarded as a mainstream medical speciality in the USA. In both surveys, alternative therapies were used mainly for chronic conditions such as back pain, allergies, anxiety, depression and headaches. Extrapolating the results to the entire population of the USA suggested a 47.3 per cent total increase in visits to alternative practitioners, from 427 million to 629 million (which was more than the number of visits to all US primary care physicians). Personal expenditure on alternative therapies was estimated at US$ 2.7 billion in 1997.

BOX 13.4   GLOBAL MARKET FOR CAM

Traditional and alternative medicine: facts and figures

General

- Up to 80% of people in [developing countries] use traditional or complementary/alternative medicine (TM/CAM) as part of primary health care.
- Traditional medicine has been fully integrated into the health systems of China, North and South Korea and Vietnam.
- The global market for traditional therapies stands at US$ 60 billion a year and is steadily growing.
- In the USA, expenditure on complementary or alternative medicine stands at US$ 2.7 billion per year.

Australia

- Traditional Chinese medicine has been practised in Australia since the 19th century. Approximately AU$ 1 billion is spent on complementary/alternative medicine.

China

- Traditional Chinese medicine is fully integrated into China's health system.
- 95% of Chinese hospitals have units for traditional medicine.
- Traditional medicine accounts for 30–50% of total consumption.
- There are 800 manufacturers of herbal products with a total annual output of US$ 1.8 billion.

Indonesia

- 40% of Indonesia's population uses traditional medicine; 70% in rural areas.
- At the end of 1999, there were 723 manufacturers of traditional medicines, 92 of which were large-scale industries.

Japan

- In 2000 the herbal medicine market in Japan was worth US$ 2.4 billion.
- An October 2000 survey showed that 72% of registered western-style doctors use kampo medicine (the Japanese adaptation of Chinese medicine) in their clinical services.

(Source: adapted from WHO, 2002)

CAM and the economy

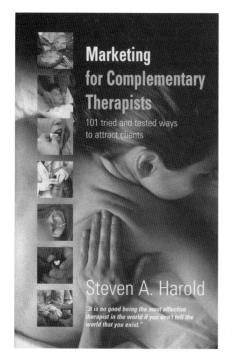

There is now a secondary growth industry giving advice and providing services that support the growing CAM industry

CAM is a growth market and has attracted the attention of big business. The public's appetite for CAM products has created significant business opportunities, as seen in the most recent Mintel survey discussed earlier. A significant proportion of CAM revenue comes from OTC products and remedies. Traditionally, the big pharmaceutical companies have shied away from herbal manufacture, one reason being that medicines derived from natural sources cannot be easily patented. As a result of existing licensing requirements, many herbal products and food supplements occupy a dubious legal status between foods and medicines.

In the UK, as elsewhere, the manufacture of CAM products is being brought closer into line with medicine-licensing regulations. In 2000, for example, the Indian government drew up regulations for good manufacturing practice for traditional Indian systems of medicine such as ayurveda, siddha and unani, so that the industry could compete in international markets. The Department of Indian Systems of Medicine identified drug standardisation and quality control as the most important changes affecting the future of the Indian systems of medicines (Sharma, 2000).

The health and leisure sector is also cashing in on the public's enthusiasm for CAM. Many gyms routinely offer a variety of CAM therapies from aromatherapy or massage to reflexology, and sell a range of 'sports-enhancing' food and vitamin supplements. Therapies such as 'lymph massage' and 'acu-pressure massage' have been added to what used to be described as 'beauty treatments', but are more likely these days to be described as 'health and beauty' treatments. As therapies grow in popularity, accompanying products appear on the market. Selling CAM-related products is not limited to specialist health outlets but extends to multi-level mainstream retailing. For example, sticking the word 'aromatherapy' on a label can be used to sell expensive air-fresheners or bottles of shampoo. Yoga equipment can now be bought with an accompanying manual and DVD in chain bookstores. Shiatsu massage machines are sold in department stores alongside portable foot spas and air purifiers.

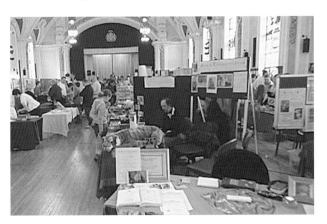

Health fairs are popular with people selling products associated with various CAM therapies

Health product suppliers have always relied on the available media to advertise their wares. CAM products and services continue to be advertised through the regular print media. In addition, since the mid-1990s, the internet has become a fertile ground for selling CAM and CAM-related products. The internet offers people more privacy and choice; however, there is no quality control over what is sold and how.

Retailing CAM

CAM poses a challenge to economic beliefs and practices in health care in the following ways.

- Placing purchasing power directly in the hands of the service user, rather than sanctioning access to a CAM practitioner through a GP, thus increasing consumer freedom to buy individualised health.
- Giving professional status to practitioners who may not have undergone a conventional medical education, thus increasing their ability to charge fees for services.
- Shifting the locus of treatment away from the institutionalised clinic setting.
- Diverting significant business away from orthodox health care.
- Implicitly rejecting hi-tech, costly interventions and pharmaceutical medicines in favour of alternative approaches.

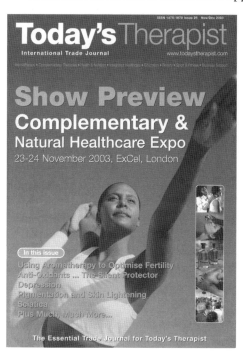

Today's Therapist is a trade journal aimed at the commercial development of the CAM market

Finance and individual CAM practitioners

Part of the lure of professionalism is that traditionally it denotes high status and salary. Is this true for CAM professions? Newly qualified chiropractors can expect to be earning up to £100,000 within five years of qualifying. Certainly, chiropractors are among the most highly paid practitioners. The majority of private CAM practitioners claim not to earn large salaries (although, as noted in Chapter 12, there are several reasons why surveys of practitioners' earnings vary considerably). Little is known about practitioners' earnings in less well established therapies. An internal survey of acupuncturists commissioned by the British Acupuncture Council in 2000 confirmed that 33 per cent of members responding earned less than £20,000 per year (see Box 13.5).

BOX 13.5   BRITISH ACUPUNCTURE COUNCIL SURVEY COSTS AND CHARGES

- Almost two members in five (38 per cent) have an annual income of up to £10,000 from acupuncture; one in three (32 per cent) earns between £10,000 and £20,000; while almost a quarter (23 per cent) earn over £20,000. Just under one member in twenty (4 per cent) is in receipt of state benefits.
- Seven in ten practitioners (70 per cent) say acupuncture is their main source of personal income. However, almost half (47 per cent) have another job as well as their practice.
- The average charged for an initial treatment is £36, and for a follow-up treatment, £26.

(Source: adapted from Ernst and White, 2000)

As more training courses are developed for potential CAM practitioners, the therapists of the future are entering a competitive market where earnings may not be as high as the students imagined. Indeed, what can explain the relatively low income levels of many CAM practitioners? Is it a matter of oversupply with so many newly qualified practitioners competing for a fixed number of fee-paying clients? Or is the apparently huge demand for CAMs expressed in the various surveys not actually matched by the public's readiness or ability to pay more than a limited amount for these services? For those struggling to earn enough money to live on as private sole practitioners, the prospect of working in the NHS may be viewed in terms of economic survival. Other practitioners would regard working in the NHS as a complete sell-out of their fundamental ideals. In terms of economics, CAM practitioners already have more in common with doctors than might be obvious. Cant and Sharma (1996) note the high level of professionalisation in both orthodox and non-orthodox medical services.

Historically, though, CAM practitioners have naturally been more interested in challenging the establishment in the orthodox system than its health workers. At times when practitioners of unorthodox medicine were drawn into a more overtly political stance, they often sought to justify their position by challenging the secrecy surrounding the practice of medicine, and championing of ordinary people's right of access to medical knowledge and greater self-determination (Stone and Matthews, 1996). Have CAM practitioners stayed political? Gil-Soo Han expresses the opinion that these days, despite its rhetoric, CAM has lost much of its alternative or radical leanings:

> There is a tendency for the holistic health movement to appear to be politically conscious and to take up the banner of social medicine which calls for the control of social factors to fight and prevent disease. However, in fact, it has been at best apolitical. Indeed, the holistic health movement shares much similarity with orthodox medicine in its organizational and social pattern. It is: 'solo, fee-for-service entrepreneurial practice; knowledge of skills sold to "consumers" in commodity forms; elitist and sexist behavior on the part of practitioners; and a clear separation between practitioners and those who are served' (Berliner and Salmon, 1980, pp. 44–45; cf. Sharp and O'Leary, 1991). As in scientific medicine, the focus of treatment is on the individual rather than a larger social class. While promoting the concept of a unified whole of mind, body and spirit, holistic health practices continue to leave aside the external world in their healing process (i.e., the role of social class, economic, social and political relations). Thus, helping the individual to adjust to a socially pathological circumstance is a major goal.
>
> (Han, 2002, para. 5.21)

In her analysis of homoeopathic practice, Anne Scott gives vent to a similar opinion, suggesting that the way in which CAM practitioners are forced to compete in the marketplace makes them focus on individual clients rather than on social activism:

> Homoeopathy's individualistic emphasis can be partially explained by its location within the private health sector. Providers compete with each other to attract patients, offering their treatments as a commodity; therefore, it is not to their economic advantage to locate the causes, or treatments, for illness in factors outside their patients' immediate control.
>
> (Scott, 1998, p. 200)

Similarly, while many practitioners claim to be interested in health equality, and talk about the need to widen access to CAM services, there is a tension in that most practitioners depend on fee-paying private clients for their living. While some work in charitable institutions or offer reduced fees for low-income patients, the lack of political cohesion in CAM means that the issue of equal access has not been tackled with any enthusiasm. Antonovsky (1987), who introduced the concept of positive health, was as critical of CAM as of orthodox medicine for concentrating its energies and endeavours on the sickness end of the wellness–illness spectrum.

The opportunities for researching and auditing CAM are limited because it is provided in the private sector. Private CAM practitioners are usually not tied into systems of quality assurance and service frameworks, so it can be difficult to gauge whether CAM is effective, or how it could work better. The choice is enormous for people who can afford to visit a CAM practitioner. In the current regulatory climate, people can seek a therapist from a range of more than 200 healing modalities. For some CAM users, paying for CAM is evidence of their commitment to taking some degree of self-responsibility for their health. It has even been argued that paying directly for a therapeutic intervention may enhance the therapeutic effect (Scott, 1998). Whether or not this is wish fulfilment by private practitioners, it is not fanciful to suggest that people who pay for their own treatment have more of a vested interest in getting value for money, and may be more likely to follow health-promoting diet, exercise and lifestyle advice.

13.5   Conclusion

Historical, social, political and economic factors all account for CAM's position in the private health care sector. CAM has thrived recently in a private, unregulated area, and its level of use seems to indicate high levels of patient satisfaction. The small-scale mode of production allows private practitioners to spend more time and energy on individual patients than they could in most NHS settings. Where CAM use strays into the realm of leisure or lifestyle choices, there is strong pressure for it to remain unregulated and a matter of consumer choice.

By virtue of its popularity, CAM can no longer be regarded as 'fringe' or 'marginal'. CAM is now big business, providing many people with a viable alternative to orthodox medicine and many vested interests, including practitioners with a lucrative source of income and profit. At a time of increased consumer sophistication, people can be as critical of complementary and alternative therapists as they are of orthodox doctors. People who pay for their health care expect value for money, and want to know which therapy is most likely to benefit them and why. To maintain current levels of enthusiasm, CAM practitioners need to be able to give consumers a reason for investing in their services. In the past, therapists often traded on their ability to spend more time with people than doctors can, and to treat the 'whole patient'. However much people value these aspects of the therapeutic encounter, they will only continue to use, or return to, complementary and alternative therapists in the future if, in addition to their empathy, therapists can also deliver favourable health outcomes.

KEY POINTS

- Since the 1990s, most of the growth in the provision and use of CAM in the UK has been in the private sector.

- Although some forms of CAM in the informal sector do not involve the exchange of money, the majority of transactions involve payment for services.

- Individuals who decide to pay for CAM services have an element of control over the services they receive, but they are not well protected by consumer safety mechanisms.

- It can be complex for governments to decide which services are provided free of charge for their citizens, especially where CAM modalities are concerned.

- Therapists who provide CAM under private arrangements are considerably free from external controls, but they may not be suitably trained or regulated by statutory authorities.

- Individuals use private CAM services for a wide range of reasons, which reflect and parallel social changes within secular society.

- Regulation of the private practice of CAM is seriously underdeveloped and governments may be keen to introduce increased levels of control in the future.

- CAM is a significant growth industry in all contemporary western societies. Its earning capacity has attracted individuals to become therapists and also involved considerable investment from commercial organisations.

- The exchange of money can affect the therapeutic relationship between client and therapist either for better (people may value treatment they pay for) or for worse (the interaction is contaminated with fears of unnecessarily prolonged treatment, etc.).

- Private CAM therapists may have to balance the needs of providing a caring, therapeutic service with the realities of surviving as a small business.

- It is difficult to audit or research CAM provision in the private sector, which may lead to problems for CAM developing quality assurance or investigating efficacy or cost effectiveness, etc. Without this, CAM may well remain a marginal activity open to changes in political opinion and adverse stories in the media.

References

Andrews, G. and Hammond, R. (2004) 'Small business complementary medicine: a profile of British therapists and their pathways to practice', *Primary Health Care Research and Development*, Vol. 5, pp. 40–51.

Andrews, G., Peter, E. and Hammond, R. (2003) 'Receiving money for medicine: some tensions and resolutions for community based private complementary therapists', *Health and Social Care in the Community*, Vol. 11, No. 2, pp. 155–67.

Antonovsky, A. (1987) *Understanding the Mystery of Health. How People Manage Stress and Stay Well*, San Francisco, CA, Jossey-Bass.

Association of Colonic Hydrotherapists (2004) *The Case for Colonic Irrigation* [online], www.colonic-association.com [accessed 17 February 2004].

Astin, J. (1998) 'Why patients use alternative medicine', *Journal of the American Medical Association*, Vol. 279, No. 19, pp. 1548–53.

Berliner, H. and Salmon, J. (1980) 'The holistic alternative to scientific medicine: history and analysis', *International Journal of Health Services*, Vol. 10, No. 1, pp. 133–47.

Beyerstein, B. (2001) 'Alternative medicine and common errors of reasoning', *Academic Medicine*, Vol. 76, No. 3, pp. 230–7.

BMA (British Medical Association) (1993) *Complementary Medicine: New Approaches to Good Practice*, Oxford, Oxford University Press.

Boyle, S. and Appleby, J. (2001) 'NHS spending: the wrong target (again?)' [online], www.kingsfund.org.uk/news/news.cfm?contentID=113 [accessed 27 October 2003].

Budd, S. and Mills, S. (2000) *Professional Organisation of Complementary and Alternative Medicine in the United Kingdom 2000: A Second Report to the Department of Health*, Exeter, University of Exeter.

Cant, S. and Sharma, U. (eds) (1996) *Complementary and Alternative Medicines. Knowledge in Practice*, London, Free Association Books.

Department of Health (1983) *The Medical Act*, London, HMSO.

Department of Health (2000) *The NHS Plan: A Plan for Investment, a Plan for Reform*, London, The Stationery Office.

Dr Foster (2002) *Good Complementary Therapist Guide*, London, Vermilion.

Eisenberg, D., Davis, B. and Ettner S. (1998) 'Trends in alternative medicine use in the United States, 1990–1997: results of a follow-up national survey', *Journal of the American Medical Association*, Vol. 280, pp. 1569–75.

Ernst, E. (1997) 'Colonic irrigation and the theory of autointoxication: a triumph of ignorance over science', *Journal of Clinical Gastroenterology*, Vol. 24, No. 4, pp. 196–8.

Ernst, E. (2000) 'The role of complementary medicine', *British Medical Journal*, Vol. 321, pp. 1133–5.

Ernst, E. and White, A. (2000) 'The BBC survey of complementary medicine use in the UK', *Complementary Therapies in Medicine*, Vol. 8, pp. 32–6.

Fitzpatrick, M. (2002) 'The surrender of scientific medicine', in Jenkins, T. et al. (eds) *Alternative Medicine: Should We Swallow It?*, London, Hodder and Stoughton.

Fox, M. (2001) 'Access to complementary health care: why the NHS is the key', *Complementary Therapies in Nursing and Midwifery*, Vol. 7, pp. 123–5.

Greenhalgh, T., Helman, C. and Chowdhury, A. (1998) 'Health beliefs and folk models of diabetes in British Bangladeshis: a qualitative study', *British Medical Journal*, Vol. 316, pp. 978–83.

Han, G. S. (2002) 'The myth of medical pluralism: a critical realist perspective', *Sociological Research Online*, Vol. 6, No. 4. Available online at www.socresonline.org.uk/6/4/han.html [accessed 16 February 2004].

Harvard Medical School (2004) website: www.intelihealth.com/IH/ihtPrint/ WSIHW000/8513/34968/358752.html?d=dmtContent&hide=t&k=basePrint [accessed 17 February 2004].

Mintel (2003) *Complementary Medicines in the UK*, Press release, March, London, Mintel.

National Council Against Health Fraud (1995) *NCAHF Position Paper on Colonic Irrigation* [online], www.ncahf.org/pp/colonic.html [accessed 16 February 2004].

Porter, R. (1989) *Health for Sale: Quackery in England 1660–1850*, Manchester, Manchester University Press.

Scott, A. (1998) 'Homoeopathy as a feminist form of medicine', *Sociology of Health and Illness*, Vol. 20, No. 2, pp. 191–214.

Sharma, R. (2000) 'India introduces regulations for making traditional medicines', *British Medical Journal*, Vol. 321, p. 134.

Sharp, R. and O'Leary, J. (1991) 'Making sense of New Age therapies: towards a preliminary conceptualization', Draft paper for the Australian Sociological Association Conference, Perth, December 1991.

Siahpush, M. (1999) 'Postmodern attitudes about health: a population-based exploratory study', *Complementary Therapies in Medicine*, Vol. 7, pp. 164–9.

Stone, J. (2002) *An Ethical Framework for Complementary and Alternative Therapists*, London, Routledge.

Stone, J. and Matthews, J. (1996) *Complementary Medicine and the Law*, New York, Oxford University Press.

Thomas, K. J., Nicholl, J. P. and Coleman, P. (2001) 'Use of and expenditure on complementary medicine in England – a population-based survey', *Complementary Therapies in Medicine*, Vol. 9, No. 1, pp. 2–11.

World Health Organization (2002) *Traditional and Alternative Medicine*, Fact sheet no. 271, June [online], www.who.int/medicines/organization/trm/ factsheet271.doc [accessed 16 February 2004].

Chapter 14 Integration of CAM with mainstream services

Tom Heller

Contents

AIMS

- To explore some of the issues relating to the integration of CAM with the statutory health care system.
- To debate the pros and cons for CAM and orthodox medical systems of possible integration using a single 'integrative' approach.

14.1 Introduction

In this chapter the focus switches to the provision of complementary and alternative medicine (CAM) within, or financed by, statutory or mainstream services. The main focus is still on issues of integration with a state-run, publicly funded and bureaucratically organised form of biomedicine, particularly the UK's National Health Service (NHS).

Previous chapters frequently discussed the acceptability of various types of CAM to people with a wide range of health-related problems. People with the opportunity, and the necessary finances, to use complementary or alternative medicine are increasingly using this type of therapy (Thomas et al., 2001a). In the UK, the majority of people seem to use CAM **in addition to** the orthodox (modern, scientific) approaches that are usually provided through statutory health care providers working within the NHS. The expression of this spectrum of choice could be considered an example of **integration** at the level of the individual person. People, as individuals, seem to be able to encompass the use of different types of health care for their own perceived needs and for their own range of reasons and belief systems (Rayner and Easthope, 2001). Astin (2000) suggests that there may be congruence of philosophy or values between the people who use CAM and the philosophical values underlying the therapies they use. However, does this potential congruence of interest extend to whole systems of health care? Can monolithic health care systems, such as the current NHS, relate to the different philosophical approaches within CAM?

Of course, the concept of integration is very complex as well as involving real practical problems. In this context it becomes almost impossible to talk about the views of the particular interest groups as if they were in any way homogeneous. For example, some general practitioners (GPs) have become major advocates for the integration of CAM within their practices, while others remain vehemently opposed to any erosion of their interests; and the majority are probably somewhere between these polarities, their attention focused on entirely different issues (Russo, 2000). Also, some CAM modalities appear to be more amenable to integration. For example, osteopathy, with its visible regulatory and training structure, might work fairly easily alongside orthodox medical practice, while more spiritual, esoteric or energy-based practices struggle for any common interest or compatibility with the routine practice of orthodox biomedicine.

Integration does not only imply practical ways of working together. The philosophy underpinning various CAM approaches might make it extremely problematic to incorporate certain ways of thinking into the quasi-rational, or 'scientific', world of biomedicine. For example, there is a world of difference between the usual linear decision-making processes of a health worker trained in orthodox medicine and people who espouse one of the 'energy-based' CAM modalities. The following quotation is far removed from the thinking of a 'typical' British GP:

> At our most elemental ... we are not a chemical reaction, but an energetic charge. Human beings and all living things are a coalescence of energy in a field of energy connected to every other thing in the world. This pulsating energy field is the central engine of our being and our consciousness, the alpha and omega of our existence. There is no 'me' and 'not-me' duality to our bodies in relation to the universe, but one underlying energy field.
>
> (McTaggart, 2001, p. 5)

The NHS system is rapidly changing and there are already many demands on it. These include the effects of requirements for evidence-based medicine, inter-professional team development and the changing roles of doctors in decision making in the NHS relative to professional managers. At the same time, the roles of people using the service and 'consumer groups' are changing and government rhetoric about local control is growing. There are also pressures for a greater emphasis on preventing major disease and on health or lifestyle education. The most important policy document setting out the hopes and aspirations for the development of the NHS in England and Wales is *The NHS Plan* (Department of Health, 2000). The background to all these policy directives is a major funding crisis in which competing priorities jockey for attention at a time when there are national and international pressures to reduce expenditure on public services and to introduce privatisation, as well as pressures from the public to increase expenditure. There also appears to be a lack of policy from central government about the local integration of CAM services. Many of the basic policy documents emanating from the Department of Health in England, or its equivalent in other UK countries, fail to mention CAM as a 'problem' to be funded or, indeed, as a solution to any of the difficulties currently facing the NHS.

Despite these institutional pressures within the statutory services, many surveys show that a large proportion of people are in favour of increased access to complementary or alternative health care (for example, Ong and Banks, 2003). There are also growing demands by some CAM practitioners and their advocates that this should be made freely available using finance from the NHS itself (Peters, 2000).

A statutory health care service such as the NHS develops its own structures, procedures and political imperatives. There are also many powerful forces acting on it from outside. In particular, the various interest groups shaping the current NHS may have difficulty encompassing the concepts that underpin the visions and philosophies of health within CAM approaches. Doctors and other health worker groups, managers and administrators (and, of course, political decision makers), whose actions and policies determine the ways in which the organisation functions, may remain largely unsympathetic to the demands of competing therapeutic approaches.

This chapter also considers issues about the integration of CAM within biomedicine in general. Are there philosophical problems of integration between such different systems of health care, or are any problems simply those associated with the current trend towards the bureaucratisation of biomedicine? How far are they inherent in the delivery of any kind of CAM and biomedicine, and how far might they be specific to certain contexts of delivery such as the NHS? Throughout the NHS there are increasingly tight controls over the practice of clinical medicine, despite doctors' claims for 'clinical autonomy'. This is evident in the introduction of protocol-based clinical procedures and the tight control over the actions of clinical workers by imposing targets and cash-limited budgets. Is this creating an atmosphere and ethos in which the integration of CAM is becoming increasingly problematic?

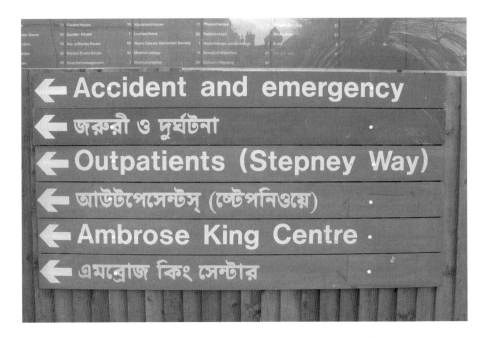

Is there room in the NHS for additional, CAM therapies?

The NHS uses large amounts of public finance and it is important to recognise the problems and opportunities involved in moving towards any further integration of CAM facilities with the statutory services. Therefore, some of the theoretical and practical issues that are involved in the integration of CAM services within the NHS will be considered next.

14.2   Is integration a good idea?

Both orthodox medicine and complementary and alternative medicine have their staunch advocates. Doctors and other health care workers who have been trained within the scientific community may find it too difficult to accept the concepts underpinning many CAM therapies:

> I cannot understand how those doctors who recommend or even practise complementary therapies can reconcile the meaningless pseudoscience that underpins aromatherapy and flower remedies with their medical training and their conscience. ... I do not object to the existence of complementary therapy. On the whole, it is harmless. All I ask is that we recognise it for what it is – a sophisticated and heavily marketed lifestyle product – and stop trying to call it medicine.
>
> (Dr Lorna Gold, GP, quoted in Dr Foster, 2002, pp. 12, 13)

Other doctors take a more pragmatic approach:

> The benefit for doctors [of including complementary practitioners within their team] is that they end up with better, happier and frequently less demanding patients because the holistic nature of complementary medicine means that patient perception and attitude is affected by treatment as well as the bare symptoms.
>
> (Dr Mike Dixon, GP, quoted in Dr Foster, 2002, p. 9)

Even some distinguished physicians remain baffled at the popularity of CAM approaches and contemplate the strategies that conventional medicine should take in response:

> How can it be that alternative practices, shrouded in mystery, grow and flourish, while a century and half of effort by scientific medicine to demystify disease and its treatment – our spectacular success in defining pathophysiology, standardizing tests and treatment, and purifying drugs – is seen as inadequate, even dangerous? Where did we go wrong? ... We could decide, for example, that alternative medicine, as an antirational, quasi-religious movement, is retrogressive and as such a direct threat to scientific medicine. ... Or we could recognize that these paradoxes reflect legitimate cries for help from our patients, dowsing rods, so to speak, that point to important gaps ... deeply embedded in our present system of conventional care.
>
> (Davidoff, 1998, pp. 1068, 1070)

ACTIVITY IS INTEGRATION A GOOD OR A BAD THING?

Allow 15 minutes

Think for a few minutes about the concept of integrating complementary and alternative therapies within NHS services.

- What is your opinion of this potential integration?
- Write a list of the points in favour of integration.
- Write a list of the points that might be raised against integration.

Comment

Many people who read a book like this will be broadly sympathetic to the widespread introduction of CAM therapies. Although most of the people who have done this activity approved of the idea of integrating CAM therapies within the NHS, a wide range of opinions were expressed. They listed the following points in favour of integration.

- Many people want the opportunity to use CAM but cannot afford to pay.
- The NHS should include all the therapies and treatments that people want to use.

- CAM reaches parts that routine NHS treatments cannot, and helps those who have not been helped by other approaches.
- CAM might save resources by reducing pressure on more expensive services.
- CAM might improve the continuity of care and may be more cost-effective than orthodox treatments.
- Administering CAM can be really good for NHS staff: 'If you give a good massage, you feel better yourself.'

However, there were also the following objections to integration.

- NHS money is already in short supply: would the provision of more CAMs take money away from other services?
- Many CAM treatments have not been properly tested: how do we know whether they work?
- What safeguards are there that CAM therapists have been properly trained and are not undertaking dangerous interventions?

Interestingly, many of the concerns expressed above about the integration of CAM within the NHS correspond with the issues raised by doctors (see Box 14.1). Of course, many of these concerns could also apply to orthodox medical practice.

BOX 14.1   DOCTORS' COMMON CONCERNS ABOUT COMPLEMENTARY MEDICINE

- Patients may see unqualified complementary practitioners.
- Patients may risk missed or delayed diagnosis.
- Patients may stop or refuse effective conventional treatment.
- Patients may waste money on ineffective treatments.
- Patients may experience dangerous adverse effects from treatment.
- The mechanism of some complementary treatments is so implausible they cannot possibly work.

(Source: Zollman and Vickers, 1999, p. 1558)

Integrating CAM therapies within statutory services may present both CAM therapists and conventional medical practitioners and other health workers with a series of challenges. Some medical practitioners (such as the GP Lorna Gold quoted above) may be unaware of the growing evidence base for CAM and remain reluctant to accept that complementary or alternative approaches to health and disease have any place within health service provision. Gold seems able to accept CAM in rather patronising and pejorative terms as a 'lifestyle' choice for some people to use. Other GPs, such as Michael Fitzpatrick, are even more forthright, claiming that 'I believe that the shift of medical practice away from the treatment of disease towards a wider intervention in personal life in the cause of enhancing health and happiness is bad for patients, bad for doctors and bad for society' (Fitzpatrick, 2002, p. 58).

Leonard Leibovici, a Professor of Medicine in Israel, writes:

> The explanations of the practitioners of alternative medicine are giving our patients a set of magical rules to control the physical world. ... They are saying that herbs are beneficial and can do no harm; a substance that causes complaints similar to those observed in a patient will cure them if diluted to an infinitesimal concentration; "we will adjust your Qi force"; these are phenomena that work only on the living human, and not on any other component of the physical world. I would guess that none of us are firm believers in magic. Honouring our patients, are we ready to offer them these explanations?
>
> (Leibovici, 1999, p. 1631)

However, not all members of the medical profession share these views. Easthope et al. (2000) suggest that doctors working in primary care have a generally more favourable attitude towards complementary therapies than those working in hospitals. Also, their survey showed that younger doctors have a more open attitude towards holistic ideals than older doctors who remain sceptical of claimed cure rates and see complementary therapies as having harmful side effects.

Resistance to the notion of integration does not come only from within the ranks of the medical profession. One strand of thought within the complementary and alternative therapy movement resists the drift towards further integration with statutory services, or indeed continued dialogue with the medical establishment. Some therapists believe that the systems of health and therapeutic endeavour that they practise are so far removed from the style, approach and philosophy of current mainstream medical practice that they have nothing to gain from any association with official or statutory services. In particular, in their opinion the power dimension within the therapeutic relationship in the system they practise is substantially different from that practised by orthodox doctors. The orthodox style that they claim relies on professional dominance may be potentially harmful to some people who seek help. They also fear control and contamination of their approach by the powerful people – managers and doctors – who currently control the NHS services.

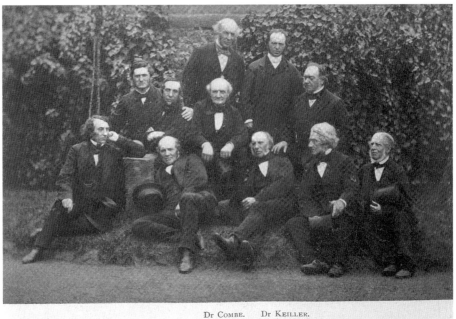

Dr Combe.   Dr Keiller.
Dr Warburton Begbie.   Dr J. Simson.   Dr Sellar.
Dr Heron Watson.
Dr Omond.   Dr Andrew Wood.   Dr Inglis.   Mr Benjamin Bell.   Dr William Brown.

Although many doctors were firmly opposed to alternative views on health and illness, this attitude has softened more recently

Although they recognise the pragmatic advantage to working alongside, and receiving finance from, the NHS, on balance they remain opposed to any further movement towards greater integration. Jonas and Levin summarise one of the fundamental problems:

> At the same time, important characteristics of CAM are at risk of being lost in its 'integration' with conventional care. The most important of these is an emphasis on self-healing as the lead approach for both improving wellness and treating disease. All of the major CAM systems approach illness by first trying to support and induce the self-healing processes of the patient. If this can stimulate recovery, then the likelihood of adverse effects and the need for high-impact/high-cost interventions are reduced.
>
> (Jonas and Levin, 1999, p. 10)

14.3   Integration or domination?

Luff and Thomas (1999) looked at possible models of complementary therapy integration within NHS primary care (or general practice). The results of their study were overwhelmingly positive, both professionals and people

attending the services reporting very high levels of satisfaction. However, for
some of the CAM therapists:

> their enthusiasm was not without reservations. Specifically there were
> concerns about the extent to which practitioners and therapies would be
> forced to compromise with the existing power structure and ethos of the
> NHS. The specific concerns about integration within the NHS for
> complementary practitioners centred around perceptions of control that
> practitioners would have in terms of their clinical integrity and professional
> status and possible changes in the working practices of complementary
> practitioners that might undermine therapeutic integrity. Briefly, the
> underlying question was integration at what price?
>
> (Luff and Thomas, 1999, p. 15)

Several issues are commonly encountered when complementary therapies are
available within primary care settings in the UK (Luff and Thomas, 1999).
These are both negative and positive. The benefits include the improved care
of people who attend for help and the many perceived benefits experienced
by the CAM practitioners themselves (Russo, 2000). The constraints or
negative effects are related to the different cultural divides between CAM
and allopathic approaches to the treatment regimes and to perceived loss of
autonomy by CAM practitioners when working within the NHS.

An American case study

In the USA, Schneirov and Geczik (2002) researched the dynamics involved
when a complementary medicine clinic was sited in a major, urban,
mainstream hospital. Their analysis led them to conclude that two
contradictory forces are at work within the alternative health movement.
One force concerns the movement towards involvement and engagement
with the dominant health care system. This component of the alternative
health movement is keen to enhance their credentials and status, and
'contest for resources, form coalitions, influence legislation, reform particular
professions, fight for the existence of new professions and educate the public'
(p. 202). They note that the alternative health clinic they studied was
successful in achieving a certain amount of institutional recognition even
within an orthodox system that contained 'highly specialised medical
expertise, sophisticated medical technology, and complex bureaucratic rules
and procedures and the pressure to generate income' (p. 205). However, the
alternative clinic was not given a 'free ride', and the researchers attempted to
discover the motivation behind official acceptance of the different form of
practice within its portals:

> the clinical director [of the official service] believes that the clinic creates a
> 'warm and fuzzy feeling' for the hospital, and can provide the hospital with
> some positive publicity. At any rate, the work done at the clinic is thought

to be 'harmless'. At the same time, the clinic is under increasing pressure to produce academically credible research to justify their clinical practices and to prove to the business side of the hospital that the clinic can be financially stable and self-sufficient within a few years.

(Schneirov and Geczik, 2002, p. 206)

The study's authors characterised another force within the alternative health movement as its **submerged networks**. These networks might develop critiques of contemporary health care practice that fundamentally challenge the routine practices of orthodox health care workers. These systems also provide the link to the radical roots of the alternative health care movement that are indeed alternative and lie outside conventional codes and institutional arrangements:

a cultural laboratory where patients and health activists can experience new authority relations, new ideas and new identities that embody a critique of the health care system, medical expertise, the administrative state and consumer culture.

(Schneirov and Geczik, 2002, pp. 202–3)

Within the clinic the healers' approach to healing is shared by many of the complementary and alternative practitioners, which could be considered to contradict many of the values inherent in much 'scientific' or orthodox medical practice. That is, they emphasise:

illness as imbalance, treating the cause of the disease and not symptoms, illness as an opportunity for self-growth and self-discovery, the use of natural and non-pharmaceutical agents, an emphasis on mobilizing the innate healing capacities of the body, and promoting a more egalitarian relationship between patient and practitioner ...

(Schneirov and Geczik, 2002, p. 203)

However, the healers within the alternative clinic recognise that there are certain advantages over and above any financial security that they gain from their involvement with mainstream services and the values that they embody:

Record keeping, clinical research, the credentializing and licensing process for practitioners gives the [alternative] clinic credibility with patients and makes it possible for the clinic leadership to learn from past practices ... The hospital setting itself gives alternative medicine credibility ...

(Schneirov and Geczik, 2002, p. 212)

In any social movement there are probably similar tensions and opportunities for mutual learning between the more institutional strands and the 'submerged' or more radical networks. For instance, in the UK there is a thriving culture and sub-culture between and among complementary and alternative therapists in informal settings, in various published journals and, of course, on the internet. A dual approach, with both forces active, is important for the growth and survival of the alternative health movement: indeed, the debates and tensions between these two forces remains an important learning point for both camps. However:

> The danger here is that alternative health activists will get caught up in this process of institutionalization and as a result lose their movement character as a kind of anarchic flow of information, remedies, and modalities which are potentially innovative, pathbreaking and at times dangerous.
>
> (Schneirov and Geczik, 2002, p. 218)

Some prominent activists within the UK's alternative health scene express similar fears, as shown in the following activity.

ACTIVITY   DOCTORS IN CHARGE?

Allow 20 minutes

Read the extract from a letter to the editor of the *British Medical Journal* (BMJ) in Box 14.2. It was written by David St George, who at that time was Director of the Centre for Integrative Sciences in Complementary and Alternative Therapies in London.

- In what ways do you agree with the sentiments expressed in the letter? Which parts of it do you disagree with?

- Write a short letter (a maximum of 250 words) of your own to the editor of the BMJ, expressing your opinions on the subject.

Comment

Many of the people who have done this activity recognised some of David St George's concerns. However, several had quite different points of view. For some it was a good idea for doctors to remain in charge of health and therapeutic endeavours, while for others it was obviously not a route they would want to follow. Most thought some independence from the medical establishment was important, so that complementary practitioners thrive and continue to develop their ideas. One person commented:

> From my own practice experience I would like to see greater integration, but a more "regulated" integration so that safety and standards of care remain a priority. There are health professionals, e.g. nurses and

physiotherapists, working in NHS settings who are qualified in CAM ... however, standards of training vary ... Some have just done weekend courses in aromatherapy and reflexology and others might decide to introduce CAM without it being the policy of their Trust.

BOX 14.2   LETTER TO THE BMJ

EDITOR – ... It is precisely because of the limitations of biomedical knowledge and treatment that doctors (particularly general practitioners) began to open the door to complementary practitioners. During the late 1980s and early 1990s some general practitioners and complementary therapists developed pragmatic forms of collaboration, which represents 'integration' on a more equal professional footing. In these arrangements, general practitioners often referred patients to complementary therapists for their opinion and advice, rather than with certainty that a particular treatment would help the patient. Also, they found that complementary therapists could make an important contribution to patient care, even in the absence of a clear cut orthodox medical diagnosis. ...

The expansion of complementary therapies over recent decades has been widespread, consumer driven, and at the grass roots. We are now witnessing the establishment finally waking up to the potential threat from alternative healing practices if they continue to flourish unchecked. Despite the pious claim to be restoring the soul to medicine, what the *BMJ* theme issue [on integrated medicine] really signifies is orthodox medicine's attempt to shore up its monopoly by bringing the professions working in complementary therapy under its wing.

(Source: St George, 2001, p. 1484)

14.4   Integrated or integrative medicine?

There are many powerful advocates of the integration of complementary and alternative forms of medicine with scientific western systems. HRH Prince Charles is a well known supporter of this approach and has established a foundation bearing his name to promote the development of links between western orthodox medicine and other approaches (Prince of Wales's Foundation for Integrated Health, 2003).

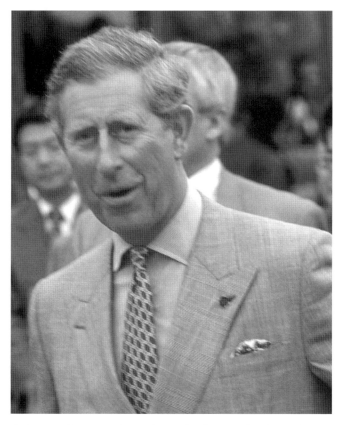

HRH Prince Charles has remained a staunch advocate for the development of integrated medicine

Other enthusiasts from the orthodox medical profession, as well as prominent members of the alternative and complementary therapist community, have ensured that the push towards further integration continues. However, for some practitioners and enthusiasts there is another step, after increasing integration, which seems to involve the development of a type of medicine that is an amalgamation of all previous branches and traditions (Oumeish, 1998). This is known as **integrative medicine** in the USA, although usually it is called **integrated medicine** in the UK.

ACTIVITY   WHAT IS INTEGRATED OR INTEGRATIVE MEDICINE?

Allow 15 minutes

Read the following quotations and then write a short description of your own understanding of 'integrated' and 'integrative' medicine.

Maizes and Caspi (1999, p. 148), claim that:

> integrative medicine shifts the paradigm from sickness to health, keeps the patient in the central focus of care, and multiplies the number of strategies available to the patient. It is a new kind of medicine that shifts the experience for both patient and provider.

Read and Czauderna (2001, p. 1485) state that:

> Integrated medicine attempts to combine the best of both systems, but it is not just about adding a bit of acupuncture to the aspirin; it is about restoring an understanding of the patient, his or her attitudes, beliefs, personal history, and life situation to health care.

Rees and Weil (2001, p. 119) claim that this form of medicine:

> is practising medicine in a way that selectively incorporates elements of complementary and alternative medicine into comprehensive treatment plans alongside solidly orthodox methods of diagnosis and treatment.

Dalen (1998, p. 2180) surveys the scene surrounding the integration of 'conventional' and 'unconventional' medicine strictly from the standpoint of a mainstream physician who is only comfortable using the techniques developed within western 'scientific' medicine:

> The leaders of integrative medicine must sort through the myriad of proposed unconventional therapies to determine which should be subjected to appropriately designed clinical trials. ... If a therapy that arose from outside the mainstream of modern Western medicine can pass the same level of scrutiny that we expect of conventional therapies, it should be integrated into mainstream medicine and added to the therapeutic armamentarium of the well-trained, conventional physician. We can do no less for our patients!

Comment

Although on one level a system that incorporates both types of medicine – as long as they are effective – would seem to be a logical and necessary step, this unification presents certain problems. Indeed, these notions of incorporating and selecting only certain therapies are most problematic for some CAM therapists. They feel that this leaves the powerful physicians from orthodox medical practices firmly in charge, picking the therapies, or bits of therapies, that they want to incorporate within their own system to their own advantage, and probably to the detriment of the alternative therapists – and ultimately to the users.

Degrees of integration

The integration of CAM with statutory services is not an 'all or nothing' phenomenon. There are degrees of integration and a wide variance of policies that might lead to greater or lesser integration (Hess, 2002). Integration can happen at the individual level, where many people seem able to 'pick and mix' the therapies that they believe work for them (Astin, 2000). As this chapter has demonstrated, integration can happen at a practitioner level: for example, in pain clinics and within palliative care and primary care settings. Professional groupings can also encompass the notion of integration: for example, anaesthetists and physiotherapists who use acupuncture. In addition, integration can also be part of strategic or governmental policy and, finally, at national and international level, whole countries may base their health care on various integrations between different medical and health care systems (Bodeker, 2001).

Bombardieri and Easthope (2000) propose four indicators of 'convergence', which are listed in Box 14.3.

BOX 14.3   LEVELS OF INTEGRATION, OR 'CONVERGENCE', BETWEEN CAM AND ORTHODOX PRACTITIONERS

1   The use by alternative practitioners of techniques commonly used by orthodox doctors.
2   The referral by alternative practitioners to general practitioners.
3   The referral by general practitioners to alternative practitioners.
4   The use of alternative therapies by medical practitioners.

(Source: Bombardieri and Easthope, 2000, p. 485)

It is important to recognise the central importance within current orthodox medical practice of so-called **evidence-based medicine** (EBM), which forms the basis of the treatment that health care workers are expected to provide. According to the central tenets of EBM, if the treatment has been shown not to work and proved to be ineffective in a randomised controlled trial (RCT), it should not be a part of contemporary, orthodox medical practice. Of course, many treatments are commonly used that have never been subjected to an RCT. There are also other serious concerns about the slavish implementation of EBM within the practice of orthodox medicine (Feinstein and Horowitz, 1997).

David Peters, a clinical director, recognises the importance of this feature of current medical practice but proposes an entirely different approach:

> At a time when 'evidence based medicine' has such enormous currency, we should bear in mind that some innovations are needs-driven and develop without a formal evidence based rationale. Are there parallels between the way CTs [complementary therapies] have been adopted by the mainstream and how counselling or hospice care were incorporated? ... these social inventions took root not as a result of clinical trials, but rather because they met previously unspoken needs ...
>
> (Peters, 2000, pp. 59, 60)

14.5 Integration and the NHS

It is hard to uncover evidence of coherent policy about the integration of complementary or alternative medicine from the decision makers in the NHS (Russo, 2000). Almost none of the recent official policy or strategy documents from the Department of Health equivalents in Scotland, Wales and Northern Ireland give firm guidelines for the way in which local NHS organisations should, or should not, move towards further integration. Indeed, many of the key health strategy documents do not mention complementary or alternative approaches to health.

As discussed earlier in this book, the House of Lords published an influential report on complementary and alternative therapy (House of Lords, 2000). This report made three important recommendations for the provision of CAM therapies in the NHS (see Box 14.4). In response to this report there has been some government support for research into various aspects of CAM provision, but there appears to be little central guidance or official recognition of the ways in which CAM could contribute to the health of the nation, or indeed help to resolve some of the problems in the current NHS.

BOX 14.4   RECOMMENDATIONS FROM HOUSE OF LORDS REPORT (2000)

42 We recommend that those practising privately-accessed CAM therapies should work towards integration between CAM and conventional medicine, and CAM therapists should encourage patients with conditions that have not been previously discussed with a medical practitioner to see their GP. We also urge CAM practitioners and GPs to keep an open mind about each other's ability to help their patients, to make patients feel comfortable about integrating their healthcare provision and to exchange information about treatment programmes and their perceptions of the healthcare needs of patients.

43 We recommend that all NHS provision of CAM should continue to be through GP referral (or by referral from doctors or other healthcare professionals working in primary, secondary or tertiary care).

44 We recommend that only those CAM therapies which are statutory [*sic*] regulated, or have a powerful mechanism of voluntary self-regulation, should be made available, by reference from doctors and other healthcare professionals working in primary, secondary or tertiary care, on the NHS.

(Source: House of Lords, 2000)

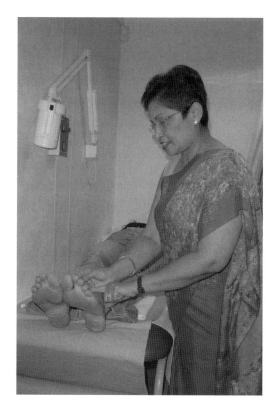

People seem to appreciate the time and attention they receive during a consultation with a complementary medicine practitioner

Local policy initiatives and developments

In the absence of national guidelines, many local NHS trusts, primary care organisations and individual units have developed their own responses to any specific proposals they have received for integrating CAM with their services. Advocates of and enthusiasts for CAM are remarkably persistent and imaginative when pressing the case for local provision and for uncovering sources of finance to establish CAM services. Often, however, the funding for these developments is from external charitable donations, or the creative manipulation of non-recurrent budgets, rather than from central funding streams. Frequently, CAM services seem to rely on short-term funding arrangements and can be the first to be threatened with closure when financial constraints affect local services.

In some hospital units there has been a significant development of CAM. Complementary and alternative forms of therapy seem to be accepted as almost the norm in certain areas of service provision, for example in NHS pain clinics and palliative care settings. Often CAM services seem to develop in precisely those areas where 'scientific' western medicine has had least impact. The House of Lords report outlines the areas in secondary care where CAM development seems greatest:

> There are existing models of CAM being part of secondary care delivery, but they are limited to three or four main areas. First, where the manipulative therapies (osteopathy and chiropractic) have been integrated into orthopaedic care. Second, where acupuncture (and occasionally some of the relaxant therapies ...) have been integrated into pain clinics. Third, where acupuncture and occasionally aromatherapy have been integrated into some obstetric and cancer services, and into palliative care, rehabilitation and care of the elderly. And fourth, where homeopathy is provided within secondary care through the homeopathic hospitals.
>
> (House of Lords, 2000, para. 9.17)

CAM within general practice or primary care

In many ways the development of complementary and alternative forms of treatment has been more successful within general practice or primary care. Luff and Thomas (2000) looked at the ways in which primary care teams find the finance to support access for their patients to CAM practitioners. Most of the therapists cited in their research experienced considerable differences in how they could practise their therapy in the NHS, compared with their private work. In some cases this was a source of frustration; in others it was an interesting challenge. The main factor which caused their NHS practice to differ from their private practice was that key dimensions of the treatment had been laid down by the organisational structure, and were no longer subject to one-to-one negotiation with their patients. In general terms, the CAM practitioners were required to work more like their orthodox colleagues who were under increasing pressure to practise protocol-driven forms of medical care that are structured within centrally produced guidelines. For the CAM practitioners, the short length of the sessions, together with the fact that the patients were referred for specific problems, tended to make their work slightly more symptom or problem oriented, although they tried hard to maintain a holistic approach to their work within this framework. In some cases, it also tended to lead to less time being spent providing explanations and information, which sometimes leads to less engagement in lifestyle factors that may have impinged on the patient's health.

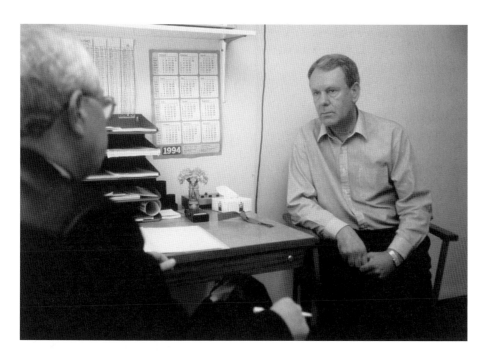

Many patients do not tell their GP that they also use complementary medicine. This may place some at unnecessary risk. In integrated settings this could be less of a problem

Despite the ad hoc basis of the primary care development of CAM services in the past, there seems to have been a steady growth in the availability of this type of service. Thomas et al. (2003) show that the proportion of general practices providing some form of access to CAM therapies rose from 39 per cent in 1995 to 50 per cent in 2001. One or more members of the primary health care team provided therapies in an estimated 29.5 per cent of practices (a rise of 38 per cent since 1995); independent CAM practitioners worked in 12.2 per cent; and 26.8 per cent of practices made NHS referrals to external CAM providers. The proportion of services supported by patient payments rose from 26 per cent in 1995 to 42 per cent in 2001.

   The way in which primary care teams and general practices receive their money has changed greatly since 1990. The further development of CAM services within primary care throughout the UK depends crucially on the attitudes and commitment of local primary care organisations (PCOs):

> Locality purchasing by Primary Care [Organisations] ... will have the potential to provide a new mechanism for delivering complementary health care services to NHS primary care patients. Whether the established services survive, or indeed expand, will depend on the success of one of two strategies; primary care providers who wish to see such services as part of the purchasing strategy for the locality must either convince the wider group of GPs and nurses in their [PCO] of their benefits and cost-effectiveness or

identify a new source of practice-specific funds to ensure provision to their own patients ... The price of greater control for primary care through increased purchasing power may produce a significant reduction in autonomy and innovation at the individual practice level and the provision of complementary or alternative health care may be one of the casualties.

(Thomas et al., 2001b, p. 29)

The relationship between people who might want to develop CAM services within primary care and their local PCO is crucial to the success or failure of such projects. In the absence of firm policy guidance and earmarked money from central sources, local decision makers have considerable discretion to accept or reject specific proposals. Even where there is a central policy about the delivery of services, there is often scope for local interpretation.

ACTIVITY   INTRODUCING CAM TO THE NHS

Allow 30 minutes

As part of the House of Lords inquiry (2000), several PCOs were asked 'What factors are important in decision-making on the provision of complementary therapies throughout your Primary Care Organisation?' Respondents were asked to identify the five most important factors. Look carefully at Figure 14.1, which sets out graphically the responses from PCOs.

- What were the most important factors that the PCOs took into consideration when deciding whether to provide CAM therapies as part of their NHS services?
- Imagine that you are the press officer for your local PCO. Write a short press release (a maximum of 350 words) based on these findings for your local newspaper, outlining why your organisation was reluctant to provide CAM for the local population.

Comment

The results show that, in considering CAM's role in NHS primary care, the most important factors are evidence of effectiveness and cost-effectiveness, followed by accreditation procedures and standards and then resource implications.

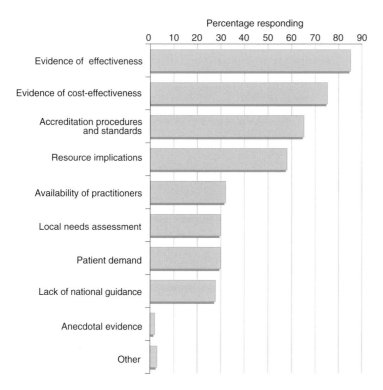

Figure 14.1 Factors affecting PCO decision making on CAM provision
(Source: House of Lords, 2000, para. 9.40)

Local PCOs are necessarily cautious about introducing services that might be controversial and could be seen to compete against established services. Most local services are heavily committed to meeting national, centrally determined targets, such as the reduction of waiting lists and various other output-based measures. In any case, there is continual financial pressure on 'regular' or orthodox services and CAM provision could be seen as having the ability to take resources away from these established 'must-do' priorities:

■ we find it difficult enough to get things funded which are evidence-based quite often ... you know, cancer, drugs or whatever, and so how can we support something [the introduction of CAM] which in theory isn't evidence-based in the way that other research is ...

■ the problem about it is that anything like that has to compete as a priority against other priorities and, in all candour it is quite hard to make a case for a big expansion in alternative medicine when it would be at the expense of an expansion in a more high profile service.

(GPs quoted in Thomas and Coleman, 2003)

So far, some of the potential barriers to integrating CAM within statutory services have been considered. These barriers originate from doctors and other health care workers who may not have the same philosophical approaches as CAM providers. Additional hurdles have been identified where national and local policy makers do not have this type of provision currently on their priority list and where there is pressure to maintain the status quo. In addition, the structures and decision-making procedures within the health service tend to create problems for people who are keen to introduce innovative services. It is always easier for large organisations such as the NHS to maintain the status quo and allocate financial support to the services and systems that are already in place. However, and despite these forms of potential hurdle, advocates and enthusiasts seem to be finding imaginative ways to ensure the provision of CAM modalities within the statutory services.

Indeed, some people see the provision of CAM not as a problem but as a solution for at least some of the problems facing the NHS (Russo, 2000). The provision of CAM may be able to help services meet their various targets for reducing waiting lists, controlling the steeply rising drugs budget or responding to patient demand and improving the outcomes for people with chronically painful conditions.

14.6   Case study: Somerset Trust for Integrated Health Care

The Trust provides subsidised NHS access to an integrated complementary health care service within a primary care context. It also evaluates and researches the service they provide. People are referred according to established protocols for a course of complementary treatment in one of four main modalities: acupuncture, osteopathy, herbalism and massage. A course of therapy consists of about three hours of treatment, usually in six half-hour appointments. Referrals are protocol-driven and evidence-based where available. The integrated musculo-skeletal medicine service is designed to ease the waiting list for the current NHS services for physiotherapy, orthopaedic and pain clinic appointments. The service has been shown to increase the range of effective treatment options, and improve patient choice and access for people who cannot afford private complementary treatment.

Care pathways have been designed for managing:

1   back pain
2   joint pains and myalgia
3   chronic pain
4   carpal tunnel syndrome.

These conditions normally generate referrals to physiotherapy and secondary care. At the point of referral, people are offered the option of referral for a course of four to six complementary therapy treatments (osteopathy or acupuncture).

The results from this project show that this approach is widely welcomed by users themselves, appears to have considerable effectiveness in a wide range of health problems, and has led to a reduced demand on other aspects of health care provision, particularly referrals to secondary care.

The complementary therapies that people were referred to seem to be particularly effective for short-term and severe conditions, and for musculo-skeletal conditions such as frozen shoulders or painful knees. The majority of referrals were for people with longer-term health conditions such as chronic arthritis. There is some evidence that people with experience of complementary health, and with an active approach to their own health management, have a better outcome, although people who ask for complementary medicine themselves did no better. Indeed, the outcome for self-requesting people seems poorer than for those who are referred by their GP.

The provision of complementary medicine in general practice is not an easy option. It is very difficult to find a way of funding such a service, although from this study, there appears to be evidence that such a service is, at least, cost-neutral (on account of savings made elsewhere) and, at best, cost effective. It is also demanding in terms of administrative time, and, with demand for the service outstripping supply, can easily lead to long waiting lists.

However, the benefits of such a service seem considerable, both for the users and for other staff at the practice, particularly since it provides another treatment option for people for whom conventional treatment has been ineffective. The people receiving the service were also very satisfied.

Implementing this kind of service currently appears to be limited by the lack of funding. The complementary health service in this case study is now being maintained through a charity, with funding from patients' donations and outside grants. While this is encouraging as a sign of general public and patient support for a service, long-term NHS funding needs to be realised if the service is to have a secure financial basis. Other obstacles to further expansion of services of this kind within an NHS setting include the difficulty for health professionals in accessing good quality information about these therapies, particularly information about the evidence base that is beginning to evolve. Funding for research also remains very limited, and there is an urgent need for research which would investigate further some of the tentative results from the present study: particularly more research into the cost-effectiveness of CAM therapies within a primary care setting.

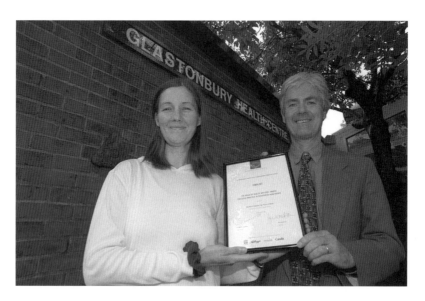

The Central Somerset Gazette reported the honour bestowed on the Glastonbury Health Centre Project (Photo courtesy of Mid Somerset Newspapers)

Further research at the Glastonbury Health Centre by Dione Hills revealed that both therapists and patients enjoy a high level of satisfaction:

> even if they had little prior experience of complementary therapies, [patients] generally appreciated the service. In addition to any improvement that it made to the particular condition from which they suffered, they also liked the opportunity that the service provided for them to talk over the problem from which they were suffering, and to see this in a wider context of their general emotional and social situation. They often received advice on how to manage their health problem, through use of self-massage, relaxation or exercise, and even if the treatment itself had not made a significant difference, the self-management techniques gave them a sense of greater control over their health.
>
> (Hills, 2003, personal communication)

However, the shortness of the sessions and the limited number were sources of frustration, particularly for people with chronic conditions, which had only just begun to respond to treatment by the time the series of sessions came to an end:

> [Therapists] were strongly committed to their particular chosen 'therapy' … almost all had some ambivalence towards the commercial side of working in private practice, and several experienced considerable professional isolation working as independent practitioners.
>
> (Hills, 2003, personal communication)

In this context the opportunity of working in an NHS setting, with a guaranteed weekly income (although small) and the opportunity for regular meetings with other therapists, was warmly welcomed. Some of the expectations that the therapists brought to their work in the NHS, however, were unfulfilled. There had not been the level of professional interchange, particularly with the GPs, that they had expected.

In terms of background and orientation, all the therapists were strongly committed to a holistic approach to their work, which involved linking the specific health problem that was being presented to other factors in the patient's life, including their emotional and psychological state and general lifestyle. In this respect, and partly because they worked in the 'private' sphere, they tended towards a strongly 'individualised' approach to health, seeing the individual as having responsibility for their general health and wellbeing: an approach which has been closely linked with a 'consumer-oriented' view of health. This sometimes tends to overlook the wider social and structural factors that could impinge on the individual's health and wellbeing, over which the individual might have little control.

This approach was attacked in the context of the NHS practice, where many of the referred patients were socially and economically disadvantaged and had social and psychological problems which could be, directly or indirectly, attributed to this disadvantage. In the context of the Glastonbury project, it is interesting to consider how far the training and background of the CAM professionals prepared them for work in a bureaucratic public setting.

There were also differences in terms of the kind of health problems the therapists were working with in the NHS practice, and the kind of patients they saw, as regards age, background and attitude to their own health. Patients were seen as being more likely to have emotional and social problems and to take a passive approach towards their health problems. These both had implications for the treatment that the practitioners could provide, although the level of variation differed considerably from therapist to therapist. Several therapists saw this as placing different kinds of demand on them, in terms of both the skills they brought to the work and the personal pressures. At least two therapists thought this had implications for the kind of professional support and supervision that they felt they needed.

14.7 Conclusion

The integration of complementary and alternative medicine within mainstream medical services is fraught with challenges. For some advocates of an integrated approach the recent drive towards integration has been entirely welcome. Enthusiasts of integration are encouraged to develop more joint projects and lobby for widespread funding for CAM therapies through statutory NHS funding (Prince of Wales's Foundation for Integrated Health, 2003). This movement is resisted by certain elements within the medical profession, and by some other health care workers, who resent the inherent challenge to their powerful monopoly position and possible undermining of the dominance of the 'scientific' approach to medicine. The move towards further integration is also resisted by certain people within the CAM movement itself. They fear that further integration will always be based on the terms and conditions imposed by the powerful medical elites. In their opinion, the unique qualities and values inherent in the various branches of CAM will be eroded and contaminated by close association with the medical mainstream.

The system of statutory health care provision, controlled by managers and administrators, is constantly under enormous financial pressure. Budgets are already stretched and targets are hard enough to reach. Why would they want to introduce even more complexity and further drains on their budgets?

However, pressure from advocates and enthusiasts continues unabated. People who use CAM are enthusiastic about the effects it has on their health and demand access through the NHS system that ostensibly is 'theirs'. The general public pay the taxes that provide the finance for the system and, increasingly, consumer and local community interests are represented on the decision-making bodies that control local health services. Innovative and imaginative ways are being found to increase access to various CAM therapies through NHS resources.

KEY POINTS

- There is considerable pressure from the general public to provide access to complementary and alternative forms of treatment through NHS channels.
- The pressure for integration is often resisted by certain powerful elements within the medical and health care establishment.
- The concept of integration is also not universally accepted by practitioners of CAM therapies, some of whom are wary of close association with mainstream medical approaches.
- Within the NHS, integration is accepted as part of certain hospital services such as NHS pain clinics.
- Primary care providers generally accept CAM therapies to a greater extent than do hospital services.
- Integrated CAM projects within the NHS often struggle for sustained funding.
- Integrated projects should be prepared to monitor and audit how they work.

References

Astin, J. (2000) 'The characteristics of CAM users: a complex picture', in Kellner, M., Wellman, B., Pescosolido, B. and Saks, M. (eds) *Complementary and Alternative Medicine: Challenge and Change*, London, Harwood Academic Publishers.

Bodeker, G. (2001) 'Lessons on integration from the developing world's experience', *British Medical Journal*, Vol. 322, pp. 164–7.

Bombardieri, D. and Easthope, G. (2000) 'Convergence between orthodox and alternative medicine: a theoretical elaboration and empirical test', *Health*, Vol. 4, No. 4, pp. 479–94.

Dalen, J. (1998) '"Conventional" and "unconventional" medicine: can they be integrated?', *Archives of Internal Medicine*, Vol. 158, pp. 2179–81.

Davidoff, F. (1998) 'Weighing the alternatives: lessons from the paradoxes of alternative medicine', *Annals of Internal Medicine*, Vol. 129, No. 12, pp. 1068–70.

Department of Health (2000) *The NHS Plan*, London, HMSO. Available online at www.publications.doh.gov.uk/nhsplan/summary.htm [accessed 2 August 2004].

Dr Foster (2002) *Good Complementary Therapist Guide*, London, Vermilion.

Easthope, G., Tranter, B. and Gill, G. (2000) 'General practitioners' attitudes toward complementary therapies', *Social Science and Medicine*, Vol. 51, pp. 1555–61.

Feinstein, A. and Horowitz, R. (1997) 'Problems in the "evidence" of "evidence-based medicine"', *American Journal of Medicine*, Vol. 103, pp. 529–35.

Fitzpatrick, M. (2002) 'The surrender of scientific medicine', *Alternative Medicine: Should We Swallow It?*, pp. 59–76, London, Institute of Ideas/Hodder and Stoughton.

Hess, D. (2002) 'Complementary or alternative? Stronger vs. weaker integration policies', *American Journal of Public Health*, Vol. 92, No. 10, pp. 1579–81.

Hills, D. (2003) *The Patient, the Practitioner and the Organisation: Research into the Glastonbury Health Centre*, Unpublished PhD thesis.

House of Lords (2000) *Complementary and Alternative Medicine, Sixth Report of the Select Committee on Science and Technology*, London, The Stationery Office. Available online at www.parliament.the-stationery-office.co.uk/pa/ld199900/ldselect/ldsctech/123/12301.htm [accessed 18 February 2004].

Jonas, W. B. and Levin, J. S. (1999) *Essentials of Complementary and Alternative Medicine*, Philadelphia, PA, Lippincott Williams & Wilkins.

Leibovici, L. (1999) 'Alternative (complementary) medicine: a cuckoo in the nest of empiricist reed warblers', *British Medical Journal*, Vol. 319, pp. 1629–31.

Luff, D. and Thomas, K. (1999) *Models of Complementary Therapy Provision in Primary Care*, Sheffield, Medical Care Research Unit, University of Sheffield.

Luff, D. and Thomas, K. (2000) 'Sustaining complementary therapy provision in primary care: lessons from existing services', *Complementary Therapies in Medicine*, Vol. 8, pp. 173–9.

Maizes, V. and Caspi, O. (1999) 'The principles and challenges of integrative medicine', *Western Journal of Medicine*, Vol. 171, No. 3, pp. 148–9.

McTaggart, L. (2001) 'May the fields be with you', *What Doctors Don't Tell You*, Vol. 12, No. 7, p. 5.

Ong, C. K. and Banks, B. (2003) *Complementary and Alternative Medicine: The Consumer Perspective*, London, The Prince of Wales's Foundation for Integrated Health.

Oumeish, O. (1998) 'The philosophical, cultural, and historical aspects of complementary, alternative, unconventional, and integrative medicine in the Old World', *Archives of Dermatology*, Vol. 134, pp. 1373–86.

Peters, D. (2000) 'From holism to integration: is there a future for complementary therapies in the NHS?', *Complementary Therapies in Nursing and Midwifery*, Vol. 6, pp. 59–60.

Prince of Wales's Foundation for Integrated Health (2003) *Setting the Agenda for the Future*, London, PoWFIH.

Rayner, L. and Easthope, G. (2001) 'Postmodern consumption and alternative medications', *Journal of Sociology*, Vol. 37, No. 2, pp. 157–76.

Read, N. and Czauderna, J. (2001) 'Finding the time is most important', *British Medical Journal*, Vol. 322, pp. 1484–5.

Rees, L. and Weil, A. (2001) 'Integrated medicine', *British Medical Journal*, Vol. 322, pp. 119–20.

Russo, H. (2000) *Integrated Healthcare: A Guide to Good Practice*, London, The Foundation for Integrated Medicine.

Schneirov, M. and Geczik, J. D. (2002) 'Alternative health and the challenges of institutionalization', *Health*, Vol. 6, No. 2, pp. 201–20.

St George, D. (2001) 'Integrated medicine means doctors will be in charge', *British Medical Journal*, Vol. 322, p. 1484.

Thomas, K. and Coleman, P. (2003) *PCG Policy Development in Relation to Complementary or Alternative Medicine (CAM) Services*, 2nd Interim Report to the Department of Health, January 2001, Sheffield, Medical Care Research Unit, University of Sheffield.

Thomas, K., Nicholl, J. and Coleman, P. (2001a) 'Use and expenditure on complementary medicine in England: a population based survey', *Complementary Therapies in Medicine*, Vol. 9, pp. 2–11.

Thomas, K. J., Nicholl, J. P. and Fall, M. (2001b) 'Access to complementary medicine via general practice', *British Journal of General Practice*, Vol. 51, pp. 25–30.

Thomas, K., Coleman, P. and Nicholl, J. (2003) 'Trends in access to complementary or alternative medicines (CAMs) via primary care in England: 1995–2001', *Family Practice*, Vol. 20, pp. 575–7.

Zollman, C. and Vickers, A. (1999) 'ABC of complementary medicine. Complementary medicine and the doctor', *British Medical Journal*, Vol. 319, pp. 1558–61.

Chapter 15 Information sources and complementary and alternative medicine

Tom Heller and Julie Stone

Contents

AIMS

- To describe some of the ways in which CAM is portrayed in the media.
- To discuss the problems with the quality and accuracy of CAM-related information in a variety of media.

15.1 Introduction

This chapter encourages you to consider some of the numerous ways in which information about complementary and alternative medicine (CAM) is created, developed and disseminated by a variety of producers and controllers of information. The ways in which this information is received, interpreted and acted on by 'consumers' of information are also explored.

ACTIVITY   FINDING OUT ABOUT CAM

Allow 15 minutes

Imagine that a friend has just rung you to let you know about a mutual acquaintance who unfortunately has developed a significant health problem. You know little about this particular condition but, during the conversation, you offer to find out more.

Make a list of all the possible sources of information you could turn to in order to inform yourself and your friend about this specific condition.

Comment

You may have considered the networks of people you could ask for advice. Knowledge and experience about health issues are widely distributed throughout the community. Your list of networks and individuals may have included:

- other friends with wider knowledge about health issues
- another friend with personal experience of this condition
- your GP or another approachable health worker
- a local self-help group which focuses on this issue
- a national organisation or telephone helpline specific to this condition
- NHS Direct or other generic health information sources.

You may also have thought of published or more widely disseminated sources of written information, including:

- local library
- health promotion department of local health authority
- health library
- advice column in newspaper
- past issues of a health magazine.

However, in recent years, the most significant source of information and knowledge has been the internet.

15.2 Health information and the internet: internauts and cyberchondriacs

The history of the growth of the internet continues to be explored and researched. Some of the originators of this electronic phenomenon – self-styled 'internauts' – created the necessary concepts and technology initially as part of the Cold War effort to ensure continued US military technological superiority (Leiner et al., 1979).

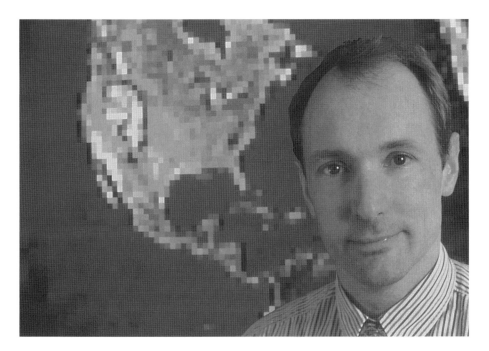

Tim Berners Lee is credited with inventing the World Wide Web. The original idea of the web was that it should be a collaborative space: that is, by writing something together, and as people worked on it, they could iron out misunderstanding

However, since its early days as a tool in the development of the defence industry, the capacity of the internet to transform many other aspects of the exchange of information throughout society has become increasingly apparent:

> The Internet is at once a world-wide broadcasting capability, a mechanism for information dissemination, and a medium for collaboration and interaction between individuals and their computers without regard for geographic location.
>
> (Leiner et al., 1979, p. 1)

Of course, academics, researchers, health workers and commercial manufacturers of health products, shortly followed by consumers, quickly seized upon the medical uses of such exchanges of information.

The internet is constantly changing and developing, and the multitude of uses to which its enormous capacity can be directed are continually shifting and expanding. For this reason, it is difficult to determine precisely statistics about its use within the medical sphere. Estimates for 2001 suggest that 25 million people in the UK had access to the web (Powell, 2002) and that 14 million used it regularly (NetRatings Inc., 2001). Worldwide, over 500 million people have logged on (Nua Internet Surveys, 2001). They have access to over three billion web documents (Google Inc., 2001), and at least

2 per cent of websites are health-related (Kiley, 1999). Indeed, accessing health information is a common reason for going online: surveys show that 50 to 75 per cent of web users have looked for health information (Murero et al., 2001; Tatsumi et al., 2001; Taylor, 2001) and have accessed such information more than three times a month (Taylor, 2001).

ACTIVITY   USING THE INTERNET

Allow 20 minutes

If you have access to the internet, think for a few minutes about the various ways in which you have used it over the last few weeks. Write a list of the different reasons why you accessed the web.

Next to each entry on your list, indicate approximately how long you spend on this activity each week.

Finally, indicate on your list how much of this activity relates to health issues for yourself or other people.

Comment

You may use the internet rarely, or you may be in danger of letting it take over your life!

Your list may have included the following reasons for accessing the web:

- email at work
- email to personal and family contacts
- access to information about 'what's on' locally
- contact specialist electronic library for access to journals
- contact library to reserve books
- online news service to read news items
- search the web for information about health issues
- online banking
- buying books from online bookstores.

Although there are numerous reasons for using the internet, health-related use is very high on the list for many people. In the USA by 2002, 73 million adults were using the internet to look for health information, compared with 52 million in 2000 (Fox and Rainie, 2002). The regular users of the internet for health-related purposes vary considerably:

> [They] research prescription drugs, explore new ways to control their weight, and prepare for doctors' appointments, among other activities. Many say the Internet has helped them or someone they know and very few report harmful effects from acting on bad information they found online.

... The typical health seeker starts [her hunt for medical information] at a [general] search site, not a medical site, and visits two to five sites during an average visit. She [women are more likely than men to look for health information online] spends at least thirty minutes on a search. She feels reassured by advice that matches what she already knew about a condition and by statements that are repeated at more than one site. She is likely to turn away from sites that seem to be selling something or don't clearly identify the source of the information. And about one third of health seekers who find relevant information online bring it to their doctor for a final quality check.

(Fox and Rainie, 2002, p. 4)

Health seekers: using the internet for health information

A major survey of health-related users of the internet in the USA reported that 'health seekers' value the convenience, anonymity and volume of online information (Fox and Rainie, 2002). Naturally, people use the internet at different points during the course of their illness or at different times for their health care needs, as described in Box 15.1. The California Healthcare Foundation categorises users in three ways: the well, the newly diagnosed, and the chronically ill and their care givers (Cain et al., 2000). Members of the 'well' group occasionally search for information about short-term medical conditions. The 'newly diagnosed' tend to engage in intensive searches for specific information, valuing the ease of access and broad range of information. The 'chronically ill and their care givers' regularly search for information about new treatments, nutrition advice and alternative therapies. In addition, the newly diagnosed and chronically ill groups both value and use online communities and chat rooms. Several studies have shown the importance of the web in providing social support, particularly to people with chronic health problems such as diabetes (Glasgow et al., 1998; Zrebiec and Jacobson, 2001) or with HIV (Reeves, 2000).

BOX 15.1   SEARCHING FOR HEALTH INFORMATION ON THE INTERNET

Gunter Eysenbach and Christian Köhler (2002) researched the different ways in which consumers search for health information on the internet. Firstly, they discovered that many searchers use rather random or idiosyncratic techniques for their searches. For example, none of them use medical portals or official sites of medical societies or recognised libraries – they all use standard search engines such as Google. Many of the subjects also do not understand the way in which they could use combinations of words to refine their searches. Although their search technique is often 'suboptimal',

> internet users successfully find health information to answer questions in less than six minutes. Participants in focus groups said that, when assessing the credibility of a website, they primarily look for the source, a professional design, a scientific or an official touch, language, and ease of use. However, in the observational study, no participants checked any 'about us' sections of websites, disclaimers or disclosure statements. In the post-search interviews, it emerged that very few participants notice and remember which websites they retrieve information from.

However, caution is needed about over-ambitious claims for the medical uses of the internet:

> Although many people use the Internet for health information, use is not as common as is sometimes reported. Effects on actual health care utilization are also less substantial than some have claimed. Discussions of the role of the Internet in health care and the development of policies that might influence this role should not presume that use of the Internet for health information is universal, or that the Internet strongly influences health care utilization.
>
> (Baker et al., 2003, p. 2400)

Access to health information is also associated with socioeconomic and demographic characteristics. People with little money are less likely to have easy access to the internet. Many surveys also show that women are more likely than men to seek health care information online, and the highest proportion of use is among people aged between 30 and 64 (Fox and Rainie, 2002). Age can also be a barrier to access: the use of the internet for seeking health information declines with age (Licciardone et al., 2001; Smith-Barbaro et al., 2001). However, despite the much-discussed 'digital divide' between the higher income, more educated 'have-nets' and the lower income, less educated 'have-nots', there is no evidence of differences in seeking health information by income group once they have online access (Pingree et al., 1996; Brodie et al., 2000).

15.3 Quality of health information on the internet

The freedom and relative accessibility of the internet is both its strength and its weakness. If anybody, or almost anybody, can publish material on the web with apparent ease, how is it possible to avoid valuable information being diluted by extraneous information (Al-Shahi et al., 2002)? Indeed, the problems associated with the quality of health information on the internet have challenged many authors since its inception.

ACTIVITY   POTENTIAL PROBLEMS WITH HEALTH INFORMATION ON THE INTERNET

Allow 15 minutes

Think for a few minutes about the possible ways in which information published on the internet might cause problems for 'consumers'.

Have you ever encountered problems yourself with information that you have retrieved from the internet? Write a short list of any problems you have had.

Comment

Your list may include the following concerns.

- Who is publishing the material?
- There is no quality filter on the information.
- Information is uncontrolled and unmonitored.
- Even 'official looking' pages may be inaccurate or dangerous.
- How much of the information is really evidence based?
- 'Quacks' can publish information about unproven remedies.
- Sources may give false reassurance or inaccurate information.
- The material might be out of date, or apply only to certain geographical regions.
- Information may include fraudulent as well as genuine practices.

The concern for quality is certainly reflected in the published work of numerous academics and 'authorised' researchers. Cline and Haynes (2001) collected examples from published criticisms of health information on the internet, including authors who claimed that such information was:

> 'bad and even dangerous' (McKinley et al., 1999), 'inaccurate, erroneous, misleading, or fraudulent' (McLeod, 1998), 'incomplete, misleading and inaccurate' (Silberg et al., 1997) and 'incomplete, contradictory or based on insufficient scientific evidence' (Abelhard and Obst, 1999). 'Not only is information incomplete, often it is not evidence based' (Pereira and Bruera, 1998; Pandolfini et al., 2000). 'Science and snake oil may not always look all that different on the Net' (Silberg et al., (1997). Dow et al. (1996) warned that 'fringe, non-scientific therapies may be touted ... as valid'.
>
> (Cline and Haynes, 2001, p. 679)

Although such concerns are frequently aired, other commentators seem to adopt a more relaxed approach, suggesting that the problems with internet sources of information are shared with all media:

> Health information in other media has not received the same degree of attention, even though the public is exposed to misleading and inaccurate information from a variety of sources (Payne et al., 2000; Slaytor and Ward, 1998) ... An alternative is to take a 'non-exceptionalist' approach to online health information. Many of the issues arising from the internet that cause concern are common to all types of information, with readability and accuracy of content causing the most anxiety. Solutions to these concerns are seldom restricted to a single method of delivering information (Powsner et al., 1998) ... Concerns about the quantity of available information and how it is delivered and accessed are valid, but these are separate from the issue of quality and should not deflect attention from the standards that need to apply across all information types and media (Silberg et al., 1997).
>
> (Shepperd and Charnock, 2002, pp. 556, 557)

However, there are scarcely any examples of people being harmed as a result of using the internet as a source of information about health issues. Crocco et al. (2002) systematically reviewed the literature and found one article that described two cases in which improper internet searches are thought to have led to emotional harm and another in which harm might have resulted from the improper use of medication purchased on the internet. Weisbord et al. (1997) similarly report a single potentially serious health problem with a pharmaceutical product bought on the internet.

There are still potential problems: inaccurate online health information has even been described as 'an epidemic' (Coiera, 1998). One study found that over 50 per cent of health information websites offer unreliable information (Abelhard and Obst, 1999). Other studies have discovered considerable problems with information about specific health conditions: the Federal Trade Commission in the USA found over 400 websites and Usenet newsgroups containing false or deceptive claims and products for six different diseases (Federal Trade Commission, 1997).

Pandolfini and Bonati (2002, p. 583), while acknowledging some of the problems associated with electronic forms of information, suggest that the quality of public health oriented health information on the web continues to improve: 'The quality of health information on the internet has improved over the past few years despite concerns over poor quality and its possible consequences.'

15.4 CAM and the internet

The discussion so far about general health information and the internet also applies to the ways in which CAM therapists and consumers use and potentially have problems with electronic sources of information.

There are some additional complications in the commercial nature of many of the sites purporting to offer advice about CAM and health-related issues. Sagaram et al. (2002) explored 216 pages of CAM information on the internet found by various methodical searches. Of these, 78 per cent were authored by commercial organisations whose purpose involved commerce 69 per cent of the time, and 52.3 per cent had no references to published material or research reports to back up their assertions:

> We conclude that consumers searching the web for health information are likely to encounter consumer-oriented CAM advertising, which is difficult to read and is not supported by the conventional literature.
>
> (Sagaram et al., 2002, p. 672)

Martin-Facklam et al. (2002) report similar findings in an evaluation of websites that purported to give information about the herbal medication St John's Wort. Of the 208 randomly selected sites, only 45 correctly listed the indication for its use (depression), and only 46 identified at least one drug interaction. Absence of financial interest was associated with the provision of correct information.

A study by Bonakdar (2002) highlights potentially even more serious claims on websites claiming herbal cures for cancer. Although there are official regulatory standards for the claims that can be made for health care products, 'A majority of sites [in the study] claim cancer cures through herbal supplementation with little regard for current regulations' (p. 522).

Some ways of finding reliable online health information are described in Box 15.2.

BOX 15.2   HOW TO FIND THE BEST HEALTH INFORMATION ONLINE

Don't search alone, even if you are an experienced web user. If the world of online health is new to you or you are dealing with a frightening or poorly understood new diagnosis, ask a web savvy friend or family member to sit by your side and show you the ropes the first few times you go online.

Double check the information you find online. Check several sites to make sure they all give the same or similar information. If you still have doubts, post a question at an online discussion group. Alternatively, email a question to an online health professional or to the webmaster of a site devoted to your condition.

If you are dealing with a serious illness, consider joining an online support group and be on the lookout for other online patient helpers who share your concerns. Knowing that your online disease mates are walking the same path and are seeking both to give and to receive support will help most online self helpers feel comfortable in establishing meaningful online relationships based on trust and mutual concern.

Use the internet to get referrals to the doctors and treatment centres you need. You can often use sites devoted to specific diseases to find the top specialists and treatment centres for your condition. You may even be able to correspond directly with leading specialists and researchers by email.

Use the internet to supplement your face to face doctor visits, not to replace them. It is not always easy to interpret what you find. A frank and open discussion with your doctors may help to clear up some of your uncertainties and help you either confirm or reconsider some of your tentative conclusions. The best case scenario is for doctors and patients to work together, as a coordinated team.

Use the internet to help evaluate the information and advice you get at your doctor's office. If you have doubts about your care, ask other online patients or your online support group to review the treatment you have received. They may suggest questions to raise with your doctor on your next visit.

Tell your doctor what you have found online, and use your increased knowledge to become a more assertive patient. The better you communicate your needs, the better your doctor will be able to respond to them. Be assertive rather than aggressive; expressing your feelings and your views honestly and openly while showing respect for your medical professional.

Let your doctor see how your online research can be helpful to your care. If you have already mastered the basics of your condition, let your doctors know that they can skip the usual explanations. If you have found a good review article on your condition in a medical journal, leave your doctor a copy with the parts relevant to your situation highlighted.

If some doctors aren't quite ready to become net friendly doctors, try to understand. Many doctors feel so overwhelmed by clinical responsibilities, paperwork demands, and their own pressing financial concerns that it can be difficult for them to see the benefit of spending additional time exchanging emails with patients or discussing information you have found online. While no conscientious doctors should be threatened by a patient or a family member who wants to know all they can about their illness, many doctors are still uneasy at having their opinions questioned and uncomfortable with the idea that 'their' patients are consulting other sources for information and advice.

(Source: Ferguson, 2002)

15.5　CAM and the printed media: infotainment, style and lifestyle

The massive surge of consumer interest in CAM has been reflected, if not actively encouraged, by the media. There has been an explosion of interest in CAM across all sections of the print media, including tabloid and broadsheet newspapers, magazines (specialised journals, health and lifestyle magazines and women's magazines) and books (particularly of the mind, body and spirit variety). There has also been an increase in the number of scientific and specialised journals on CAM, although consumers access them less frequently (Schmidt et al., 2001). Many well known CAM practitioners write books about their therapy; yet not many eminent doctors write about biomedicine for the general public, and those who do are given little credit for it by their colleagues. Perhaps CAM gurus need to write to publicise their therapy – or their way of doing it.

The press and public responsibility

In 1949, the report of the Royal Commission on the press took the view that the press is more than just another business (Ross, 1949). It has a public task and a corresponding public responsibility, being the most important instrument for instructing the public on the chief issues of the day. This report noted that the democratic form of society demands that its members participate actively and intelligently in the affairs of their community, whether local or national. It assumes that they are sufficiently well informed about the issues of the day to make the broad judgements required by an election, and to maintain, between elections, the necessary vigilance in those whose governors are their servants, not their masters. Democratic society was deemed to need a clear and truthful account of events and of their background and their causes; a forum for discussion and informed criticism; and a means whereby individuals and groups can express a point of view or advocate a cause. The Royal Commission was concerned to see that the press should show truthfulness and diversity and avoid sensationalism. This view was repeated by successive Royal Commissions and is summarised below.

- Truthfulness was said to be the avoidance of excessive bias, which included the deliberate suppression or omission of relevant facts and the exaggerated or highly emotive presentation of facts.
- Diversity was seen as the requirement that the number and variety of newspapers should be such that the press gives an opportunity for all important points of view to be effectively presented. This was stated in terms of the varying standards of taste, public opinion and education among the principal groups of the population.
- Sensationalism was seen as giving crime, scandal, entertainment and human interest undue attention. The Commission was also concerned that the layout of newspapers should not dangerously stimulate public excitement during tense times.

Health journalism, including journalistic coverage of CAM, should be set broadly within the above principles. However, newspapers are designed to sell as many copies as possible and this market pressure inevitably influences journalism. Chris Shumway, an expert on ethical issues for online professionals, explains that, historically, once the media free-market, with its capital-intensive rotary presses, was in place, newspapers looked to how they could maximise revenue:

The huge investment in plant meant that a mass market had to be found for press output in order to recoup the investment and pay shareholders' dividends. That entailed a movement towards entertaining readers, toning down any potentially offensive content ... Today's 'public sphere' is so dominated by the mass media, almost all obeying the capitalist imperative to maximize profits, that news in some media organs is non-existent, tabloidized infotainment in others, sensationalist, phoney and mendacious in most and commoditized in all but a very few.

(Shumway, 2004a)

ACTIVITY   CAM AND THE MEDIA

Allow 45 minutes

Over the next few days collect as many examples as you can of how the various media you come into contact with treat CAM issues. Stay aware of any journal articles, news reports and items on the television and radio that cover the subject of CAM.

Then look at your collection and write a short analysis of the types of articles and items that you became aware of.

In what ways does your collection portray CAM? Is it all positive, or are there critical or cynical reports too? How influential do you think this continued interest in CAM has become?

Comment

In one small-scale study, Ernst and Weihmayr (2000) set out to determine the frequency and tone of newspaper reporting on medical topics in the UK and Germany. They examined four UK broadsheet newspapers and four German newspapers on eight randomly chosen working days in 1999 and analysed the content of all the medical articles. A total of 256 newspaper articles were evaluated and four articles in the German papers and 26 in the UK newspapers referred to CAM. All of the UK articles were positive in their attitude towards CAM, whereas only one German article had a positive attitude to CAM. On the other hand, the attitudes towards conventional medicine in the UK newspapers were more critical than in the German ones. Ernst and Weihmayr acknowledge that this analysis was limited by the small sample size, the short observation period and the subjectivity of some of the end points. Yet the study suggests that, compared with German newspapers, British newspapers report more frequently on medical matters and generally have a more critical attitude. The proportion of articles about complementary medicine seems considerably larger in the UK (15 versus 5 per cent) and, in contrast to articles on medical matters in general, reporting on complementary medicine in the UK is overwhelmingly positive. Given that both health care professionals and the general public gain their knowledge of complementary medicine predominantly from the media, the authors concluded that these findings may be important.

So, is news coverage of CAM in the UK overwhelmingly positive? The journalist John Diamond (1953–2001) explained, in the opening chapter of his final book *Snake Oil and Other Preoccupations* (2001), that he was writing it because there were 'precious few' books on the failings of alternative medicine, a phenomenon he describes as:

> a business which gets regular and often uncritical coverage in most of our popular papers and magazines, which regularly makes – or allows to be made on its behalf – remarkable claims for its abilities, which are often untested, let alone proven ... and which from time to time kills its customers as a direct result of the advice or actions of its practitioners.
>
> (Diamond, 2001, p. 3)

The accuracy of media coverage of CAM is a recurrent concern. Ernst (2001) warns that inaccurate journalism may lead to harm. He cites a regular column in the *Sunday Times* entitled 'What's the Alternative?' as just one example of a column giving potentially harmful advice. In this instance, it recommended using the herbal remedy skullcap to relax young children during a long-haul flight, despite the fact it is known to cause complications such as liver damage. Ernst criticises journalists for rarely doing enough background research, for writing about issues without a full medical understanding of them, and for seeking expert quotations that only fit in with the storyline. This problem was also noted by the Prince of Wales's Foundation for Health in their evidence to the House of Lords:

> Newspapers and television companies are in the business of selling their newspapers and programmes and that very often is what determines the story. This weekend, for example, there has been the continuing saga of St John's Wort published in a number of Sunday papers, and one of the stories I saw I helped the journalist with. I gave a lot of information to that journalist and none of it appeared in the story simply because it did not suit the very scaremongering angle this particular story took, which is unfortunate because there is a genuine story there. There are definite issues around the use of this herb and we need to be aware of them, but in some of the stories the driving need is to sell the newspaper and unfortunately reasoned debate does not always sell newspapers.
>
> (House of Lords, 2000, para. 8.38)

The writer and academic Edzard Ernst draws a similar conclusion, accepting that journalists 'are charming people simply struggling to make a living', and recognising that:

they want to sell their goods and it seems obvious that a juicy story sells better than the scientist's standard and boring conclusion 'we need more research'. Yet, there must be an acceptable compromise between sensationalism and accurate information.

(Ernst, 2001, p. 246)

ACTIVITY   THE JOURNALISTIC SPECTRUM

Allow 20 minutes

Read the articles in Boxes 15.3 and 15.4, which appeared in the same newspaper in the same week.

Make notes on the different styles and assumptions made in each article. How might the readers of this newspaper begin to discover for themselves which article gives helpful or harmful advice?

Comment

It can be difficult for people to discriminate between helpful and harmful advice. Some commentators have raised the idea of kite-marking CAM information produced by the media, but it is hard to see how kite-marking could operate in a competitive commercial environment. Of course, people need to be discerning in weighing up the truth of what they read in the newspapers. What they read about health is no exception.

BOX 15.3   QUACK TALES

I am delighted to be able to present you with the head of an American doctor, who has been struck off after the complementary therapies he was peddling turned out to be not just ineffective but downright dangerous.

Dr James E. Johnson MD – because Americans always manage to make doctors sound like soap stars – has had his licence revoked after a string of increasingly bizarre and dangerous attempts to cure what he believed was a yeast infection. He started with garlic but his patient was in a hurry and so he decided to speed things along by administering hydrogen peroxide, a popular pseudoscientific therapy.

On this occasion the hydrogen peroxide was given intravenously, through a peripherally-inserted central catheter into a vein in her arm, travelled all the way up through her armpit and on into her chest where it sat snugly next to her heart. After a few 'treatments' her arm became red and painful, and she became dizzy with a headache. Johnson diagnosed a 'mini-stroke' and, like a good complementary therapist, initiated intramuscular vitamin C injections. The injection site for these became red and inflamed but instead of using antibiotics which, he told his patient, were 'incompatible' with hydrogen peroxide, he prescribed charcoal poultice compresses. With painful inevitability, things deteriorated further.

By the time his credulous patient managed to dredge up the reserves of self confidence necessary to rethink her values and approach a conventional doctor, an ultrasound scan revealed that she had developed an abscess the size of a baseball, which was surgically removed in hospital, after which she mercifully recovered.

For decades, optimistic alternative therapists have been claiming that hydrogen peroxide therapy can treat cancer and various infections (latterly including Aids), as well as improving tissue oxygenation: a quick hunt around the alternative therapy section of any bookshop, or the internet, will produce entertaining examples. The fundamental misunderstandings seem to be, as far as it is possible to untangle these things, that H_2O_2 is water with a bit of extra oxygen, that this can be used by cells as normal oxygen, or as some form of special oxygen [to] inhibit enzymes in tumour cells, or produce 'glyoxylide' which has alleged healing properties but has never been isolated. It can be jolly dangerous, and several pseudoscientists have been successfully disciplined for lying about it ever since Dr Koch, its inventor, was first censured by the FDA in 1942.

(Source: Goldacre, 2003)

BOX 15.4   ASK EMMA

[Question] I had a lumpectomy and removal of lymph glands two months ago, and am awaiting radiotherapy. I'm on tamoxifen, 20 mg daily, which, I believe, suppresses oestrogen. Should I take supplements, and is there a natural way I can retain my femininity?

[Answer] Many natural therapies have been found to help people with cancer. You could benefit from supplements, herbs, acupuncture, yoga and other therapies, but it is hard to give advice without knowing more about you, your symptoms, current supplements, diet and history of conventional and complementary treatments. Excellent support, advice and resources are available from New Approaches To Cancer (0800 389 2662; anac.org.uk), a charity happy to suggest therapies complementary to conventional treatment or to help you, if you choose, to take a completely alternative approach.

(Source: Mitchell, 2003)

The press is currently voluntarily self-regulated, and the print media are accountable to the Press Complaints Commission (PCC). However, the ability of the PCC to govern the industry has repeatedly been called into question. Until recently, the PCC's committee entirely comprised editors, with no lay input whatsoever. The body has been criticised for having 'no teeth', and for being unable to exert control over newspapers which are in breach of their responsibilities (Select Committee for Culture, Media and Sport, 2003).

Lifestyle journalism

In the past, stories about CAM tended to be on the health pages of a newspaper. Since the early 1990s, several newspapers have had a specific alternative health section: for example, *The Observer's* 'Barefoot Doctor'. What is interesting about this phenomenon is the apparent shift of CAM from news to entertainment in the form of 'lifestyle' journalism. Information about CAM is now more likely to be situated in a glossy supplement alongside articles about food, wine and property, interspersed with advertisements for cars and luxury goods. In other words, CAM can be branded, not as a form of health care, but as part of a desirable consumer lifestyle. What differentiates lifestyle reporting from news reporting is the proximity to advertising and the promotion of therapies and therapeutic practice as something that can be bought to make people's lives better. Consumerism is the 'new democracy' in which everyone is supposedly free to buy into a lifestyle (although some are obviously more free than others).

Doel and Segrott (2003) compared the literature on CAM published by patient groups with that in various lifestyle magazines and found that:

> An initial comparison of lifestyle magazines with the publications of patient groups might suggest that the former are frivolous, distracting, and ultimately pacifying. They refer 'anxious' and 'incompetent' readers to expert authority and to object pathways. ... the readers of health and lifestyle magazines are not necessarily expected to submit to use, need, or functionality. They are primarily called upon to participate actively in working with the untold possibilities of the practices and materials presented to them, and the innumerable ways in which they could be taken up. ... In accordance with the logic of consumer culture, an interest in CAM does not need to commence with a particular illness or disease: either because the focus is on the treatment itself ... or because the emphasis is on health, well-being, and pleasure ... . '**Special treat** – Mother's Day doesn't necessarily mean flowers and chocolates. Pamper the special lady in your family with a relaxing beauty or holistic treatment' (*Natural Health & Well-being* 2001, page 7.)

(Doel and Segrott, 2003, pp. 748, 749)

The same trend exists in marketing CAM books, which now account for a significant percentage of health titles, generally found in the 'Mind, Body and Spirit' section of larger bookshops. At the time of writing, a quick search on an online book sales website revealed over 1000 titles listed under 'complementary and alternative health'. In addition, titles are mass-marketed: for example, Patrick Holford's *Optimum Nutrition* is currently on sale at supermarkets alongside Jamie Oliver's cookery books. It is interesting how even bookshops are diversifying in order to increase their market share. This phenomenon exists in CAM: for example, supermarkets, bookshops and chemists are selling not only books on yoga but also 'yoga kits' so that, as well as buying the book, consumers can buy a mat, a book and a demonstration video.

15.6 CAM as news

There is a smaller, although still important, interest in CAM in the broadcast media. In theoretical terms, the media in the UK operate within a 'public service' model, in contrast to the US 'free-market' model. This means it has a responsibility to produce news that is accurate and unbiased. However, broadcasters are primarily in the business of attracting audiences, in exactly the same way as newspapers are. The financial pressure on broadcasters to attract high ratings ensures that companies produce material that is likely to appeal to the widest audience. In a free-market system, such as in the USA, the programmes are targeted at the largest audience share possible, in order to 'give the public what they want'. However, in the UK, which is governed by a public service model, the output is less distorted. The media agencies responsible for broadcasting standards are less firmly located in the commercial sector, and regulatory bodies are in place to ensure that the broadcasting companies observe rules, including those about taste, decency, respect for human dignity and privacy (for example, the Independent Television Commission or ITC). In the British broadcasting system, the capitalist imperative to make programmes that appeal to more popular audiences is less evident than in the USA. This is partly because the BBC is financed by the licence payers and partly because of the requirements for certain types of output within a 'public service' system: requirements which apply to the independent broadcasters as well.

> Nevertheless, it is not the case in the UK that broadcasters are free of financial pressures. The independent companies clearly have to keep their advertisers (and the terrestrial broadcasters are now under greater pressure because of competition from satellite) and therefore need to keep ratings high. ... It is this pressure to respond to the capitalist imperative that has led to increasing criticism of ITV companies for moving towards 'tabloid TV'... more 'edutainment' and 'infotainment' etc.
>
> (Shumway, 2004b)

CAM and celebrity

Any discussion of CAM and the media would be incomplete without an analysis of the increasing visibility of celebrity involvement in, and influence on, health matters. Media fascination with celebrity is at an all-time high, reflecting the public's seemingly insatiable appetite for insights into the lives of the rich and famous. This obsession includes a desire for inside knowledge about the celebrities' health, and the treatments they seek out. There are now several journals dedicated to celebrity health, including EMAP's *Celebrity Bodies*, launched in March 2001. Similar titles include Time's *InStyle* and Condé Nast's *Glamour*. There is even a website dedicated to discussing health issues, 'combining healthcare expertise and celebrity experiences in a caring supportive community' (Spotlight Health, 2004). On this site, celebrities share their experiences of ill health, and there is an accompanying medical commentary, together with chat rooms for the public to share the experience.

There is no shortage of celebrities endorsing various CAM approaches (Stone and Matthews, 1996). Indeed, the writer and healer the 'Barefoot Doctor' has become a celebrity in his own right, with his highly successful 'Urban Warrior' books, offering 'high-speed spirituality for people on the run' (Russell, 2001). When considering celebrity endorsement, the royal family deserves a special mention (Stone and Matthews, 1996). There has been a long tradition of royal patronage of CAM in the UK. The cause of complementary medicine has been furthered by always having 'friends in high places'. Members of the royal family are prominent among the users and enthusiastic supporters of complementary medicine. Prince Charles has an ongoing influence in this field through the Prince of Wales's Foundation for Integrated Health, the charitable organisation and policy body of which he is President (PoWFIH, 2004).

ACTIVITY   CELEBRITY HEALTH AND CAM

Allow 15 minutes

In your opinion, why are so many members of the general public interested in celebrities and their health?

List some of the ways in which you think celebrity endorsement of a disease or treatment may be both helpful and unhelpful.

Comment

It is hard to pinpoint why people are so fascinated with celebrity illness but the following reasons are possibilities.

- **Sense of identification:** members of the general public believe they know celebrities – they care about them and share their sorrows as if they are their own.
- **Voyeurism:** it is an opportunity to see behind the public face.
- *Schadenfreude***:** the desire to see people who may be thought to 'have it easy' laid low by suffering.
- **Interest** in how rich people, who can buy the best of everything, treat their illnesses.

Although fawning on celebrities might cause a sense of despair, there are ways in which press attention can be put to good use. Celebrities are in a privileged position to foster awareness about a medical condition, and to assist charities and fundraisers in securing money for treatment and research. Their courage and openness can be highly influential in removing the stigma of certain diseases (sport star Michael Jordan and AIDS) and for instilling hope (the late actor Christopher Reeve and his improved mobility after a riding accident). Celebrities, such as actor Michael J. Fox, can mobilise political power for the improved treatment for Parkinson's disease more than any number of 'ordinary' sufferers. However, a fundamental criticism of journalism about celebrity health is that it is designed to entertain and titillate, rather than to inform.

15.7   Conclusion

Complementary and alternative health issues are now important components of many different types of media product. Most newspapers and journals in developed western societies carry frequent stories about the use and misuse of complementary and alternative therapies and, of course, the internet has enormous quantities of material about CAM.

Passive consumers, and even proactive information seekers, using these media can easily be confused and distracted by the enormous quantity of material they are exposed to. In all media, the problems of quality control remain predominant. How do people accessing this information know whether it is accurate and reliable? On the one hand, some observers believe that members of the general public are fully aware of the problems of reliability of the information in the media and can be left with the responsibility to decide for themselves what to believe, what advice to act on and what action to take. On the other hand, others, including some professional bodies and government agencies, want to control and govern the information that is available in this way.

The quality and reliability of information available on the web and through written and broadcast media is certainly very variable. This chapter should have clarified some of the issues involved in the accuracy and safety of health-related messages.

> **KEY POINTS**
>
> ■ There is an enormous range of information on CAM that is available through a wide range of media.
>
> ■ Information on a multitude of subjects, including CAM, has grown exponentially since the development of the internet.
>
> ■ The quality of health information on the internet is variable and causes concern among some health-related interest groups.
>
> ■ CAM is a subject of great interest in the printed media.
>
> ■ Journalists writing about CAM and other health issues always have to be aware of the subjects that are attractive to their audience and that will help sell their products.
>
> ■ The search for markets for written and broadcast material may distort or contaminate the reliability of health information in media reports on CAM.
>
> ■ Seeking reliable health information from most media sources requires considerable discernment and skill.

References

Abelhard, K. and Obst, O. (1999) 'Evaluation of medical Internet sites', *Methods of Information in Medicine*, Vol. 39, pp. 75–9.

Al-Shahi, R., Sadler, M., Rees, M. and Bateman, D. (2002) 'The Internet', *Journal of Neurology, Neurosurgery and Psychiatry*, Vol. 73, pp. 619–28.

Baker, L., Wagner, T. H., Singer, S. and Bundorf, M. K. (2003) 'Use of the Internet and e-mail for health care information: results from a national survey', *Journal of the American Medical Association*, Vol. 289, No. 18, pp. 2400–6.

Bonakdar, R. (2002) 'Herbal cures on the web: non-compliance with the Dietary Supplement Health and Education Act', *Family Medicine*, Vol. 34, No. 7, pp. 522–7.

Brodie, M., Flournoy, R. E., Altman, D. E., Blendon, R. J., Benson, J. M. and Rosenbaum, M. D. (2000) 'Health information, the Internet and the digital divide', *Health Affairs*, Vol. 19, No. 6, pp. 255–65.

Cain, M., Mittman, R., Sarasohn-Kahn, J. and Wayne, J. (2000) *Health E-people: The Online Consumer Experience*, Oakland, CA, California Healthcare Foundation and the Institute for the Future. Available online at www.chcf.org/documents/ihealth/HealthEPeople.pdf [accessed 23 February 2004].

Cline, R. J. W. and Haynes, K. M. (2001) 'Consumer health information seeking on the Internet: the state of the art', *Health Education Research*, Vol. 16, No. 6, pp. 671–92.

Coiera, E. (1998) 'Information epidemics, economics, and immunity on the internet', *British Medical Journal*, Vol. 317, pp. 1469–70.

Crocco, A., Villasis-Keever, M. and Jadad, A. (2002) 'Analysis of cases of harm associated with use of health information on the Internet', *Journal of the American Medical Association*, Vol. 287, pp. 2869–971.

Diamond, J. (2001) *Snake Oil and Other Preoccupations*, London, Vintage.

Doel, M. A. and Segrott, J. (2003) 'Beyond belief? Consumer culture, complementary medicine, and the dis-ease of everyday life', *Society and Space*, Vol. 21, pp. 739–59.

Dow, M. G., Kearns, W. and Thornton, D. H. (1996) 'The Internet II: future effects on cognitive behavioral practice', *Cognitive and Behavioral Practice*, Vol. 3, pp. 137–57.

Ernst, E. (2001) 'Complementary/alternative medicine and the media', *Focus on Alternative and Complementary Therapies*, Vol. 6, No. 4, pp. 245–6.

Ernst, E. and Weihmayr, T. (2000) 'UK and German media differ over complementary medicine', *British Medical Journal*, Vol. 321, p. 707.

Eysenbach, G. and Köhler, C. (2002) 'How do consumers search for and appraise health information on the world wide web? Qualitative study using focus groups, usability tests, and in-depth interviews', *British Medical Journal*, Vol. 324, pp. 573–7.

Federal Trade Commission (1997) *Surf Days: Detection and Defence* [online], www.ftc.gov/reports/fraud97/surfdays.htm [accessed 6 August 2004].

Ferguson, T. (2002) 'From patients to end users: quality of online patient networks needs more attention than quality of online health information', *British Medical Journal*, Vol. 324, pp. 555–6. Available online at www.bmj.com/cgi/content/fuli/324/7337/555/DC1 [accessed 27 May 2003].

Fox, S. and Rainie, L. (2002) 'Vital decisions: how Internet users decide what information to trust when they or their loved ones are sick', Washington, DC, Pew Internet & American Life Project. Available online at: www.pewinternet.org/reports/toc.asp?Report=59 [accessed 27 May 2003].

Glasgow, R., Barrera, M., McKay, H. and Boles, S. (1998) 'Social support and health among participants in an Internet-based diabetes support program: a multi-dimensional investigation', *Diabetes*, Vol. 47, p. 1263.

Goldacre, B. (2003) 'Quack tales', in 'Bad Science', *The Guardian*, 29 May.

Google Inc. (2001) 'Google offers immediate access to 3 billion Web documents', Press release, Mountain View, CA, Google Inc. Available online at www.google.com/press/pressrel/3billion.html [accessed 23 February 2004].

House of Lords (2000) *Complementary and Alternative Medicine*, Select Committee on Science and Technology, Sixth Report 1999–2000, London, The Stationery Office.

Kiley, R. (1999) Editorial – 'Internet statistics', *Health Information on the Internet*, Vol. 10, pp. 1–2.

Leiner, B. M., Cerf, V. G., Clark, D. D., Kahn, R. E., Kleinrock, L., Lynch, D. C., Postel, J., Roberts, L. G. and Wolff, S. (1979) *A Brief History of the Internet* [online], www.isoc.org/internet/history/brief.shtml [accessed 23 February 2004].

Licciardone, J., Smith-Barbaro, P. and Coleridge, S. (2001) 'Use of the Internet as a resource for consumer health information: results of the Second Osteopathic Survey of Health Care in America (OSTEOSURV-II)', *Journal of Medical Internet Research*, Vol. 3, No. 4, p. 31.

Martin-Facklam, M., Kostrzewa, M., Schubert, F., Gasse, C. and Haefeli, W. (2002) 'Quality markers of drug information on the Internet: an evaluation of sites about St John's Wort', *American Journal of Medicine*, Vol. 113, No. 9, pp. 740–5.

McKinley, J., Cattermole, H. and Oliver, C. (1999) 'The quality of surgical information on the Internet', *Journal of the Royal College of Surgeons in Edinburgh*, Vol. 44, pp. 265–8.

McLeod, S. D. (1998) 'The quality of medical information on the internet: a new public health concern', *Archives of Ophthalmology*, Vol. 116, pp. 1663–5.

Mitchell, E. (2003) 'Ask Emma', *The Guardian*, 24 May.

Murero, M., D'Ancona, G. and Karamanoukian, H. (2001) 'Use of the Internet by patients before and after cardiac surgery: telephone survey', *Journal of Medical Internet Research*, Vol. 3, No. 3, p. 27.

NetRatings Inc. (2001) 'Internet usage statistics for the month of December 2001 (United Kingdom)' [online], www.epm.netratings.com/uk/web/NRpublicreports.usagemonthly [accessed 24 January 2002].

Nua Internet Surveys (2001) 'How many online? August 2001' [online], www.nua.com/surveys/how_many_online/index.html [accessed 24 January 2002].

Pandolfini, C. and Bonati, M. (2002) 'Follow up of quality of public oriented health information on the world wide web: systematic re-evaluation', *British Medical Journal*, Vol. 324, pp. 582–3.

Pandolfini, C., Impicciatore, P. and Bonati, M. (2000) 'Parents on the Web: risks for quality management of cough in children', *Paediatrics*, Vol. 105, p. e1.

Payne, S., Large, S., Jarrett, N. and Turner P. (2000) 'Written information given to patients and families by palliative care units: a national survey', *The Lancet*, Vol. 355, p. 1792.

Pereira, J. and Bruera, E. (1998) 'The Internet as a resource for palliative care and hospice: a review and proposals', *Journal of Pain and Symptom Management*, Vol. 16, No. 1, pp. 59–68.

Pingree, S., Hawkins, R. P., Gustafson, D. H., Boberg, E. W., Bricker, E. and Wise, M., et al. (1996) 'Will the disadvantaged ride the information superhighway? Hopeful answers from a computer-based health crisis system', *Journal of Broadcasting and Electronic Media*, Vol. 40, pp. 331–53.

Powell, J. (2002) 'The WWW of the World Wide Web: Who, What and Why?', *Journal of Medical Internet Research*, Vol. 4, No. 1, p. 4. Available online at www.jmir.org/2002/1/e4/ [accessed 27 May 2003].

PoWFIH (Prince of Wales's Foundation for Integrated Health) (2004) website: www.fihealth.org.uk [accessed 2 August 2004].

Powsner, S. M., Wyatt, J. C. and Wright, P. (1998) 'Opportunities for and challenges of computerisation', *The Lancet*, Vol. 352, pp. 1617–22.

Reeves, P. (2000) 'Coping in cyberspace: the impact of Internet use on the ability of HIV-positive individuals to deal with their illness', *Journal of Health Communication*, Vol. 5, Supplement, pp. 47–59.

Ross, W. (1949) *Chair: Royal Commission on the Press 1947–1949*, Cmnd 7700, London, HMSO.

Russell, S. (2001) *Return of the Urban Warrior: Barefoot Doctor. High Speed Spirituality for People on the Run*, London, Thorsons.

Sagaram, S., Walji, M. and Bernstam, E. (2002) 'Evaluating the prevalence, content and readability of complementary and alternative medicine (CAM) web pages on the internet', *Proceedings of the American Medical Informatics Association Symposium*, pp. 672–6.

Schmidt, K., Pittler, M. and Ernst, E. (2001) 'A profile of journals of complementary and alternative medicine', *Swiss Medical Weekly*, Vol. 131, No. 39–40, pp. 588–91.

Select Committee for Culture, Media and Sport (2003) *Privacy and Media Intrusion*, 16 June, London, House of Commons.

Shepperd, S. and Charnock, D. (2002) 'Against internet exceptionalism', *British Medical Journal*, Vol. 324, pp. 556–7.

Shumway, C. (2004a) 'The Internet as public sphere' [online], www.cultsock.ndirect.co.uk/MUHome/cshtml/media/internet4.html [accessed 2 August 2004].

Shumway, C. (2004b) 'De Fleur's model of the taste-differentiated model' [online], www.cultsock.ndirect.co.uk/MUHome/cshtml/media/de_fleur.html [accessed 17 June 2004].

Silberg, W., Lundberg, G. and Musacchio, R. (1997) 'Assessing, controlling, and assuring the quality of medical information on the internet: caveant lector et viewor – let the reader and viewer beware', *Journal of the American Medical Association*, Vol. 277, pp. 1244–5.

Slaytor, E. and Ward, J. (1998) 'How risks of breast cancer and benefits of screening are communicated to women: analysis of 58 pamphlets', *British Medical Journal*, Vol. 317, pp. 263–4.

Smith-Barbaro, P., Licciardone, J., Clarke, H. and Coleridge, S. (2001) 'Factors associated with intended use of a Web site among family practice patients', *Journal of Medical Internet Research*, Vol. 3, No. 2, p. 17.

Spotlight Health (2004) website: www.spotlighthealth.com [accessed 2 August 2004].

Stone, J. and Matthews, J. (1996) *Complementary Medicine and the Law*, Oxford, Oxford University Press.

Tatsumi, H., Mitani, H., Haruki, Y. and Ogushi, Y. (2001) 'Internet medical usage in Japan: current situation and issues', *Journal of Medical Internet Research*, Vol. 3, No. 1, p. 12.

Taylor, H. (2001) *The Harris Poll #19: Cyberchondriacs Update* [online], www.harrisinteractive.com/harris_poll/index.asp?PID=229 [accessed 15 February 2002].

Weisbord, S., Soule, J. and Kimmel, P. (1997) 'Poison on line – acute renal failure caused by oil of wormwood purchased through the Internet', *New England Journal of Medicine*, Vol. 337, p. 1483.

Zrebiec, J. F. and Jacobson, A. M. (2001) 'What attracts patients with diabetes to an internet support group? A 21-month longitudinal website study', *Diabetic Medicine*, Vol. 18, No. 2, pp. 154–8.

Index